Genetic Disorders Sourcebook

Genetic Disorders Sourcebook

Edited by **Luke Stanton**

hayle medical

New York

Published by Hayle Medical,
30 West, 37th Street, Suite 612,
New York, NY 10018, USA
www.haylemedical.com

Genetic Disorders Sourcebook
Edited by Luke Stanton

International Standard Book Number: 978-1-63241-228-7 (Hardback)

Printed in China.

Contents

Preface

Various studies have approached the subject by analyzing it with a single perspective, but the present book provides diverse methodologies and techniques to address this field. This book contains theories and applications needed for understanding the subject from different perspectives. The aim is to keep the readers informed about the progress in the field; therefore, the contributions were carefully examined to compile novel researches by specialists from across the globe.

Genes are the building blocks of heredity. Human genetics is a rapidly evolving field in medical science. This book presents an overview on recent developments in some of the genetic diseases. It discusses various genetic disorders, dealing with epidemiology, etiology, molecular basis and new treatment measures for these diseases. Experts from different countries in Europe, Asia, and America have contributed in the compilation of this book. The content serves readers with different and valuable content, offering a welcome personalized overview on various subjects. This book does not provide a strictly systematic view of human genetic disorders. However, it is a valuable reference for medical practitioners, researchers, biologists and students in various fields of medical science.

Indeed, the job of the editor is the most crucial and challenging in compiling all chapters into a single book. In the end, I would extend my sincere thanks to the chapter authors for their profound work. I am also thankful for the support provided by my family and colleagues during the compilation of this book.

Editor

Chapter 1

Laminopathies

Tomás McKenna, Jean-Ha Baek and Maria Eriksson

Additional information is available at the end of the chapter

1. Introduction

1.1. The nuclear envelope

The nucleus is the defining characteristic organelle of the eukaryotes, and contains the nuclear genome. It is segregated from the cellular cytoplasm by the bilayer nuclear envelope (Figure 1), which consists of concentric inner and outer nuclear membranes, between which lies the perinuclear space. The outer nuclear membrane is contiguous with the rough endoplasmic reticulum, like which it is studded with protein producing ribosomes, and the perinuclear space is contiguous with the lumen of the endoplasmic reticulum. Transport across the nuclear envelope is accommodated by nuclear pore complexes (NPCs). The NPCs are the site where the inner and outer nuclear membranes are connected, as their shared lipid bilayers are united at that point. These NPCs are large, complex and heterogeneous protein structures, made up of multiple copies of approximately 30 different proteins, called nucleoporins [1]. NPCs span the inner and outer nuclear membranes, and allow the regulated relocation of molecules between the nucleoplasm and cytoplasm. While smaller molecules, such as small metabolites or proteins under 40 kDa, are passively transported through the NPCs, larger molecules such as mRNAs, tRNAs, ribosomes and signalling molecules can be actively transported from the nucleus, while signalling molecules, proteins, lipids and carbohydrates are actively transported both into and out of the nucleus [2,3].

The inner nuclear membrane is embedded by various inner nuclear membrane proteins, such as LAP1, LAP2 and MAN1, which are involved in cell cycle control, linking the nucleus to the cytoskeleton and chromatin organisation [4,5]. Underlying and connected by various nuclear envelope proteins to the inner nuclear membrane are the nuclear lamina, a thin (30-100nm) and densely woven fibrillar mesh of intermediate filaments, composed of evolutionarily conserved lamins A, B1, B2 and C, and lamin associated proteins. These proteins are closely associated with the NPCs (Figure 1). This assembly of outer nuclear membrane, inner nuclear membrane, NPCs, and the lamina can be thought of as complex interface, coupling the nuclear genome to the rest of the cell, allowing for a sophisticated means of regulated traffic between inner and outer nuclear space, while compartmentalising DNA replication, RNA transcription and mRNA editing from translation at the ribosomes [3].

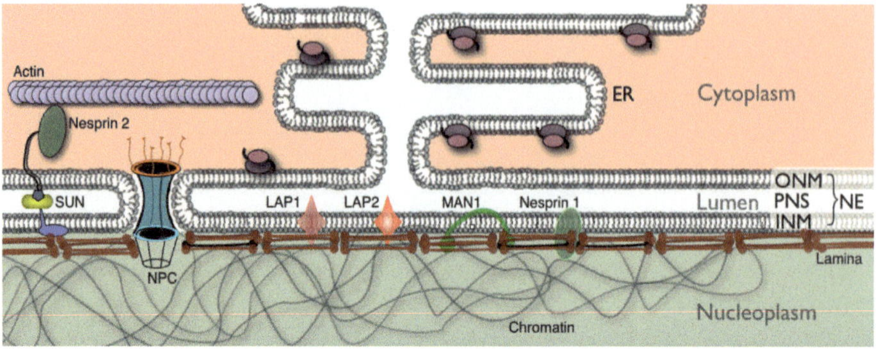

Figure 1. Structure of the nuclear envelope and associated proteins. The nuclear A-type and B-type lamins underlay the nucleoplasmic side of the inner nuclear membrane, and provide stability to the nucleus, an organisational binding platform for chromatin, and facilitate localisation and binding of nuclear pore complexes as well as a large family of nuclear envelope proteins. ONM, outer nuclear membrane; PNS, perinuclear space; INM, Inner nuclear membrane; NE, Nuclear envelope; NPC, Nuclear pore complex; ER, Endoplasmic reticulum, The structures on the ER represent ribosomes.

The nuclear lamins are type V intermediate filaments (IFs), and are closely related to the cytoplasmic intermediate filaments (types I-IV, which include the keratins), differing by the presence of a nuclear localisation signal (NLS) located in the initial section of the tail domain [6]. Physically, these lamins have the characteristic tripartite assemblage of intermediate filaments; a short globular N-terminal head domain and a long C-terminal tail domain containing an immunoglobin-like domain, separated by a conserved central alpha-helical rod domain (Figure 4). Coiled-coil homodimers of A- and B-type lamins are formed by interaction between adjacent heptad hydrophobic repeats on the central rod domain, and charged residues along the centre of this dimer promote further assembly between dimers, leading to assembly of filamentous fibrils, whereas the N and C terminal endings facilitate head-to-tail polymerisation [6-8]. The nuclear lamina has been shown to have a major role in nuclear structure, heterochromatin organisation and gene regulation [8-11].

1.2. The lamins

The *LMNA* gene (Online inheritance in man: 150330) is located on chromosome 1q21.2-q21.3 and is composed of 12 exons. Exon 1 codes the N-terminal head domain, exons 1-6 code the central rod domain, and exons 7-9 code the C-terminal tail domains. Exon 7 also contains the 6 amino acid NLS, necessary for importation of the protein into the nucleus by nuclear transport through NPCs [6,12,13]. Exons 11 and 12 specifically code lamin A, and the CaaX motif of prelamin A (the immature form of lamin A) is located in exon 12. The CaaX motif is a series of four amino acids at the C-terminus of a protein, consisting of a cysteine, two of any aliphatic amino acid, and a terminal amino acid. It is important for the post-translational processing including farnesylation. The motif is identified by the prenyltransferases, farnesyltransferase, or geranylgeranyltransferase-I, and is modified and removed during maturation of lamin A [14]. Lamin C does not contain a CaaX motif, and terminates in an alternative six amino-acid C-terminal end (VSGSRR) (Figure 4).

LMNA produces the major lamin A and C proteins (Figure 4), and the minor AΔ10 and C2 proteins by alternative splicing within exon 10, and they are differentially expressed in a developmentally and tissue specific way [13,15]. Lamin AΔ10 is identical to lamin A, except exon 10 is absent [16], and lamin C2 (which is expressed exclusively in germ cells) is identical to lamin C, except an alternative exon, 1C2, located in intron 1 of *LMNA*, codes for the N-terminal head domain [17,18]. A TATA-like promotor sequence (TATTA) for RNA polymerase attachment, and a CAT-box for RNA transcription factor attachment, lie 236 and 297 base pairs upstream of the ATG initiation codon [6,13].

A-type lamins are expressed only in differentiated cells, suggesting that they have a role in stabilising differential gene expression [15,16,19,20]. The main products in somatic cells are lamins A and C, with C2 and AΔ10 being less common isoforms, lamin C2 being specific to the testes [6,13,16,21]. The first 566 amino acids of lamins A and C are identical. However, at the C-terminals lamin A has 98 unique amino acids, and as with lamin B1 and B2, ends in a CaaX box motif, whilst lamin C has 6 unique terminal amino acids.

The second family of lamins, the B-type lamins, consist of lamin B1 encoded by the *LMNB1* gene, and lamin B2 and B3, encoded by the *LMNB2* gene. At least one of these B-type lamins are expressed in all cell types [13,22-25]. Lamin B3 is a minor variant, arising from differential splicing and alternative polyadenylation of *LMNB2* and is expressed in male germ cells [24]. B-type lamins have a CAAX motif and are constitutively farnesylated, whereas lamin A loses its farnesyl group once targeted to the lamina [26].

The maturation process for lamin A, lamin B1 and B2 is detailed below, with these post-translational modifications taking place in the nucleus [27].

- Prenylation: A farnesyl or geranylgeranyl isoprenoid group is covalently attached to the cysteine of the CaaX motif of prelamin A, lamin B1 and B2 by farnesyltransferase or geranylgeranyltransferase-I, respectively.
- Cleavage: The terminal -aaX amino acids are removed by RCE1 and FACE1 for prelamin A, and by RCE1 alone for lamin B1 and B2.
- Methylation: The now exposed C-terminal farnesylcysteine undergoes a methylation step, performed by a carboxymethyltransferase, isoprenylcysteine carboxyl methyltransferase (ICMT) [28]. This is the final post-translational step for B-type lamins, therefore they retain the farnesylcysteine α-methyl ester at the C-terminus.
- Second cleavage (for prelamin A only): FACE1 cleaves the carboxy-terminal 15 amino acids, including the farnesylcysteine methyl ester group, at the NM [29]. This final modifi-

cation step completes the post-translational modification of prelamin A to mature lamin A. This maturation is thought to aid localisation of lamin A to the nuclear rim [30,31].

2. Laminopathies

Diseases caused by mutations in the *LMNA* gene are collectively known as primary laminopathies [32], whereas mutations in genes coding for B-type lamins (*LMNB1* and *LMNB2*), prelamin A processing proteins (such as *ZMPSTE24*), or lamin-binding proteins (such as *EMD, TMPO, LBR* and *LEMD3*) are known as secondary laminopathies [33,34]. At present, 458 different mutations from 2,206 individuals have been identified in the *LMNA* gene (www.umd.be/LMNA/). These mutations can be *de novo* or heritable, with a gain- or loss-of-function effect, and with severity ranging from minor arrhythmia arising in adolescence to a neonatally lethal tight skin condition [35]. Unlike with the *LMNA* gene, there are only a few mutations found affecting B-type lamins [36]. This is most likely due to the wide-ranging and non-redundant functions of lamin B1 in early growth and development [29].

Laminopathies are caused by a heterogeneous set of pleiotropic mutations affecting universally expressed genes. However, their effects can be tissue specific to a degree, allowing for categorisation into five groups (Table 1). Striated muscles are affected in muscular dystrophies, peripheral nerves are affected in neuropathies, adipose tissue in lipodystophies, several tissues affected with premature development of multiple markers of senescence in segmental progeriod diseases, and finally diseases displaying symptoms from more than one category are known as overlapping syndromes.

2.1. Muscular dystrophies

Within this following section, selected muscular dystrophies will be detailed, while Table 2 shows a complete listing of known muscular dystrophy laminopathies, at the time of writing.

2.1.1. Emery-dreifuss muscular dystrophy

Emery-Dreifuss muscular dystrophy (EDMD), first described in 1955 [37], is the most prevalent laminopathy, affecting 1 in 100,000 births. It is also a prototypical laminopathy, occurring both as a primary and secondary laminopathy. The most commonly occurring form is autosomal dominant (AD-EDMD). It also occurs as an autosomal recessive (AR-EDMD) or X-linked (XL-EDMD) form [38,39]. Mutations in the emerin gene are responsible for XL-EDMD [40-43], while mutations in the *LMNA* gene have been found to cause AD-EDMD, AR-EDMD and sporadic EDMD [44-47]. It most commonly occurs with nonsense mutations, although there has also been a report of at least one case with a premature stop codon in exon 1 of *LMNA* resulting in loss-of-function and haploinsufficiency as the genetic mechanism (Figure 4). The similarities in the clinical features of EDMD irrespective of whether the causative mutation is affecting emerin or lamin A/C indicates a close functional relationship between these proteins. Emerin mediates linkage between membranes and the cytoskeleton, and is closely linked to lamins [40].

Laminopathy	Acronym	OMIM	Locus	Gene
Muscular dystrophy				
Cardiomyopathy, dilated, 1A	CMD1A	115200	1q22	*LMNA*
Emery-Dreifuss muscular dystrophy 1, X-linked	EDMD1	310300	Xq28	*EMD*
Emery-Dreifuss muscular dystrophy 2, AD	EDMD2	181350	1q22	*LMNA*
Emery-Dreifuss muscular dystrophy 3, AR	EDMD2	181350	1q22	*LMNA*
Emery-Dreifuss muscular dystrophy 4, AD	EDMD4	612998	6q25.1-q25.2	*SYNE1*
Emery-Dreifuss muscular dystrophy 5, AD	EDMD5	612999	14q23.2	*SYNE2*
Emery-Dreifuss muscular dystrophy 6, X-linked	EDMD6	300696	Xq26.3	*FHL1*
Heart-hand syndrome, Slovenian type	HHS-S	610140	1q22	*LMNA*
Malouf syndrome	MLF	212112	1q22	*LMNA*
Muscular dystrophy, congenital	MDC	613205	1q22	*LMNA*
Muscular dystrophy, limb-girdle, type 1B	LGMD1B	159001	1q22	*LMNA*
Lipodystrophy				
Acquired partial lipodystrophy	APLD	608709	19p13.3	*LMNB2*
Lipodystrophy, familial partial, 2	FPLD2	151660	1q22	*LMNA*
Mandibuloacral dysplasia with type A lipodystrophy	MADA	248370	1q22	*LMNA*
Mandibuloacral dysplasia with type B lipodystrophy	MADB	608612	1p34.2	*ZMPSTE24*
Neuropathies				
Adult-onset autosomal dominant leukodystrophy	ADLD	169500	5q23.2	*LMNB1*
Charcot-Marie-Tooth disease, type 2B1	CMT2B1	605588	1q22	*LMNA*
Segmental progeroid diseases				
Hutchinson-Gilford progeria syndrome	HGPS	176670	1q22	*LMNA*
Restrictive dermopathy	RD	275210	1p34.2/1q 22	*ZMPSTE24/LMNA*
Atypical Werner syndrome	AWRN	277700	8p12	*RECQL2*
Overlapping syndromes				
Hydrops-Ectopic calcification-moth-eaten skeletal dysplasia	HEM	215140	1q42.12	*LBR*
Pelger-Huet anomaly	PHA	169400	1q42.12	*LBR*
Reynolds syndrome	RS	613471	1q42.12	*LBR*
Buschke-Ollendorff syndrome	BOS	166700	12q14.3	*LEMD3*
Melorheostosis with osteopoikilosis	MEL	155950	12q14.3	*LEMD3*

Table 1. A summary of primary and secondary laminopathies, grouped into five categories. LMNA, Lamin A/C; EMD, Emerin; SYNE1, Nesprin-1; SYNE2, Nesprin-2; FHL1, four and a half LIM domains; LMNB1, lamin B1; LMNB2, lamin B2; ZMPSTE24, zinc metallopeptidase (STE24 homolog); RECQL2, Werner syndrome, RecQ helicase-like; LBR, lamin B receptor; LEMD3, LEM domain-containing protein 3.

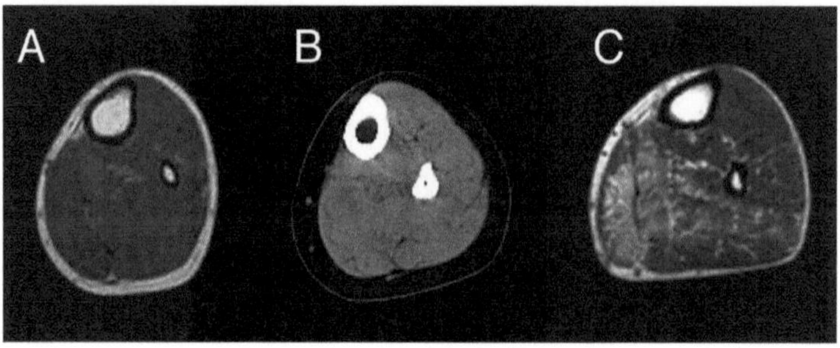

Figure 2. Lower limb imaging of skeletal muscles from patients with laminopathies. Leg muscles from an unaffected control individual (A), a 44 years old female with LGMD1B, LMNA c.673C>T, p.R225X (B), and a 50 years old male with EDMD2, LMNA c.799T>C, p.Y267H (C). While the LGMD1B muscle shows a mild involvement of the medial head of gastrocnemius and moderate involvement of soleus (B) there is a moderate to severe involvement of the same muscles in the EDMD2 patient (C). Photo courtesy of Dr. Nicola Carboni and Dr. Marco Mura, University of Cagliari, Sardinia, Italy.

EDMD is characterised by an onset in the teenage years of a slow, progressive wasting of skeletal muscle tissue in the shoulder girdle and distal leg muscles. This atrophy leads to muscle weakness around the humerus and fibula (a pattern described as scapulo-humero-peroneal), early contractures of the *pes cavus* (resulting in high arched feet), proximal muscles of the lower leg and upper arm, and the elbow and Achilles tendons. Muscle cell damage is indicated by elevated serum creatine kinase levels. Muscle pathology shows variations in muscle fibre sizes and type-1 fibre atrophy. Cardiac muscle is also affected, with problems arising in early adulthood. Atrial rhythm disturbances, atrioventricular conduction defects, arrhythmias and dilated cardiomyopathy with atrial ventricular block lead to severe ventricular dysrhythmias and death [38,48].

2.1.2. *Limb-girdle muscular dystrophy, type 1B*

Limb-girdle muscular dystrophy, type 1B (LGMD1B) is a slowly progressive variant caused by an autosomal dominant mutation of the *LMNA* gene, and is characterised by a limb-girdle pattern of muscular atrophy [49,50].

Patients display a classic limb-girdle pattern of muscle atrophy, with a proximal lower limb muscular weakness starting by age 20. By the 30s and 40s upper limb muscles also gradual weakened [49]. As in EDMD, serum creatine kinase levels were normal or elevated. The late occurrence or absence of spinal, elbow and Achilles contractures distinguishes LGMD1B from EDMD. Cardiac conduction abnormalities with dilated cardiomyopathy also occur. One neonatally lethal case of LGMD1B was found to be caused by a homozygous *LMNA* Y259X mutation [51].

2.1.3. *Dilated cardiomyopathy with conduction defect 1*

Dilated cardiomyopathy with conduction defect 1 (CMD1A) is a highly heterogeneous disease, both genetically and phenotypically, with 16 genes currently found to be causatively mutated in cases of CMD1A [52]. Five heterozygotic missense mutations in the *LMNA* gene were identified in 5 of 11 families with autosomal dominant CMD [53].

Dilated cardiomyopathy is a serious cardiac condition, in which the heart becomes weakened and enlarged, with downstream effects on the lungs, liver and other organs. Conduction problems and dilated cardiomyopathy arise, leading to frequent heart failure and sudden death events. Affected family members have little or no associated skeletal myopathy.

2.1.4. Malouf syndrome

Malouf syndrome (MLF) is an extremely rare disorder with only a handful of cases described in the literature. The disease has been found to be caused by one of two mutations in exon 1 of the *LMNA* gene. These mutations, A57P and L59R (Figure 4), have been designated as causing AWS or atypical HGPS, however genital anomalies and missing progeroid features suggest instead a distinct laminopathy [54,55].

In males primary testicular failure, and in females premature ovarian failure, is a characteristic feature of the disease. Mild to moderate dilated cardiomyopathy also occurs. Micrognathia and sloping shoulders can give an atypical progeroid phenotype, however in patients suffering from MLF there is no severe growth failure, alopecia, or atherosclerosis [54].

2.1.5. Heart-hand syndrome, Slovenian type

The heterogeneous family of genetic diseases characterised by both congenital cardiac disease with limb deformities are known as Heart–hand syndromes (HHS). The Heart-hand syndrome, Slovenian type (HHS-S) disorder has been shown to be caused by a mutation (IVS9-12T-G) in intron 9 of the *LMNA* gene. It is an exceedingly rare disorder affecting several generations of a single family in Slovenia [56].

The characteristic changes to the hands and feet include short distal, and proximal phalanges, as well as webbing or fusion of the fingers or toes. Dilated cardiomyopathy, with an adult-onset progressive conduction disorder is also present, with sudden death due to ventricular tachyarrhythmia [56,57].

2.2. Lipodystrophies

Within this section, selected lipodystrophies were detailed, while Table 2 shows a complete listing of known lipodystrophy laminopathies, at the time of writing.

2.2.1. Familial partial lipodystrophy type 2

Familial partial lipodystrophy type 2 (FPLD2; Dunnigan variety of familial partial lipodystrophy) is an autosomal dominant lipodystophy, caused by a heterozygotic mutation in the *LMNA* gene [58-60]. Mutations are clustered in exons 8 and 11, in the globular C-terminal domain region of type-A lamins, the most common of which is a substitution of arginine at position 482 with a neutral amino acid [61].

FPLD2 shows the characteristic lypodystrophy reduction or loss of subcutaneous adipose tissue in certain regions, starting in childhood, puberty or early adulthood. Patients gradually lose fat from the upper and lower limbs, buttocks and trunk. However intramuscular and bone-marrow fat are preserved. Adipose tissue may increase around the face, neck, back and intra-abdominally [62]. Insulin resistance can occur with consequent complications of diabetes, dyslipidaemia, hypertension and hepatic steatosis. Clinical features may also include abnormalities of the menstrual cycle, hirsutism, and acanthosis nigricans.

2.2.2. *Mandibuloacral dysplasia, type A and B*

Mandibuloacral dysplasia (MAD) is an autosomal recessive disease, with strongly heterogeneous clinical features. It is categorised into type A (MADA), which is caused by mutations in the *LMNA* gene and type B (MADB), which is caused by mutations in the *ZMPSTE24* gene [63-65].

Patients with MADA exhibit an acral loss of adipose tissue and a normal or increased fatty layer in the face, neck and trunk, whereas MADB is marked by a severe progressive glomerulopathy, and generalised lipodystrophy affecting the extremeties, but also the face. Growth retardation, osteolysis of the digits, pigmentary changes, mandibular hypoplasia and skeletal anomalies occur in both variants. Patients may also display some symptoms of progeria, and metabolic disorders such as insulin-resistant diabetes [63,66].

2.3. Neuropathies

2.3.1. *Adult-onset autosomal dominant leukodystrophy*

Adult-onset autosomal dominant leukodystrophy (ADLD) is an adult-onset neuropathy, caused by a heterozygous tandem genomic duplication resulting in a duplication of the lamin B1 gene, and a corresponding over-expression of lamin B1 [67,68].

ADLD is slowly progressive, with symptoms becoming apparent in the 40s and 50s, and are markedly similar to progressive multiple sclerosis. These symptoms include symmetric demyelination of the brain and spinal cord, autonomic abnormalities, as well as pyramidal and cerebellar dysfunction. Pathological examination reveals that ADLD differs from progressive multiple sclerosis with a lack of astrogliosis and a preservation of oligodendroglia in the presence of subtotal demyelination [67].

2.3.2. *Charcot-Marie-Tooth disorder*

Charcot-Marie-Tooth disorder (CMT) disorder was described simultaneously by Charcot, Marie and Tooth in 1886. Today the disease is considered a spectrum of phenotypically and genetically heterogeneous inherited neuropathies, with over 40 genes known to be associated with the disorder (www.molgen.ua.ac.be/CMTMutations). The autosomal recessive variant, CMT2B1 (AR-CMT2A or CMT4C1) (OMIM: 605588), is known to be caused by a mutation in *LMNA* [69,70]. All CMT disorders affect approximately 1 in 2,500 people, making them the most common group of inherited neuropathies [71,72]. Individuals with normal or slightly reduced sensory nerve conduction velocities (greater than 38 m/s) are categorised as type 2 (CMT2), and are diagnosed as axonal neuropathies [73]. The disease-causing mutation for CMT2B1 was identified as a homozygous *LMNA* c.829C>T mutation in exon 5 of the *LMNA* gene, causing an R298C amino acid substitution [69,70].

Sufferers of CMT2B1 display an early onset muscle wasting in the distal lower limbs (peroneal muscular atrophy syndrome), high arched feet (*pes cavus*), with a curled, claw-like appearance of the toes, as well as walking difficulties stemming from reduced tendon reflexes [74,75].

2.4. Segmental progeroid diseases

2.4.1. Hutchinson-Gilford progeria syndrome

Hutchinson-Gilford progeria syndrome (HGPS) is an extremely rare, fatal genetic disorder that displays a marked phenotype of premature senility (see chapter on Hutchinson-Gilford progeria syndrome). At least 90% of all HGPS cases are caused by a *de novo* mutation, where a single base nucleotide in exon 11 of the *LMNA* gene is substituted (c.1824C>T, p.G608G). This mutation results in an increased activation of a cryptic splice site in exon 11, which in turn increases the production and subsequent accumulation of a truncated, partially processed prelamin A protein that remains farnesylated, called progerin [76].

Individuals with HGPS are born normally but they present failure to thrive and sclerodermatous skin with loss of subcutaneous fat usually before one year of age. The early symptoms of HGPS also include short stature, and low body weight, which is followed by the occurrence of a tight skin over the abdomen and thighs beginning at the age one or two. Alopecia, scleroderma and the loss of subcutaneous fat also occur at early stages of the disease, succeeded by thin epidermis, fibrosis in the dermis and a loss of skin appendages. Patients often show micrognathia, prominent eyes and veins along with a small beaked nose. Atherosclerosis and calcification of the thoracic aorta is recurrent and death occurs in the early teenage years, most commonly due to cardiovascular complications [76-80].

2.4.2. Restrictive dermopathy

Restrictive dermopathy (RD) is a rare lethal autosomal recessive disease most often caused by loss of function mutations of the *ZMPSTE24* gene, and one case has been described with a dominant mutation in intron 11 of the *LMNA* gene (Figure 4). Similar to HGPS, progerin accumulation occurs, however at a greater level, and this accumulation has been proposed to correspond to the severity of the clinical symptoms [81].

Intrauterine growth retardation is an early sign of RD, along with decreased foetal movement. Thin, translucent, tight skin, as well as joint contractures, respiratory insufficiency, a small pinched nose, micrognathia and mouth in a characteristic fixed 'o' shape are the signs of the disease at birth. Usually respiratory failure due to the tight skin leads to a neonatal death within a few weeks of birth [81,82].

2.4.3. Atypical Werner syndrome

First described in 1904 by Otto Werner, Werner syndrome (WS) is caused by mutations in the *WRN* gene, encoding a nuclear helicase [83]. However approximately 20% of patients diagnosed with WS do not carry mutations in the *WRN* gene, and are classed as suffering from atypical Werner syndrome (AWS). A minority of these have been found to carry heterozygous mutations in the *LMNA* gene, typically at the N-terminal region [84].

WRN is known as 'progeria of the adult' and symptoms, such as pubertal growth failure, begin to emerge in the early teenage years. Then in the late teenage years or early 20s, skin atrophy and ulcers, cataracts, type 2 diabetes mellitus, osteoporosis, atherosclerosis, hair greying and alopecia follow. Lipoatrophy and a mild axonal sensorimotor polyneuropathy can also occur. There is also an increased risk of malignancies, reduced fertility and gonadal atrophy. Severe coronary, and peripheral artery disease is also present, and the most common causes of death are myocardial infarction and cancer by a median age of 54 [85,86].

2.5. Overlapping syndromes

2.5.1. Hydrops-Ectopic calcification-moth-eaten skeletal dysplasia

Hydrops-Ectopic calcification-moth-eaten (HEM) skeletal dysplasia is an extremely rare, autosomal recessive lethal chondrodystrophy, which was first described by Greenberg in 1988, in an examination of two sibling foetuses. A 7-bp, homozygous 1599–1605 TCTTCTArCTAGAAG substitution in exon 13 of the lamin B receptor gene (*LBR*), gave rise to a premature stop codon, resulting in a truncated protein and loss of *LBR* activity [87,88].

In utero radiological examination revealed ectopic calcifications, a 'moth eaten' appearance of the shortened tubular bones. Extramedullary erythropoiesis was also found in both foetuses [89].

2.5.2. Pelger-Huet anomaly

Pelger-Huet anomaly (PHA) is a benign, autosomal dominant blood disorder, with characteristic misshapen, hypolobulated nuclei and abnormally course chromatin in blood granulocytes, caused by a mutation in the *LBR* gene [89,90]. As PHA was found in relatives to two HEM cases, it is thought that these disorders may be related [91].

Heterozygous patients are clinically normal, while homozygosity has been associated with skeletal dysplasia and early lethality in animal models, although at least one case of non-lethal homozygotic PHA has been found in humans [92].

2.5.3. Reynolds syndrome

Reynolds syndrome (RP) is caused by a heterozygous mutation in the *LBR* gene, and was first described in 1971 by Reynolds *et al.* [93].

RP displays a highly heterogeneous set of clinical features similar to the elements of CREST syndrome (CREST is an acronym that stands for calcinosis, Raynaud's phenomenon, esophageal dysmotility, sclerodactyly, and telangiectasia). These symptoms include scleroderma, liver disease, telangiectasia, eosophageal varicies and Raynaud's phenomenon [94].

2.5.4. *Osteopoikilosis/Buschke-Ollendorff syndrome*

Osteopoikilosis/Buschke-Ollendorff syndrome (BOS) is a highly penetrant, benign, rare, autosomal dominant bone disorder. It is caused by a mutation in the *LEMD3* gene, which encodes the MAN1 protein, an integral protein of the inner nuclear membrane. BOS gives rise to osteopoikilosis with subcutaneous nevi or nodules [95], and is known as osteopoikilosis if no skin phenotype is present [96]. It displays an extremely variable set of clinical features even within the same family [97].

The osteopoikilosis is revealed by radiographs as numerous and widespread grain- to pea-sized areas of increased bone density, most often in the cancellous bone regions of the epiphyses and metaphyses, although they are found in almost all bones in the body, with the exception of the cranium where they are rarely found. The skin phenotype is manifested as firm lesions, which histologically are revealed to be either elastic-type (juvenile elastoma) or collagen-type (dermatofibrosis lenticularis disseminata) nevi. Joint stiffness may also be present [98].

2.5.5. *Melorheostosis with osteopoikilosis*

Melorheostosis with osteopoikilosis (MEL) has been thought to be caused by a mutation in the *LEMD3* gene [96]. It is sometimes a features of BOS, however not universally, and evidence for *LEMD3* mutations causing isolated sporadic melorheostosis has not yet been found [97].

MEL is characterised by the flowing hyperostosis of the tubular bone cortices, and sometimes accompanied by abnormalities in surrounding soft-tissue, such as muscle atrophy, joint-contractures, epidermal lesions or hemangiomas [96].

3. Linking genotype and phenotype of laminopathies

A marked change in heterochromatin is one of the most apparent features noted when examining cells affected by laminopathies, from loci of diminished or clumped heterochromatin to total loss of peripheral heterochromatin [99-103]. This alteration of normal heterochromatin, coupled with the known interactions between lamins and gene regulatory proteins, defines a major constituent for the molecular mechanism behind laminopathies [104]. Lamins have been shown to interact with proteins of the inner nuclear membrane (emerin, myne-1, nesprin, LAP1 and LAP2, LBR and MAN1), and chromatin-associated proteins (H2a, H2B, H3-H4, Ha95, HP1 and BAF) [105-109]. These associations allow for gene silencing by means of heterochromatin reorganisation, which could be a causative factor for phenotypic changes [107]. Recruiting genes selectively to the inner nuclear membrane has also been shown to result in their transcriptional repression [10]. The tissue specific gene regulatory role of lamins is thought to underlie the tissue-specific symptoms observed in laminopathies [34,110]. Tissue specific regulation of lamin A expression may also be an explanatory factor for tissue-specific symptoms. Low-level of prelamin A expression in the brain has been shown to be due to a brain-specific microRNA, miRNA-9 [111], and miR-9 overexpression has been shown to alleviate nuclear blebbing in non-neural cells [112].

A mouse model with the *LMNA* H222P mutation for EDMD, displaying muscular dystrophy and cardiomyopathy, was investigated in order to see how gene regulation and metabolic pathways are affected. This investigation revealed that the extracellular signal-regulated kinase (ERK) and c-Jun N-terminal kinase (JNK) branches of the Mitogen-Activated Protein Kinase (MAPK) pathway were activated before any histological changes were visible in the animals. This result was then *in vitro* confirmed by expressing the mutant lamin A *in vitro* [113]. This MAPK signalling change is known to be associated with cardiomyopathy [114-116]. Similar results have been demonstrated in an *EMD*-knockout mouse model for X-linked EDMD, in which MAPK pathway was activated [117].

The possibility of complex interactions between these different causative mechanisms, the complex multirole functionality of lamins, along with widely varying environmental and genetic co-factors affecting this spectrum of processes, would afford a possible explanation for the heterogeneity of disease effects amongst the sufferers of laminopathies [48,118,119]. This variance of disease is one of the most fascinating aspects of laminopathies, the disparity between how a very large family of mutations affecting many genes give rise to diseases with such interrelated clinical features, and on the other hand how even amongst members of a single family carrying the same mutation, disease manifestations are diverse and variable. In AD-EDMD, heterozygous mutations in the *LMNA* gene can give rise to diverse effects, varying from typical EDMD to no disease phenotype, while members of the same family displaying the same mutation can be disease free, or suffer from contractures and muscular atrophy [120].

The diversity of disease phenotypes in consanguineous patients with identical mutations, such as disease onset, severity and progress, indicates that laminopathies are strongly influenced by disease modifiers such as genetic or environmental factors. For example, female sufferers of FPLD2 exhibit a more pronounced phenotype than male [121], family members with BOS can have both or just one of the bone and skin manifestations of that disease. Different missense mutations at the same locus can also give rise to different laminopathies. For example, in the *LMNA* gene, R527H and R527C result in MAD [122,123], while R527P causes EMDM (Figure 4) [46]. The same missense mutation at the same locus can also give rise to different laminopathies. For example, S573L in exon 11 of the *LMNA* in one family gave rise to CDM1A, and in another FPLD2. Of five patients with the same E358K mutation in the *LMNA* gene, three were diagnosed with autosomal dominant EDMD, one with early-onset LGMD1B, and the last patient with congenital muscular dystrophy (Figure 4] [124]. Although the R644C mutation in exon 11 of *LMNA* is associated with CDM1A, three cases with this mutation, and one with an R644H mutation were found to have very high variance in their disease phenotypes, with features ranging from reduced foetal movement and a severe congenital muscular dystrophy-like phenotype, to mild skeletal muscle aberrations and severe and fatal hypertrophic cardiomyopathy [125, 126]. Even amongst members of the same family with the same single nucleotide deletion at position 959, in exon 6 of *LMNA*, one was classified as having DCM, one with EDMD and two with LGMD (Figure 4) [118]. This variation in phenotypes is a recurrent theme in the history of laminopathies, with multiple examples in the literature, which reinforces the importance of disease modifiers.

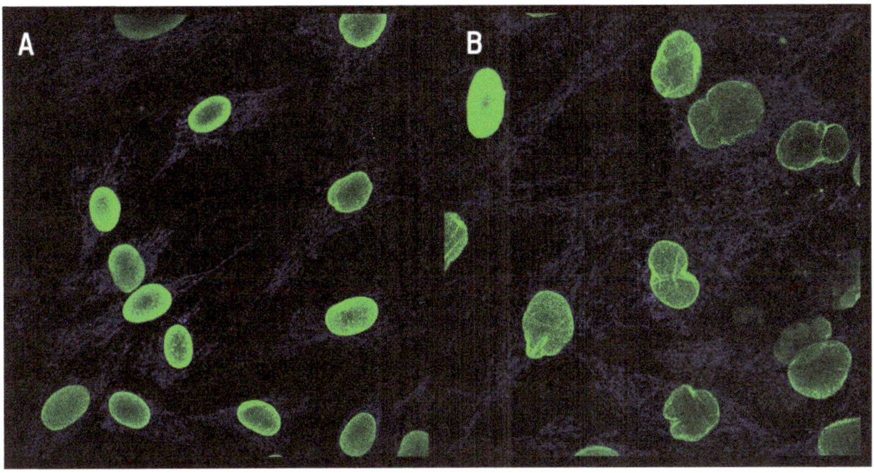

Figure 3. Nuclei showing characteristic blebbing and herniation as a result of a mutation in the LMNA gene. (A) is from sample AG06298 (unaffected HGPS parent) and (B) is from sample AG06917 (HGPS), and has the c.1824C>T, G608G mutation in the LMNA gene. Approximately 50% of the AG06917 cells display blebs. Both are primary fibroblasts hybridised with an antibody for lamin A/C (green) and mitochondria (blue). Photo courtesy of Dr. Peter Berglund.

The *LMNA* missense mutations causing FPLD have been shown to result in nuclei with abnormal shapes, herniated NE and increased fragility, and other laminopathies (including HGPS, Figure 3) have also been found to cause severe changes in nuclear morphology [76,127]. A-type lamin knockout cells display misshapen nuclei with herniations of the NE, slight clustering of NPCs, with mislocalised emerin and B-type lamins. Whereas cells expressing progerin display nuclear blebbing, thickening and honeycombing of the lamina, intranuclear lamina foci, loss of heterochromatin and NPC clustering [2,113,117,128-132]. In PHA however, normally lobulated mature neutrophils exhibit hypolobulation and fail to correctly function [90,133].

An altered nuclear integrity, leading to a weakness in cell structure and a susceptibility to mechanical stress as a constituent of the causative mechanism for laminopathies is supported by the specificity of some laminopathies, such as HGPS or EDMD, to tissues affected by high levels of mechanical stress (the skin, muscles and aortic arch), as well as the similarity of muscular dystrophies caused by mutations in genes responsible for karyoskeleton, cytoskeleton and myotubule proteins to laminopathic muscular dystrophies. The unique expression pattern of lamins in muscle cells might also illuminate a causative system for laminopathies. As no lamin B1 is expressed in muscle cells at all, when *LMNA* protein products are expressed at reduced levels, or functionally impaired, lamin B2 alone must fulfil the lamina requirements of the cell, undergirding the inner nuclear membrane, localising and supporting key proteins of the inner nuclear membrane and organising and regulating the heterochromatin [134].

Various hypotheses have been put forward to account for the muscle cell specificity of EDMD [135]. Muscle cells contain very low or undetectable amounts of lamin B1, whereas in most other cell types lamin B1 is a major lamin, leaving muscle cells more sensitive to loss of function of either emerin or lamin A/C [42,136]. Emerin may also interact with transcription factors or directly with DNA to cause specific gene regulation in muscle cells [137]. Finally, muscle cells also undergo mechanical stress, and emerin, as part of a nucleo-cytoskeletal system may have a protective role against mechanical stress [138].

Lamin A mutations have also been shown to cause premature exhaustion of somatic stem cell populations, as well as stem cell dysfunction. As adult somatic stem cell population is depleted, tissues undergoing a high rate of turnover, such as the skin, would be affected first [139,140].

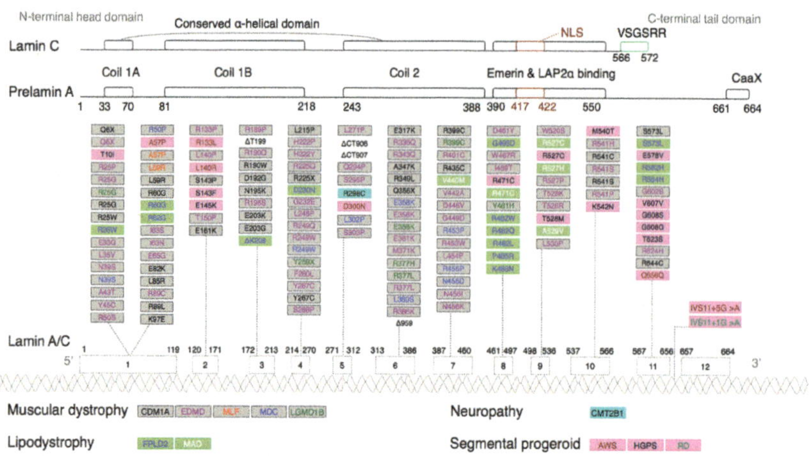

Figure 4. Distribution of laminopathy-causing mutations causing mutations in the LMNA gene. Exons 1-9 and a section of exon 10 encode Lamin C, Lamin A is a result of alternative splicing, adding exon 11 and 12, but removing the lamin C specific part of exon 10 (lamin C specific amino acids marked in green). The conserved α-helical segments of the central rod domain marked with coil 1a, coil 1b, and coil 2. Numbers refer to residues in the primary sequence. Lipodystrophy causing mutations are clustered at exon 8, which codes for an Ig-like domain. The majority (80%) of lipodystrophy cases are caused by a mutation at p.482. Similarly most (>90%) HGPS patients carry the de novo c. 1824C>T, G608G mutation, and most (85%) MAD patients carry a homozygous mutation at p.527 [76,141]. The size of introns are not to scale. CDM1A, dilated cardiomyopathy, type 1A; EDMD, Emery–Dreifuss muscular dystrophy; MLF, Malouf Syndrome; MDC, Muscular dystrophy, congenital; LGMD1B, limb girdle muscular dystrophy, type 1B; FPLD, Dunnigan familial partial lipodystrophy; MAD, mandibuloacral dysplasia; CMT2B1, Charcot–Marie–Tooth disorder, type 2B1; AWS, atypical Werner syndrome; HGPS, Hutchinson–Gilford progeria syndrome;

A consistent relationship between mutation location on the *LMNA* gene and its subsequent effect is difficult to pin down, as shown in figure 4, mutations causing muscular dystrophies are spread all along the gene. However the majority of mutations causing lipodystrophies are located at codon R482, which is conserved across human, mouse, rat and chicken lamin A/C genes [7]. Additionally, the vast majority of segmental progeriod cases are caused by mutations at G608, which affect splicing [34]. The position of the mutation on the *LMNA* gene relative to the NLS seems to play a significant role in the type of laminopathy induced. When laminopathies were segregated on the basis of which organs they showed clinical pathology in, it was found that there was a strong correlation between the position of the mutation relative to the NLS, and the group the resultant laminopathy was sorted into. For example laminopathies with mutations upstream (N-terminally) of the NLS were more likely to display cardiomyopathy and muscle atrophy, while laminopathies with mutations downstream of the NLS (C-Terminally) were more likely to have progeriod symptoms [32]. The tissue-specificity of the mutations may then be correlated with whether the mutation affects the conserved structurally important rod-domain that lies upstream of the NLS, or if it affects the region downstream of the NLS which has been shown to associate with chromatin and/or transcription factors (Figure 4) [142].

It was suspected that a duplication of the *LMNB1* gene was the cause behind ADLD as *LMNB1* was the only gene in the duplicated region expressed in the brain, as well as detection of increased levels of lamin B1 in the brains of affected individuals. The role of *LMNB1* was confirmed by over-expressing lamin B1 in *Drosophila melanogaster*, and in HEK293 cells, which showed a strong phenotype, and nuclear folding and blebbing respectively [67,68].

Finally, a link between levels of progerin produced in laminopathies that exhibit an accumulation of the mutant lamin A/C precursor, and both the severity and age of onset of the phenotype has been shown. RD is considered to be similar but more severe than HGPS, with a correspondingly higher rate of prelamin A accumulation [143,144]. Two cases of a Werner syndrome-like form of progeria displayed a progeria-like aspect with middle age onset coronary artery disease, with a level of progerin that was one quarter of that seen in HGPS cells [85]. Further proof of the toxicity of accumulated progerin is shown by the decrease of progerin levels in cell cultures by treatment with rapamycin, with a resultant rescue of the phenotype [145]. As allele dependant differences in expression of the *LMNA* gene have been observed, with one allele accounting for 70% and the other accounting for 30% of the expressed lamin A and C transcripts, one explanation for phenotype variation might depend on which allele the disease-causing mutation is located [146].

These details paint a complex picture of a heterogeneous family of mutations resulting in varying and overlapping phenotypes, with a diversity in severity and age of onset resulting from tissue specific gene regulation, site of mutation and various genetic and possibly environmental co-factors.

4. Mouse models

Mouse models have yielded invaluable knowledge about the functions of the *LMNA* gene and about the molecular effects of mutations that cause laminopathies. Possibilities for treatment have also been explored with mouse models for these diseases. Various methods have been used to produce strains of mice with similar phenotype to those shown in human laminopathies. Most of the available relevant models have been summarized in the table below (Table 2).

Mice that were thought to completely lack A-type lamin expression were created in order to study a model with no expressed lamin A/C. These *Lmna*-null mice are phenotypically normal at birth, but develop a condition similar to EDMD. By two to three weeks of age they display a growth retardation and arrest. Skeletal abnormalities including kyphosis occur, and a loss of white adipose tissue was noted. Cardiac myopathies also develop, and death occurred within eight weeks. An analysis of mouse embryonic fibroblasts (MEFs) showed misshapen, herniated nuclei. Mice heterozygous for *Lmna* were phenotypically normal [101]. The phenotype for *Lmna* knockout mice showed neuropathic features, decreased axon density paired with increased axon diameter and non-myelinated axons, features that are markedly similar to human axonopathies [70,101]. The only known case of an *LMNA*-null human, with homozygous nonsense mutations in *LMNA*, resulted in a perinatal lethality, exhibiting small size, retrognathia, severe limb and phalangeal contractures, fractures in the femur and arm, muscular dystrophy. Death was due to respiratory failure [51]. Apart from these differences in disease severity, changes in the proliferation of *LMNA*-null fibroblasts were also markedly dissimilar for human as compared to mouse. Patient fibroblasts showed a reduced proliferation [160], while MEFs showed an increased proliferative potential compared to wild-type MEFs [161]. Recently these mice have been found to express a C-terminally truncated *Lmna* gene product, missing residues 461–657 of wild-type lamin A, which are normally encoded by exons 8–11. This expression, both on a transcriptional and protein level, perhaps explains the difference in fibroblast proliferative potential between human *LMNA*-null fibroblasts and MEFs from this mouse model, as well as raising questions about the many studies that have been performed on these mice [162].

Mice with the *Zmpste24* gene knocked out were created independently by two groups [151,163]. While loss of the *ZMPSTE24* gene due to homozygous or compound heterozygous mutations in humans results in the neonatally lethal disease, RD, these mouse models did not display an equivalent phenotype. The *Zmpste24*$^{-/-}$ mice lack the ability to convert farnesylated prelamin A to mature lamin A, and so accumulate prelamin A at the nuclear rim, resulting in aberrant nuclear morphology. Normal at birth, they develop a HGPS-like condition, showing growth retardation, alopecia, kyphosis, weight loss and incisor defects. Spontaneous bone fractures also occur as the animals age and death occurs prematurely, at 20-30 weeks [150,151]. That the accumulation of prelamin A was the direct cause of the disease state was demonstrated when *Zmpste24*$^{-/-}$ mice with only one allele for the *Lmna* gene were compared to *Zmpste24*$^{-/-}$ mice with two copies of *Lmna*. The *Zmpste24*$^{-/-}$*Lmna*$^{+/-}$ mice had significantly reduced levels of prelamin A compared to *Zmpste24*$^{-/-}$*Lmna*$^{+/+}$ mice. All disease phenotype was missing, and the ratio of misshapen nuclei to normal was also reduced [103].

Mouse model	Description	Pathology	Reference
$Lmna^{-/-}$	These *Lmna* null mice were designed to produce no lamin A or C. Recently however they have been found to produce a truncated lamin A protein.	Postnatal lethality, with cardiomyopathy and muscular dystrophy	[101,147]
$Lmna^{GT-/-}$	These mice have a total loss of lamin A/C.	Growth retardation, developmental heart defects, skeletal muscle hypotrophy, decreased subcutaneous adipose tissue. Death occurs at 2 to 3 weeks *post partum*, without dilated cardiomyopathy or an obvious progeroid phenotype.	[148]
$Lmna^{LCO/LCO}$	These lamin C only mice carry a mutant Lmna allele that yields lamin C exclusively, without lamin A.	No disease phenotypes and a normal lifespan.	[132]
$Lmna^{LAO/LAO}$	Mature lamin A only mouse, bypassing prelamin A synthesis and processing.	No detectable pathology, fibroblasts show misshapen nuclei.	[149]
$Zmpste24^{-/-}$	These mice are null for the endoprotease responsible for the final cleavage step in prelamin A maturation, leading to an accumulation of farnesylated pre-lamin A.	Mice have rib fractures, osteoporosis, muscle weakness and die at 6–7 months.	[150] [99]
		Postnatal growth retardation, shortened lifespan, loss of fat layer and muscular dystrophy.	[151]
$Lmna^{N195K/N195K}$	These mice have a missense CDM1A-associated lamin A mutation, N195K.	Postnatal death associated with cardiomyopathy. MEFs showed nuclear abnormalities.	[152]
$Lmna^{H222P/H222P}$	These mice have a missense EDMD-associated lamin A mutation, H222P.	These mice show a stiff walking posture and cardiac dysfunction. Death occurs by 9 months of age. MEFs showed nuclear abnormalities.	[153]
$Lmna^{HG/HG}$	These mice carry an *Lmna*-knock in allele that produces progerin. Mice accumulate farnesyl–prelamin A.	Heterozygous mice, $Lmna^{HG/-}$, express large amounts of progerin and develop many disease phenotypes of progeria. MEFs display nuclear blebbing.	[154]
$Lmna^{L530P/L530P}$	These mice have a L530P mutation in the lamin A gene that is associated with EDMD in humans.	Homozygous mice display defects consistent with HGPS, and die within 4-5 weeks of birth.	[155]
$Lmna^{M371K}$	cDNA with mis-sense mutation expressed with a heart specific promoter.	Cardiomyopathy and early postnatal lethality	[156]
$Lmna^{G609G}$	The wild-type mouse *lmna* gene is replaced with a copy containing the c. 1827C>T;p.G609G mutation. This is the equivalent of the HGPS c.1824C>T;p.G608G mutation in the human *LMNA* gene.	Growth retardation, weight loss, cardiovascular problems and shortened lifespan.	[157]
$Lmnb1^{-/-}$	These mice have an insertional mutation in *Lmnb1*, resulting in a mutant lamin B1 protein missing several functional domains.	Mice survive embryonic development, however die at birth with lung and bone defects.	[29]
$Emd^{-/-}$	These mice do not express emerin.	Mice overtly normal but with slightly retarded muscle regeneration.	[158,159]

Table 2. Selected mouse models relevant for studying laminopathies.

A mouse model for EDMD was created by knocking out the *Emd* gene. These animals had no abnormal clinical features outside of a slightly retarded muscle regeneration, and altered motor coordination when tested on a rotarod [158,159]. The human AD-EDMD mutations in the *LMNA* gene, H222P (with a histidine substituting for a proline at residue 222) and N195K (with a lysine substituting for asparagine at residue 195), have also been used to create mouse models for AD-EDMD. Again, mice heterozygous for the mutations are indistinguishable from wild-type animals. Mice with two copies of the mutation however, showed a muscular dystrophy and cardiomyopathy phenotype [152,153].

Knock-in mouse models such as the $Lmna^{G609G}$ mouse model closely mimic the human disease HGPS. A copy of the wild-type mouse *lmna* gene was replaced with a copy containing the c.1827C>T;p.G609G mutation, the equivalent of the HGPS c.1824C>T;p.G608G mutation in the human *LMNA* gene. This gave a phenotype of growth retardation, weight loss, cardiovascular problems and curtailed lifespan, correlating neatly with the clinical features found in the human disease. However, the disease symptoms were most marked and similar in the homozygous state, whereas in humans an autosomal dominant state with only a single mutated allele confers the disease state [157].

A mouse model where only lamin-C is produced ($Lmna^{LCO}$), without producing any prelamin A or mature lamin A. These $Lmna^{LCO/LCO}$ animals were entirely healthy, with only a minimal alteration to normal nuclear shape [132]. More recently a mouse model where only mature lamin A is expressed was made. These $Lmna^{LAO/LAO}$ mice synthesis mature lamin A without any prelamin A synthesis or processing steps. They display no disease phenotype, but do have an increased level of nuclear blebbing compared to wild-type, demonstrating that bypassing prelamin A processing and directly synthesising mature lamin A has little effect on the transportation of lamin A to the nuclear envelope [149].

In order to study early post-natal development effects caused by loss of lamin A/C, an $Lmna^{GT-/-}$ model was created. This model simultaneously inactivates and reports the expression of *Lmna*. Loss of lamin A/C resulted in growth retardation, developmental defects of the heart, skeletal muscle hypotrophy, loss of subcutaneous adipose tissue and impaired *ex vivo* adipogenic differentiation. Premature death occurred at two to three week *post partum* [148].

A mouse model was created using a heart-selective promoter (α-myosin heavy chain promoter) to control the expression of human normal lamin A, and lamin A containing the EDMD causing mutation M371K. Mice expressing the wild-type human lamin A were born at slightly less than expected rates, and had a normal lifespan. However, mice expressing mutant M371K lamin A exhibited a much higher risk of prenatal death, and were born at only a fraction (0.07) of the expected frequency. Those animals that were born died within 2-7 weeks, and displayed pulmonary and cardia edema. Cardiac cells from these mice showed abnormal, convoluted nuclear envelopes with clumped chromatin and intranuclear foci of lamins [156].

Mouse models of laminopathies are limited by the gross physiological differences between rodent (mouse models being the most relevant models used to investigate laminopathies) and human. However, despite the limitations of mouse models, the advantages are legion; being able to study very rare diseases at any stage of disease, with limitless sampling, temporal and physically controlled expression of mutant protein, and with the possibilities for testing different type of treatment.

5. Treatment

Current treatments for laminopathies are largely symptomatic, controlling the secondary effects of the disease. Corrective surgery is used to treat the EDMD contractures, coronary artery bypass surgery for HGPS, pacemaker installation or heart transplantation for DCMI or LGMD1B patients [164]. FPLD2 patients with diabetes mellitus and hypertension are treated with antidiabetic drugs, angiotensin converting enzyme inhibitors, calcium channel blockers and beta blockers [52,165,166]. The administration of a recombinant methionyl human leptin has been tried with some success in patients suffering from FPLD, giving rise to improved fasting glucose concentrations, insulin sensitivity, and triglyceride levels [167,168]. The impairment of pre-adipocyte differentiation, an impairment which is brought about by the negative effects of prelamin A accumulation on the rate of DNA-bound SREBP1, may also be treated with troglitazone, a PPAR-gamma ligand which promotes the adipogenic program [169].

Curative treatment for laminopathies that are autosomal-recessive involving loss-of-function of a protein, such as EDMD-AR, would require the expression of a healthy wild-type allele in the affected tissue. However, autosomal dominant laminopathies require a more complex treatment, in which the production, modification and/or the effect of the mutant protein also need to be eliminated. For example, in a phase II clinical trial with HGPS patients, lonafarnib, a farnesyl transferase inhibitor (FTI) is being given as treatment (see chapter on Hutchinson-Gilford progeria syndrome) [170]. FTI is normally used as an anti-tumour treatment, but it also reduces the amount of progerin produced by inhibiting the farnesylation of prelamin A. Previous experiments with FTIs in cell cultures showed marked improvements, with a reduction of misshapen nuclei [171]. With mouse models for HGPS an improvement in disease phenotype was noted, although no total reversal was apparent [172-176]. This may be due to the fact that although FTI treatment inhibits the farnesylation of prelamin-A by farnesyl transferase, a secondary modification pathway, a geranylgeranylation by geranylgeranyltransferase, allows prelamin A to be processed into progerin despite the FTI treatment [177]. However, a combination of statins (a potent HMG-CoA reductase inhibitor, used to inhibit the production of cholesterol in the liver) and bisphosphonates (a class of drugs used to treat osteoporosis), was used to inhibit the synthesis of farnesyl pyrophosphate, a co-substrate of farnesyltransferase and a precursor of a substrate for geranylgeranyltransferase I. This combination inhibits prenylation, and when used to treat laminopathies, resulted in an increased longevity, reduced oxidative stress, cellular senescence and improved phenotype in mice [61,154,172,178,179]. A triple drug trial was initiated in 2009 to examine the efficacy of treatment involving an FTI, a statin and a bisphosphonate, however the results of this trial have not yet been made public.

Long-term treatment with FTIs is not without risks. All CaaX box/motif proteins would have their farnesylation processing inhibited, which would mean an inhibition of lamin-B maturation. Non-farnesylated lamins might also accumulate in the cell, with unexpected effects. In a mice model where non-farnesylated prelamin-A was solely expressed, with the CaaX motif/box mutated to SAAX, a cardiomyopathy was observed to occur [180]. In HIV treatment, acquired lipodystrophy is a possible side-effect of the use of HIV protease inhibitors, which cause pre-lamin A accumulation [181]. This pre-lamin accumulation was also observed in fibroblasts from FPLD2 patients, further hinting at the toxicity of pre-lamin A accumulation [61].

Rapamycin, an immunosuppressant antibiotic drug, has also been examined as a possible treatment in laminopathies. Rapamycin treatment in HGPS cell cultures resulted in reduced nuclear blebbing and decreased rates of senescence, as well as a marked reduction of progerin and prelamin A levels, a restoration of wildtype LAP2α, BAF and trimethylated H3K9 organisation, and a rescue of the normal chromatin phenotype. These effects come about by means of autophagic degradation of prelamin A, triggered by inactivation of the inhibitory mammalian target of rapamycin (mTOR) dependent pathway [145,182]. In an *Lmna*$^{-/-}$ mouse model treatment with rapamycin was shown to improve cardiac and skeletal muscle function, as well as improving the survival rate [183]. In the *Lmna*$^{H222P/H222P}$ mouse model, rapamycin treatment was shown to improve cardiac function [184]. This mouse model has also been treated with other inhibitors of MAPK/ERK kinase (MEK) (the mitogen-activated protein kinase (MAPK kinase) that activates extracellular signal-regulated protein kinase (ERK)), in order to see if administration would alleviate or prevent the cardiomyopathy. The MEK-inhibitor treated animals were indistinguishable from wild-type animals, while untreated control animals displayed reduced ejection fraction, indicating a dilated cardiomyopathy. Interestingly, abnormal elongation of heart cell nuclei was noted in untreated control animals, but was not observed in the treatment group [113,185]. As with FTIs, the long-term treatment of patients with rapamycin would entail the acceptance of know side-effects, such as lung toxicity, insulin resistance, cataracts and testicular degeneration [186-189].

Pre-lamin A antisense oligonucleotides were used to reduce pre-lamin A levels, with a resultant decrease in misshapen nuclei. The most common HGPS point mutation causes an increased usage of a cryptic splice site in exon 11, CAG#GTGGGC, which is also used at near-undetectable levels in wild-type cells. Antisense morpholino oligonucleotides directed to this site resulted in an improvement of HGPS fibroblast disease phenotype [190]. RNA interference has also been used to successfully improve proliferation and nuclear morphology, as well as reducing senescence in fibroblasts expressing mutant lamin A [191]. In another experiment exon 11 splice donor site antisense oligonucleotides were also used to promote the alternative splice pathway, leading to an increased in progerin production in fibroblast cells, and short hairpin RNA (shRNA) were then used to diminish this production in fibroblasts, leading to an improvement of phenotype [192]. Morpholinos have also been used to target the cryptic splicing event in mouse. The use of antisense morpholinos to the exon 10 lamin A splice donor site and the c.1827C>T;p.G609G mutation of the *LMNA* transcript was shown to reduce progerin levels, partially restore a wild-type phenotype and extend lifespan of a mouse model for HGPS [157].

In light of the recent Glybera Gene therapy [193], future gene therapies for the treatment of the cardiomyopathy prevalent in muscular dystrophies may also be an area of interest [194-196].

6. Conclusion

During the last decade the number of diseases found to be caused by mutations in lamin or lamin associated genes has increased significantly. These phenotypically diverse diseases have been categorised both phenotypically and genetically, and today research is focused on both deciphering the pathogenic mechanisms behind their pathophysiological processes, as well as understanding how such diverse pathologies can arise from this related family of mutations. During that time the appreciated role for lamins has changed from being regarded merely as a structural scaffold for the nucleus, to a key element in DNA replication and transcription, chromatin organisation, cell replication and differentiation. Future research is sure to continue at an ever-increasing pace, especially as the development and integration of next generation sequencing technologies and technologies that allows for global analysis of the genome and epigenome into both research and clinical settings. For researchers this level of genomic interrogation brings about unprecedented access to new information about our genome, which will be valuable for the creation of maps of genetic and possibly epigenetic variation that influence disease.

The laminopathies described in this review are without a doubt, exceedingly rare. However by researching these rare conditions, it is hoped that we can shed light on their all too common clinical symptoms, such as cardiac disease, metabolic disorders such as insulin resistance, and even ageing itself.

Acknowledgements

Our work is supported by a VINNMER fellow grant from VINNOVA, and an Innovator grant from The Progeria Research Foundation. We thank the patients, and Dr. Nicola Carboni and Dr Marco Mura for contributing photos of patients. Primary fibroblast cultures were obtained from the Aging Repository of the Coriell Cell Repository.

Author details

Tomás McKenna*, Jean-Ha Baek and Maria Eriksson

*Address all correspondence to: tomas.mckenna@ki.se

Department of Biosciences and Nutrition, Center for Biosciences, Karolinska Institutet, Huddinge, Sweden

References

[1] Cronshaw JM, Krutchinsky AN, Zhang W, Chait BT, Matunis MJ. Proteomic analysis of the mammalian nuclear pore complex. Journal of Cell Biology. 2002Sep.2;158(5): 915–27.

[2] Shimi T, Butin-Israeli V, Goldman RD. The functions of the nuclear envelope in mediating the molecular crosstalk between the nucleus and the cytoplasm. Current Opinion in Cell Biology. 2012Feb.;24(1):71–8.

[3] Fried H, Kutay U. Nucleocytoplasmic transport: taking an inventory. Cell. Mol. Life Sci. 2003Aug.;60(8):1659–88.

[4] Zastrow MS, Vlcek S, Wilson KL. Proteins that bind A-type lamins: integrating isolated clues.

[5] Lin F. MAN1, an integral protein of the inner nuclear membrane, binds Smad2 and Smad3 and antagonizes transforming growth factor- signaling. Human Molecular Genetics. 2004Dec.8;14(3):437–45.

[6] Fisher D, Chaudhary N. cDNA sequencing of nuclear lamins A and C reveals primary and secondary structural homology to intermediate filament proteins. Proceedings of the .... 1986Jan.1.

[7] Stuurman N, Heins S, Aebi U. Nuclear Lamins: Their Structure, Assembly, and Interactions* 1. Journal of structural biology. 1998Aug.18;:1–25.

[8] Dechat T, Pfleghaar K, Sengupta K, Shimi T, Shumaker DK, Solimando L, et al. Nuclear lamins: major factors in the structural organization and function of the nucleus and chromatin. Genes & development. 2008Apr.1;22(7):832–53.

[9] Moir R, Spann T. The structure and function of nuclear lamins: implications for disease. Cellular and Molecular Life Sciences. 2001Jan.1.

[10] Reddy KL, Zullo JM, Bertolino E, Singh H. Transcriptional repression mediated by repositioning of genes to the nuclear lamina. Nature. 2008Mar.13;452(7184):243–7.

[11] Gruenbaum Y, Margalit A, Goldman RD, Shumaker DK, Wilson KL. The nuclear lamina comes of age. Nat Rev Mol Cell Biol. 2005Jan.;6(1):21–31.

[12] Rout MP. The Nuclear Pore Complex as a Transport Machine. Journal of Biological Chemistry. 2001Apr.5;276(20):16593–6.

[13] Lin F, Worman HJ. Structural organization of the human gene encoding nuclear lamin A and nuclear lamin C. J Biol Chem. 1993Aug.5;268(22):16321–6.

[14] Barrowman J, Hamblet C, George CM, Michaelis S. Analysis of prelamin A biogenesis reveals the nucleus to be a CaaX processing compartment. Mol. Biol. Cell. 2008Dec.;19(12):5398–408.

[15] Röber RA, Weber K, Osborn M. Differential timing of nuclear lamin A/C expression in the various organs of the mouse embryo and the young animal: a developmental study. Development. 1989Feb.;105(2):365–78.

[16] Zorenc AHG. An Alternative Splicing Product of the Lamin A/C Gene Lacks Exon 10. Journal of Biological Chemistry. 1996Apr.19;271(16):9249–53.

[17] Jahn D, Schramm S, Benavente R, Alsheimer M. Dynamic properties of meiosis-specific lamin C2 and its impact on nuclear envelope integrity. Nucleus. 2010May;1(3): 273–83.

[18] Alsheimer M, Benavente R. Change of karyoskeleton during mammalian spermatogenesis: expression pattern of nuclear lamin C2 and its regulation. Experimental Cell Research. 1996Nov.1;228(2):181–8.

[19] Stick R, Hausen P. Changes in the nuclear lamina composition during early development of Xenopus laevis. Cell. 1985May;41(1):191–200.

[20] Lehner CF, Stick R, Eppenberger HM, Nigg EA. Differential expression of nuclear lamin proteins during chicken development. Journal of Cell Biology. 1987Jul.;105(1): 577–87.

[21] Furukawa K, Inagaki H, Hotta Y. Identification and cloning of an mRNA coding for a germ cell-specific A-type lamin in mice. Experimental Cell Research. 1994Jun.;212(2): 426–30.

[22] Lin F, Worman HJ. Structural organization of the human gene (LMNB1) encoding nuclear lamin B1. Genomics. 1995May20;27(2):230–6.

[23] Biamonti G, Giacca M, Perini G, Contreas G, Zentilin L, Weighardt F, et al. The gene for a novel human lamin maps at a highly transcribed locus of chromosome 19 which replicates at the onset of S-phase. Mol. Cell. Biol. 1992Aug.;12(8):3499–506.

[24] Furukawa K, Hotta Y. cDNA cloning of a germ cell specific lamin B3 from mouse spermatocytes and analysis of its function by ectopic expression in somatic cells. The EMBO journal. 1993Jan.;12(1):97–106.

[25] Pollard KM, Chan EK, Grant BJ, Sullivan KF, Tan EM, Glass CA. In vitro posttranslational modification of lamin B cloned from a human T-cell line. Mol. Cell. Biol. 1990May;10(5):2164–75.

[26] Kitten GT, Nigg EA. The CaaX motif is required for isoprenylation, carboxyl methylation, and nuclear membrane association of lamin B2. Journal of Cell Biology. 1991Apr.;113(1):13–23.

[27] Lutz RJ, Trujillo MA, Denham KS, Wenger L, Sinensky M. Nucleoplasmic localization of prelamin A: implications for prenylation-dependent lamin A assembly into the nuclear lamina. Proceedings of the National Academy of Sciences of the United States of America. 1992Apr.1;89(7):3000–4.

[28] Holtz D, Tanaka RA, Hartwig J, McKeon F. The CaaX motif of lamin A functions in conjunction with the nuclear localization signal to target assembly to the nuclear envelope. Cell. 1989Dec.22;59(6):969–77.

[29] Vergnes L, Péterfy M, Bergo MO, Young SG, Reue K. Lamin B1 is required for mouse development and nuclear integrity. Proceedings of the National Academy of Sciences of the United States of America. 2004Jul.13;101(28):10428–33.

[30] Hennekes H, Nigg EA. The role of isoprenylation in membrane attachment of nuclear lamins. A single point mutation prevents proteolytic cleavage of the lamin A precursor and confers membrane binding properties. 1994.

[31] Worman HJ, Fong LG, Muchir A, Young SG. Laminopathies and the long strange trip from basic cell biology to therapy. J. Clin. Invest. 2009Jul.;119(7):1825–36.

[32] Hegele R. LMNA mutation position predicts organ system involvement in laminopathies. Clinical Genetics. 2005Apr.5;68(1):31–4.

[33] Landires I, Pascale JM, Motta J. The position of the mutation within the LMNA gene determines the type and extent of tissue involvement in laminopathies. Clinical Genetics. 2007Apr.25;71(6):592–3.

[34] Broers JLV, Ramaekers FCS, Bonne G, Yaou RB, Hutchison CJ. Nuclear lamins: laminopathies and their role in premature ageing. Physiological Reviews [Internet]. 2006Jul.;86(3):967–1008. Available from: http://physrev.physiology.org/cgi/content/abstract/86/3/967

[35] Zaremba-Czogalla M, Dubińska-Magiera M, Rzepecki R. Laminopathies: the molecular background of the disease and the prospects for its treatment. Cell. Mol. Biol. Lett. 2011Mar.;16(1):114–48.

[36] Hegele RA, Cao H, Liu DM, Costain GA, Charlton-Menys V, Rodger NW, et al. Sequencing of the reannotated LMNB2 gene reveals novel mutations in patients with acquired partial lipodystrophy. Am. J. Hum. Genet. 2006Aug.;79(2):383–9.

[37] Emery AE, Dreifuss FE. Unusual type of benign x-linked muscular dystrophy. J. Neurol. Neurosurg. Psychiatr. 1966Aug.;29(4):338–42.

[38] Muchir A, Worman HJ. Emery-Dreifuss muscular dystrophy. Curr Neurol Neurosci Rep. 2007Jan.;7(1):78–83.

[39] Helbling-Leclerc A, Bonne G, Schwartz K. Emery-Dreifuss muscular dystrophy. Eur J Hum Genet. 2002Mar.;10(3):157–61.

[40] Manilal S, Nguyen TM, Sewry CA, Morris GE. The Emery-Dreifuss muscular dystrophy protein, emerin, is a nuclear membrane protein. Human Molecular Genetics. 1996Jun.;5(6):801–8.

[41] Nagano A, Koga R, Ogawa M, Kurano Y, Kawada J, Okada R, et al. Emerin deficiency at the nuclear membrane in patients with Emery-Dreifuss muscular dystrophy. Nat Genet. 1996Mar.;12(3):254–9.

[42] Manilal S. Distribution of emerin and lamins in the heart and implications for Emery-Dreifuss muscular dystrophy. Human Molecular Genetics. 1999Feb.1;8(2):353–9.

[43] Meinke P, Nguyen TD, Wehnert MS. The LINC complex and human disease. Biochem. Soc. Trans. 2011Dec.;39(6):1693–7.

[44] Scharner J, Brown CA, Bower M, Iannaccone ST, Khatri IA, Escolar D, et al. Novel LMNA mutations in patients with Emery-Dreifuss muscular dystrophy and functional characterization of four LMNA mutations. Hum. Mutat. 2011Feb.;32(2):152–67.

[45] Lassuthová P, Baránková L, Kraus J, Maríková T, Seeman P. Emery-Dreifuss muscular dystrophy: a novel mutation in the LMNA gene. Pediatr. Neurol. 2009Aug.;41(2): 127–30.

[46] Bonne G, Di Barletta MR, Varnous S, Bécane HM, Hammouda EH, Merlini L, et al. Mutations in the gene encoding lamin A/C cause autosomal dominant Emery-Dreifuss muscular dystrophy. Nat Genet. 1999Mar.;21(3):285–8.

[47] Felice KJ, Schwartz RC, Brown CA, Leicher CR, Grunnet ML. Autosomal dominant Emery-Dreifuss dystrophy due to mutations in rod domain of the lamin A/C gene. Neurology. 2000Jul.25;55(2):275–80.

[48] Canki-Klain N, Récan D, Milicić D, Llense S, Leturcq F, Deburgrave N, et al. Clinical variability and molecular diagnosis in a four-generation family with X-linked Emery-Dreifuss muscular dystrophy. Croat. Med. J. 2000Dec.;41(4):389–95.

[49] Muchir A, Bonne G, van der Kooi AJ, van Meegen M, Baas F, Bolhuis PA, et al. Identification of mutations in the gene encoding lamins A/C in autosomal dominant limb girdle muscular dystrophy with atrioventricular conduction disturbances (LGMD1B). Human Molecular Genetics. 2000May22;9(9):1453–9.

[50] Yuan W-L, Huang C-Y, Wang J-F, Xie S-L, Nie R-Q, Liu Y-M, et al. R25G mutation in exon 1 of LMNA gene is associated with dilated cardiomyopathy and limb-girdle muscular dystrophy 1B. Chin. Med. J. 2009Dec.5;122(23):2840–5.

[51] van Engelen BGM, Muchir A, Hutchison CJ, van der Kooi AJ, Bonne G, Lammens M. The lethal phenotype of a homozygous nonsense mutation in the lamin A/C gene. Neurology. 2005Jan.24;64(2):374–6.

[52] Song K, Dubé MP, Lim J, Hwang I, Lee I, Kim J-J. Lamin A/C mutations associated with familial and sporadic cases of dilated cardiomyopathy in Koreans. Exp. Mol. Med. 2007Feb.28;39(1):114–20.

[53] Fatkin D, MacRae C, Sasaki T, Wolff MR, Porcu M, Frenneaux M, et al. Missense mutations in the rod domain of the lamin A/C gene as causes of dilated cardiomyopathy and conduction-system disease. New England journal of medicine. 1999Dec. 2;341(23):1715–24.

[54] McPherson E, Turner L, Zador I, Reynolds K, Macgregor D, Giampietro PF. Ovarian failure and dilated cardiomyopathy due to a novel lamin mutation. Am. J. Med. Genet. 2009Feb.15;149A(4):567–72.

[55] Garg A, Subramanyam L, Agarwal AK, Simha V, Levine B, D'Apice MR, et al. Atypical Progeroid Syndrome due to Heterozygous Missense LMNA Mutations. Journal of Clinical Endocrinology & Metabolism. 2009Dec.3;94(12):4971–83.

[56] Renou L, Stora S, Yaou RB, Volk M, Sinkovec M, Demay L, et al. Heart-hand syndrome of Slovenian type: a new kind of laminopathy. Journal of Medical Genetics. 2008Jun.25;45(10):666–71.

[57] Sinkovec M, Petrovič D, Volk M, Peterlin B. Familial progressive sinoatrial and atrioventricular conduction disease of adult onset with sudden death, dilated cardiomyopathy, and brachydactyly. A new type of heart-hand syndrome? Clinical Genetics. 2005Jun.17;68(2):155–60.

[58] Morel CF. A LMNA Splicing Mutation in Two Sisters with Severe Dunnigan-Type Familial Partial Lipodystrophy Type 2. Journal of Clinical Endocrinology & Metabolism. 2006Apr.18;91(7):2689–95.

[59] Shackleton S, Lloyd DJ, Jackson SN, Evans R, Niermeijer MF, Singh BM, et al. LMNA, encoding lamin A/C, is mutated in partial lipodystrophy. Nat Genet. 2000Feb.;24(2):153–6.

[60] Saha B, Lessel D, Hisama FM, Leistritz DF, Friedrich K, Martin GM, et al. A Novel LMNA Mutation Causes Altered Nuclear Morphology and Symptoms of Familial Partial Lipodystrophy (Dunnigan Variety) with Progeroid Features. Mol Syndromol. 2010Sep.;1(3):127–32.

[61] Caron M, Auclair M, Donadille B, Béréziat V, Guerci B, Laville M, et al. Human lipodystrophies linked to mutations in A-type lamins and to HIV protease inhibitor therapy are both associated with prelamin A accumulation, oxidative stress and premature cellular senescence. Cell Death Differ. Nature Publishing Group; 2007Jul.6;14(10):1759–67.

[62] GARG A, Wilson R, Barnes R, Arioglu E, Zaidi Z, Gurakan F, et al. A gene for congenital generalized lipodystrophy maps to human chromosome 9q34. Journal of Clinical Endocrinology & Metabolism. 1999Sep.;84(9):3390–4.

[63] Garavelli L, D'Apice MR, Rivieri F, Bertoli M, Wischmeijer A, Gelmini C, et al. Mandibuloacral dysplasia type A in childhood. Am. J. Med. Genet. 2009Oct.;149A(10):2258–64.

[64] Agarwal AK, Fryns J-P, Auchus RJ, Garg A. Zinc metalloproteinase, ZMPSTE24, is mutated in mandibuloacral dysplasia. Human Molecular Genetics. 2003Aug.15;12(16):1995–2001.

[65] Garg A, Cogulu O, Ozkinay F, Onay H, Agarwal AK. A novel homozygous Ala529Val LMNA mutation in Turkish patients with mandibuloacral dysplasia. Journal of Clinical Endocrinology & Metabolism. 2005Sep.;90(9):5259–64.

[66] Zirn B, Kress W, Grimm T, Berthold LD, Neubauer B, Kuchelmeister K, et al. Association of homozygous LMNA mutation R471C with new phenotype: mandibuloacral dysplasia, progeria, and rigid spine muscular dystrophy. Am. J. Med. Genet. 2008Apr.15;146A(8):1049–54.

[67] Padiath QS, Saigoh K, Schiffmann R, Asahara H, Yamada T, Koeppen A, et al. Lamin B1 duplications cause autosomal dominant leukodystrophy. Nat Genet. 2006Oct.; 38(10):1114–23.

[68] Schuster J, Sundblom J, Thuresson A-C, Hassin-Baer S, Klopstock T, Dichgans M, et al. Genomic duplications mediate overexpression of lamin B1 in adult-onset autosomal dominant leukodystrophy (ADLD) with autonomic symptoms. Neurogenetics. 2011Feb.;12(1):65–72.

[69] Bouhouche A, Benomar A, Birouk N, Mularoni A, Meggouh F, Tassin J, et al. A locus for an axonal form of autosomal recessive Charcot-Marie-Tooth disease maps to chromosome 1q21. 2-q21. 3. Am. J. Hum. Genet. Elsevier; 1999;65(3):722–7.

[70] de Sandre-Giovannoli A, Chaouch M, Kozlov S, Vallat J-M, Tazir M, Kassouri N, et al. Homozygous defects in LMNA, encoding lamin A/C nuclear-envelope proteins, cause autosomal recessive axonal neuropathy in human (Charcot-Marie-Tooth disorder type 2) and mouse. Am. J. Hum. Genet. 2002Mar.;70(3):726–36.

[71] Skre H. Genetic and clinical aspects of Charcot-Marie-Tooth's disease. Clinical Genetics. Wiley Online Library; 1974;6(2):98–118.

[72] Krajewski KM, Lewis RA, Fuerst DR, Turansky C, Hinderer SR, Garbern J, et al. Neurological dysfunction and axonal degeneration in Charcot-Marie-Tooth disease type 1A. Brain. 2000Jul.;123 (Pt 7):1516–27.

[73] Garcia CA. A clinical review of Charcot-Marie-Tooth. Ann. N. Y. Acad. Sci. 1999Sep. 14;883:69–76.

[74] De Jonghe P, Timmerman V, Van Broeckhoven C. 2nd Workshop of the European CMT Consortium: 53rd ENMC International Workshop on Classification and Diagnostic Guidelines for Charcot-Marie-Tooth Type 2 (CMT2–HMSN II) and Distal Hereditary Motor Neuropathy (Distal HMN–Spinal CMT) 26–28 September 1997, Naarden, The Netherlands. Neuromuscular Disorders. Elsevier; 1998;8(6):426–31.

[75] Gemignani F, Marbini A. Charcot-Marie-Tooth disease (CMT): distinctive phenotypic and genotypic features in CMT type 2. J. Neurol. Sci. 2001Feb.15;184(1):1–9.

[76] Eriksson M, Brown WT, Gordon LB, Glynn MW, Singer J, Scott L, et al. Recurrent de novo point mutations in lamin A cause Hutchinson–Gilford progeria syndrome. Nature. Nature Publishing Group; 2003Apr.25;423(6937):293–8.

[77] Salamat M, Dhar PK, Neagu DL, Lyon JB. Aortic calcification in a patient with hutchinson-gilford progeria syndrome. Pediatr Cardiol. 2010Aug.;31(6):925–6.

[78] Rodríguez JI, Pérez-Alonso P, Funes R, Pérez-Rodríguez J. Lethal neonatal Hutchinson-Gilford progeria syndrome. Am. J. Med. Genet. 1999Jan.29;82(3):242–8.

[79] Gillar PJ, Kaye CI, McCourt JW. Progressive Early Dermatologic Changes in Hutchinson-Gilford Progeria Syndrome. Pediatr Dermatol. 1991Sep.;8(3):199–206.

[80] Merideth MA, Gordon LB, Clauss S, Sachdev V, Smith ACM, Perry MB, et al. Phenotype and course of Hutchinson–Gilford progeria syndrome. New England journal of medicine. Mass Medical Soc; 2008;358(6):592–604.

[81] Smigiel R, Jakubiak A, Esteves-Vieira V, Szela K, Halon A, Jurek T, et al. Novel frameshifting mutations of the ZMPSTE24 gene in two siblings affected with restrictive dermopathy and review of the mutations described in the literature. Am. J. Med. Genet. 2010Feb.;152A(2):447–52.

[82] Mok Q, Curley R, Tolmie J, Marsden R. Restrictive dermopathy: a report of three cases. Journal of Medical Genetics. 1990Jan.1.

[83] Yu CE, Oshima J, Fu YH, Wijsman EM, Hisama F, Alisch R, et al. Positional cloning of the Werner's syndrome gene. Science. 1996Apr.12;272(5259):258–62.

[84] Chen L, Lee L, Kudlow BA, Santos Dos HG, Sletvold O, Shafeghati Y, et al. LMNA mutations in atypical Werner's syndrome. The Lancet. Elsevier; 2003;362(9382):440–5.

[85] Hisama FM, Lessel D, Leistritz D, Friedrich K, McBride KL, Pastore MT, et al. Coronary artery disease in a Werner syndrome-like form of progeria characterized by low levels of progerin, a splice variant of lamin A. Am. J. Med. Genet. 2011Dec.;155A(12):3002–6.

[86] Hisama FM, Kubisch C, Martin GM, Oshima J. Clinical utility gene card for: Werner syndrome. Eur J Hum Genet. Nature Publishing Group; 2012Jan.18;20(5):1–3.

[87] Wassif CA, Brownson KE, Sterner AL, Forlino A, Zerfas PM, Wilson WK, et al. HEM dysplasia and ichthyosis are likely laminopathies and not due to 3beta-hydroxysterol Delta14-reductase deficiency. Human Molecular Genetics. 2007May15;16(10):1176–87.

[88] Waterham HR, Koster J, Mooyer P, Noort G, Kelley RI, Wilcox WR, et al. Autosomal Recessive HEM/Greenberg Skeletal Dysplasia Is Caused by 3β-Hydroxysterol Δ 14-Reductase Deficiency Due to Mutations in the Lamin B Receptor Gene. Am. J. Hum. Genet. Elsevier; 2003;72(4):1013–7.

[89] Konstantinidou A, Karadimas C, Waterham HR, Superti-Furga A, Kaminopetros P, Grigoriadou M, et al. Pathologic, radiographic and molecular findings in three fetuses diagnosed with HEM/Greenberg skeletal dysplasia. Prenat. Diagn. 2008;28(4):309–12.

[90] Hoffmann K, Dreger CK, Olins AL, Olins DE, Shultz LD, Lucke B, et al. Mutations in the gene encoding the lamin B receptor produce an altered nuclear morphology in granulocytes (Pelger-Huët anomaly). Nat Genet. 2002Aug.;31(4):410–4.

[91] Waterham HR, Koster J, Mooyer P, Noort Gv GV, Kelley RI, Wilcox WR, et al. Autosomal Recessive HEM/Greenberg Skeletal Dysplasia Is Caused by 3β-Hydroxysterol Δ 14-Reductase Deficiency Due to Mutations in the Lamin B Receptor Gene. Am. J. Hum. Genet. 2003Apr.;72(4):1013–7.

[92] Oosterwijk JC. Congenital abnormalities reported in Pelger-Huet homozygosity as compared to Greenberg/HEM dysplasia: highly variable expression of allelic phenotypes. Journal of Medical Genetics. BMJ Group; 2003Dec.1;40(12):937–41.

[93] Reynolds TB, Denison EK, Frankl HD, Lieberman FL, Peters RL. Primary biliary cirrhosis with scleroderma, Raynaud's phenomenon and telangiectasia. New syndrome. Am. J. Med. 1971Mar.;50(3):302–12.

[94] Gaudy-Marqueste C, Roll P, Esteves-Vieira V, Weiller PJ, Grob JJ, Cau P, et al. LBR mutation and nuclear envelope defects in a patient affected with Reynolds syndrome. Journal of Medical Genetics. 2010Jun.3;47(6):361–70.

[95] Berlin R, Hedensiö B, Lilja B, Linder L. Osteopoikilosis—-a Clinical and Genetic Study. Acta Medica Scandinavica. Wiley Online Library; 1967;181(3):305–14.

[96] Hellemans J, Preobrazhenska O, Willaert A, Debeer P, Verdonk PCM, Costa T, et al. Loss-of-function mutations in LEMD3 result in osteopoikilosis, Buschke-Ollendorff syndrome and melorheostosis. Nat Genet. 2004Oct.17;36(11):1213–8.

[97] Zhang Y, Castori M, Ferranti G, Paradisi M, Wordsworth BP. Novel and recurrent germline LEMD3mutations causing Buschke-Ollendorff syndrome and osteopoikilosis but not isolated melorheostosis. Clinical Genetics. 2009Jun.;75(6):556–61.

[98] Schena D, Germi L, Zamperetti MR, Colato C, Girolomoni G. Buschke-Ollendorff syndrome. Int. J. Dermatol. 2008Nov.;47(11):1159–61.

[99] Liu B, Wang J, Chan KM, Tjia WM, Deng W, Guan X, et al. Genomic instability in laminopathy-based premature aging. Nat Med. 2005Jul.;11(7):780–5.

[100] Scaffidi P, Misteli T. Reversal of the cellular phenotype in the premature aging disease Hutchinson-Gilford progeria syndrome. Nat Med. 2005Apr.;11(4):440–5.

[101] Sullivan T, Escalante-Alcalde D, Bhatt H, Anver M, Bhat N, Nagashima K, et al. Loss of A-type lamin expression compromises nuclear envelope integrity leading to muscular dystrophy. Journal of Cell Biology. 1999Nov.29;147(5):913–20.

[102] Goldman A, Erdos M, Eriksson M, Collins FS. Accumulation of mutant lamin A causes progressive changes in nuclear architecture in Hutchinson–Gilford progeria syndrome. Proceedings of the National Academy of Sciences. 2004Jan.1.

[103] Fong LG, Ng JK, Meta M, Coté N, Yang SH, Stewart CL, et al. Heterozygosity for Lmna deficiency eliminates the progeria-like phenotypes in Zmpste24-deficient mice. Proceedings of the .... 2004.

[104] Arancio W. A Bioinformatics Analysis of Lamin-A Regulatory Network: A Perspective on Epigenetic Involvement in Hutchinson–Gilford Progeria Syndrome. Rejuvenation Research. 2012Apr.;15(2):123–7.

[105] Padmakumar VC, Libotte T, Lu W, Zaim H, Abraham S, Noegel AA, et al. The inner nuclear membrane protein Sun1 mediates the anchorage of Nesprin-2 to the nuclear envelope. Journal of Cell Science. 2005Aug.1;118(Pt 15):3419–30.

[106] Mislow JMK, Kim MS, Davis DB, McNally EM. Myne-1, a spectrin repeat transmembrane protein of the myocyte inner nuclear membrane, interacts with lamin A/C. Journal of Cell Science. 2002Jan.1;115(Pt 1):61–70.

[107] Maraldi NM, Lattanzi G. Linkage of lamins to fidelity of gene transcription. Crit. Rev. Eukaryot. Gene Expr. 2005;15(4):277–94.

[108] Lattanzi G, Cenni V, Marmiroli S, Capanni C, Mattioli E, Merlini L, et al. Association of emerin with nuclear and cytoplasmic actin is regulated in differentiating myoblasts. Biochem Biophys Res Commun. 2003Apr.11;303(3):764–70.

[109] Lattanzi G, Columbaro M, Mattioli E, Cenni V, Camozzi D, Wehnert M, et al. Pre-Lamin A processing is linked to heterochromatin organization. J. Cell. Biochem. 2007Dec.1;102(5):1149–59.

[110] Vlcek S, Foisner R. Lamins and lamin-associated proteins in aging and disease. Current Opinion in Cell Biology. 2007Jun.;19(3):298–304.

[111] Jung HJ, Sun T, Pleasure S, Young S, al E. Regulation of prelamin A but not lamin C by miR-9, a brain-specific microRNA. Proceedings of the .... 2012.

[112] Nissan X, Blondel S, Navarro C, Maury Y, Denis C, Girard M, et al. Unique Preservation of Neural Cells in Hutchinson- Gilford Progeria Syndrome Is Due to the Expression of the Neural-Specific miR-9 MicroRNA. Cell Reports. 2012Jul.;2(1):1–9.

[113] Muchir A, Pavlidis P, Decostre V, Herron AJ, Arimura T, Bonne G, et al. Activation of MAPK pathways links LMNA mutations to cardiomyopathy in Emery-Dreifuss muscular dystrophy. J. Clin. Invest. 2007May;117(5):1282–93.

[114] Haq S, Choukroun G, Lim H, Tymitz KM, del Monte F, Gwathmey J, et al. Differential activation of signal transduction pathways in human hearts with hypertrophy versus advanced heart failure. Circulation. 2001Feb.6;103(5):670–7.

[115] Cook S. Activation of c-Jun N-Terminal Kinases and p38-Mitogen-activated Protein Kinases in Human Heart Failure Secondary to Ischaemic Heart Disease. Journal of Molecular and Cellular Cardiology. 1999Aug.;31(8):1429–34.

[116] Nicol RL, Frey N, Pearson G, Cobb M, Richardson J, Olson EN. Activated MEK5 induces serial assembly of sarcomeres and eccentric cardiac hypertrophy. The EMBO journal. 2001Jun.1;20(11):2757–67.

[117] Muchir A, Pavlidis P, Bonne G, Hayashi YK, Worman HJ. Activation of MAPK in hearts of EMD null mice: similarities between mouse models of X-linked and autosomal dominant Emery Dreifuss muscular dystrophy. Human Molecular Genetics. 2007Aug.1;16(15):1884–95.

[118] Brodsky GL, Muntoni F, Miocic S, Sinagra G, Sewry C, Mestroni L. Lamin A/C gene mutation associated with dilated cardiomyopathy with variable skeletal muscle involvement. Circulation. 2000Feb.8;101(5):473–6.

[119] Vytopil M, Ricci E, Russo Dello A, Hanisch F, Neudecker S, Zierz S, et al. Frequent low penetrance mutations in the Lamin A/C gene, causing Emery Dreifuss muscular dystrophy. Neuromuscular Disorders. 2002Dec.;12(10):958–63.

[120] Marina Raffaele di Barletta ERGGPTMMLMARTVKHOLMCTVBIHPSBRRKSGBDT. Different Mutations in the LMNA Gene Cause Autosomal Dominant and Autosomal Recessive Emery-Dreifuss Muscular Dystrophy. Am. J. Hum. Genet. Elsevier; 2000Apr.1;66(4):1407.

[121] Genschel J, Schmidt HHJ. Mutations in the LMNA gene encoding lamin A/C. Hum. Mutat. Wiley Online Library; 2000;16(6):451–9.

[122] Novelli G, Muchir A, Sangiuolo F, Helbling-Leclerc A, D'Apice MR, Massart C, et al. Mandibuloacral dysplasia is caused by a mutation in LMNA-encoding lamin A/C. Am. J. Hum. Genet. 2002Aug.;71(2):426–31.

[123] Shen JJ, Brown CA, Lupski JR, Potocki L. Mandibuloacral dysplasia caused by homozygosity for the R527H mutation in lamin A/C. Journal of Medical Genetics. 2003Nov.;40(11):854–7.

[124] Mercuri E, Poppe M, Quinlivan R, Messina S, Kinali M, Demay L, et al. Extreme variability of phenotype in patients with an identical missense mutation in the lamin A/C gene: from congenital onset with severe phenotype to milder classic Emery-Dreifuss variant. Arch. Neurol. 2004May;61(5):690–4.

[125] Mercuri E, Brown SC, Nihoyannopoulos P, Poulton J, Kinali M, Richard P, et al. Extreme variability of skeletal and cardiac muscle involvement in patients with mutations in exon 11 of the lamin A/C gene. Muscle Nerve. 2005;31(5):602–9.

[126] Genschel J, Bochow B, Kuepferling S, Ewert R, Hetzer R, Lochs H, et al. A R644C mutation within lamin A extends the mutations causing dilated cardiomyopathy. Hum. Mutat. 2001Feb.;17(2):154.

[127] Vigouroux C, Auclair M, Dubosclard E, Pouchelet M, Capeau J, Courvalin J-C, et al. Nuclear envelope disorganization in fibroblasts from lipodystrophic patients with heterozygous R482Q/W mutations in the lamin A/C gene. Journal of Cell …. 2001.

[128] Gonzalez JM, Navarro-Puche A, Casar B, Crespo P, Andres V. Fast regulation of AP-1 activity through interaction of lamin A/C, ERK1/2, and c-Fos at the nuclear envelope. The Journal of Cell Biology. 2008Nov.10;183(4):653–66.

[129] de Sandre-Giovannoli A, Bernard R, Cau P, Navarro C, Amiel J, Boccaccio I, et al. Lamin a truncation in Hutchinson-Gilford progeria. Science. 2003Jun.27;300(5628): 2055.

[130] Muchir A, Wu W, Worman HJ. Reduced expression of A-type lamins and emerin activates extracellular signal-regulated kinase in cultured cells. Biochim. Biophys. Acta. 2009Jan.;1792(1):75–81.

[131] Emerson LJ, Holt MR, Wheeler MA, Wehnert M, Parsons M, Ellis JA. Defects in cell spreading and ERK1/2 activation in fibroblasts with lamin A/C mutations. Biochimica et Biophysica Acta (BBA)-Molecular Basis of Disease. Elsevier; 2009;1792(8):810–21.

[132] Fong LG. Prelamin A and lamin A appear to be dispensable in the nuclear lamina. J. Clin. Invest. 2006Mar.1;116(3):743–52.

[133] Olins AL, Olins DE. Cytoskeletal influences on nuclear shape in granulocytic HL-60 cells. BMC Cell Biol. 2004Aug.19;5:30.

[134] Dahl KN, Booth-Gauthier EA, Ladoux B. In the middle of it all: mutual mechanical regulation between the nucleus and the cytoskeleton. Journal of biomechanics. Elsevier; 2010;43(1):2–8.

[135] Morris GE. Heart to heart: from nuclearproteins to Emery-Dreifuss muscular dystrophy. Human Molecular Genetics. 1999Sep.1;8(10):1847–51.

[136] Broers J, Machiels B, Kuijpers H, Smedts F, van den Kieboom R, Raymond Y, et al. A- and B-type lamins are differentially expressed in normal human tissues. Histochemistry and cell biology. 1997;107(6):505–17.

[137] Ostlund C, Ellenberg J, Hallberg E, Lippincott-Schwartz J, Worman HJ. Intracellular trafficking of emerin, the Emery-Dreifuss muscular dystrophy protein. Journal of Cell Science. 1999Jun.;112 (Pt 11):1709–19.

[138] Maniotis AJ, Chen CS, Ingber DE. Demonstration of mechanical connections between integrins, cytoskeletal filaments, and nucleoplasm that stabilize nuclear structure. Proceedings of the National Academy of Sciences of the United States of America. 1997Feb.4;94(3):849–54.

[139] Rosengardten Y, McKenna T, Grochová D, Eriksson M. Stem cell depletion in Hutchinson-Gilford progeria syndrome. Aging Cell. 2011Sep.8.

[140] Meshorer E, Gruenbaum Y. Gone with the Wnt/Notch: stem cells in laminopathies, progeria, and aging. The Journal of Cell Biology. 2008Apr.7;181(1):9–13.

[141] Bertrand AT, Chikhaoui K, Yaou RB, Bonne G. Clinical and genetic heterogeneity in laminopathies. Biochem. Soc. Trans. 2011Nov.21;39(6):1687–92.

[142] Herrmann H, Aebi U. Intermediate filaments: molecular structure, assembly mechanism, and integration into functionally distinct intracellular Scaffolds. Annu. Rev. Biochem. 2004;73:749–89.

[143] Reunert J, Wentzell R, Walter M, Jakubiczka S, Zenker M, Brune T, et al. Neonatal progeria: increased ratio of progerin to lamin A leads to progeria of the newborn. Eur J Hum Genet. 2012Mar.14.

[144] Moulson C, Fong L, Gardner J. Increased progerin expression associated with unusual LMNA mutations causes severe progeroid syndromes. Hum. Mutat. 2007Jan.1.

[145] Cenni V, Capanni C, Columbaro M, Ortolani M, D'Apice MR, Novelli G, et al. Autophagic degradation of farnesylated prelamin A as a therapeutic approach to lamin-linked progeria. Eur J Histochem. 2011;55(4):e36.

[146] Rodriguez S, Eriksson M. Low and high expressing alleles of the LMNA gene: implications for laminopathy disease development. PLoS ONE. 2011;6(9):e25472.

[147] Jahn D, Schramm S, Schnölzer M, Heilmann CJ, de Koster CG, Schütz W, et al. A truncated lamin A in the Lmna (-/-) mouse line: Implications for the understanding of laminopathies. Nucleus. 2012Sep.1;3(5).

[148] Kubben N, Voncken JW, Konings G, van Weeghel M, van den Hoogenhof MMG, Gijbels M, et al. Post-natal myogenic and adipogenic developmental: Defects and metabolic impairment upon loss of A-type lamins. Nucleus. Landes Bioscience; 2011May1;2(3):195–207.

[149] Coffinier C, Jung HJ, Li Z, Nobumori C, Yun UJ, Farber EA, et al. Direct Synthesis of Lamin A, Bypassing Prelamin A Processing, Causes Misshapen Nuclei in Fibroblasts but No Detectable Pathology in Mice. Journal of Biological Chemistry. 2010Jun. 25;285(27):20818–26.

[150] Bergo M, Gavino B, Ross J. Zmpste24 deficiency in mice causes spontaneous bone fractures, muscle weakness, and a prelamin A processing defect. Proceedings of the National Academy of Sciences. 2002Jan.1.

[151] Pendás AM, Zhou Z, Cadiñanos J, Freije JMP, Wang J, Hultenby K, et al. Defective prelamin A processing and muscular and adipocyte alterations in Zmpste24 metalloproteinase-deficient mice. Nat Genet. 2002May;31(1):94–9.

[152] Mounkes LC, Kozlov SV, Rottman JN, Stewart CL. Expression of an LMNA-N195K variant of A-type lamins results in cardiac conduction defects and death in mice. Human Molecular Genetics. 2005Aug.1;14(15):2167–80.

[153] Arimura T, Helbling-Leclerc A, Massart C, Varnous S, Niel F, Lacène E, et al. Mouse model carrying H222P-Lmna mutation develops muscular dystrophy and dilated cardiomyopathy similar to human striated muscle laminopathies. Human Molecular Genetics. 2005Jan.1;14(1):155–69.

[154] Yang SH, Bergo MO, Toth JI, Qiao X, Hu Y, Sandoval S, et al. Blocking protein farnesyltransferase improves nuclear blebbing in mouse fibroblasts with a targeted Hutch-

inson-Gilford progeria syndrome mutation. Proceedings of the National Academy of Sciences. 2005Jul.19;102(29):10291–6.

[155] Mounkes LC, Kozlov S, Hernandez L, Sullivan T, Stewart CL. A progeroid syndrome in mice is caused by defects in A-type lamins. Nature. 2003May15;423(6937):298–301.

[156] Wang Y, Herron AJ, Worman HJ. Pathology and nuclear abnormalities in hearts of transgenic mice expressing M371K lamin A encoded by an LMNA mutation causing Emery-Dreifuss muscular dystrophy. Human Molecular Genetics. 2006Aug. 15;15(16):2479–89.

[157] Osorio FG, Navarro CL, Cadinanos J, Lopez-Mejia IC, Quiros PM, Bartoli C, et al. Splicing-Directed Therapy in a New Mouse Model of Human Accelerated Aging. Science Translational Medicine. 2011Oct.26;3(106):106ra107–7.

[158] Melcon G, Kozlov S, Cutler DA, Sullivan T, Hernandez L, Zhao P, et al. Loss of emerin at the nuclear envelope disrupts the Rb1/E2F and MyoD pathways during muscle regeneration. Human Molecular .... 2006.

[159] Ozawa R, Hayashi YK, Ogawa M, Kurokawa R, Matsumoto H, Noguchi S, et al. Emerin-lacking mice show minimal motor and cardiac dysfunctions with nuclear-associated vacuoles. Am. J. Pathol. 2006Mar.;168(3):907–17.

[160] Muchir A, van Engelen BG, Lammens M, Mislow JM, McNally E, Schwartz K, et al. Nuclear envelope alterations in fibroblasts from LGMD1B patients carrying nonsense Y259X heterozygous or homozygous mutation in lamin A/C gene. Experimental Cell Research. 2003Dec.10;291(2):352–62.

[161] Van Berlo JH, Voncken JW, Kubben N, Broers JLV, Duisters R, van Leeuwen REW, et al. A-type lamins are essential for TGF-beta1 induced PP2A to dephosphorylate transcription factors. Human Molecular Genetics. 2005Oct.1;14(19):2839–49.

[162] Jahn D, Schramm S, Schnölzer M, Heilmann CJ, de Koster CG, Schütz W, et al. A truncated lamin A in the Lmna–/– mouse line: Implications for the understanding of laminopathies. Nucleus. 2012Sep.1;3(5).

[163] Leung GK, Schmidt WK, Bergo MO, Gavino B, Wong DH, Tam A, et al. Biochemical studies of Zmpste24-deficient mice. J Biol Chem. 2001Aug.3;276(31):29051–8.

[164] Ambrosi P, Mouly-Bandini A, Attarian S, Habib G. Heart transplantation in 7 patients from a single family with limb-girdle muscular dystrophy caused by lamin A/C mutation. International Journal of Cardiology. 2009Nov.;137(3):e75–6.

[165] Dyck JD, David TE, Burke B, Webb GD, Henderson MA, Fowler RS. Management of coronary artery disease in Hutchinson-Gilford syndrome. The Journal of Pediatrics. 1987Sep.;111(3):407–10.

[166] Savage DB, Tan GD, Acerini CL, Jebb SA, Agostini M, Gurnell M, et al. Human metabolic syndrome resulting from dominant-negative mutations in the nuclear receptor peroxisome proliferator-activated receptor-gamma. Diabetes. 2003Apr.;52(4):910–7.

[167] Javor ED, Cochran EK, Musso C, Young JR, Depaoli AM, Gorden P. Long-term efficacy of leptin replacement in patients with generalized lipodystrophy. Diabetes. 2005Jul.;54(7):1994–2002.

[168] Park JY, Javor ED, Cochran EK, Depaoli AM, Gorden P. Long-term efficacy of leptin replacement in patients with Dunnigan-type familial partial lipodystrophy. Metab. Clin. Exp. 2007Apr.;56(4):508–16.

[169] Maraldi NM, Capanni C, Lattanzi G, Camozzi D, Facchini A, Manzoli FA. SREBP1 interaction with prelamin A forms: A pathogenic mechanism for lipodystrophic laminopathies. Advances in Enzyme Regulation. Advances in enzyme ...; 2008Jan.;48(1): 209–23.

[170] Kieran MW, Gordon L, Kleinman M. New approaches to progeria. Pediatrics. 2007Oct.;120(4):834–41.

[171] Capell B, Erdos M, Madigan J, Fiordalisi J. Inhibiting farnesylation of progerin prevents the characteristic nuclear blebbing of Hutchinson- .... Proceedings of the National Academy of Sciences. 2005Jan.1.

[172] Mallampalli MP, Huyer G, Bendale P, Gelb MH, Michaelis S. Inhibiting farnesylation reverses the nuclear morphology defect in a HeLa cell model for Hutchinson-Gilford progeria syndrome. Proceedings of the National Academy of Sciences of the United States of America. 2005Oct.4;102(40):14416–21.

[173] Toth J, Yang S, Qiao X, Beigneux A, Gelb M. Blocking protein farnesyltransferase improves nuclear shape in fibroblasts from humans with .... Proceedings of the National Academy of Sciences. 2005Jan.1.

[174] Capell BC, Olive M, Erdos MR, Cao K, Faddah DA, Tavarez UL, et al. A farnesyltransferase inhibitor prevents both the onset and late progression of cardiovascular disease in a progeria mouse model. Proceedings of the National Academy of Sciences. 2008Oct.14;105(41):15902–7.

[175] Yang S. Treatment with a farnesyltransferase inhibitor improves survival in mice with a Hutchinson–Gilford progeria syndrome mutation. Biochimica et Biophysica Acta (BBA) - Molecular and Cell Biology of Lipids. 2008Jan.1;1781(1-2):36–9.

[176] Fong L, Frost D, Meta M, Qiao X, Yang S. A Protein Farnesyltransferase Inhibitor Ameliorates Disease in a Mouse Model of Progeria. Science. 2006Jan.1.

[177] Shao H Yang DAAHPSSGYLGF. Progerin elicits disease phenotypes of progeria in mice whether or not it is farnesylated. The Journal of Clinical Investigation. American Society for Clinical Investigation; 2008Oct.1;118(10):3291.

[178] Varela I, Pereira S, Ugalde AP, Navarro CL, Suárez MF, Cau P, et al. Combined treatment with statins and aminobisphosphonates extends longevity in a mouse model of human premature aging. Nat Med. 2008Jun.29;14(7):767–72.

[179] Glynn M, Glover T. Incomplete processing of mutant lamin A in Hutchinson-Gilford progeria leads to nuclear .... Human Molecular Genetics. 2005Jan.1.

[180] Davies BSJ, Barnes RH, Tu Y, Ren S, Andres DA, Spielmann HP, et al. An accumulation of non-farnesylated prelamin A causes cardiomyopathy but not progeria. Human Molecular Genetics. 2010Jun.10;19(13):2682–94.

[181] Coffinier C, Hudon SE, Farber EA, Chang SY, Hrycyna CA, Young SG, et al. HIV protease inhibitors block the zinc metalloproteinase ZMPSTE24 and lead to an accumulation of prelamin A in cells. Proceedings of the National Academy of Sciences of the United States of America. 2007Aug.14;104(33):13432–7.

[182] Cao K, Graziotto JJ, Blair CD, Mazzulli JR, Erdos MR, Krainc D, et al. Rapamycin reverses cellular phenotypes and enhances mutant protein clearance in Hutchinson-Gilford progeria syndrome cells. Science Translational Medicine. 2011Jun.29;3(89): 89ra58.

[183] Ramos FJ, Chen SC, Garelick MG, Dai D-F, Liao C-Y, Schreiber KH, et al. Rapamycin Reverses Elevated mTORC1 Signaling in Lamin A/C-Deficient Mice, Rescues Cardiac and Skeletal Muscle Function, and Extends Survival. Science Translational Medicine. 2012Jul.25;4(144):144ra103.

[184] Choi JC, Muchir A, Wu W, Iwata S. Temsirolimus activates autophagy and ameliorates cardiomyopathy caused by lamin A/C gene mutation. Science. 2012.

[185] Wu W, Muchir A, Shan J, Bonne G, Worman HJ. Mitogen-Activated Protein Kinase Inhibitors Improve Heart Function and Prevent Fibrosis in Cardiomyopathy Caused by Mutation in Lamin A/C GeneClinical Perspective. Circulation. Am Heart Assoc; 2011;123(1):53–61.

[186] Chhajed PN, Dickenmann M, Bubendorf L, Mayr M, Steiger J, Tamm M. Patterns of pulmonary complications associated with sirolimus. Respiration. 2006;73(3):367–74.

[187] Filippone EJ, Carson JM, Beckford RA, Jaffe BC, Newman E, Awsare BK, et al. Sirolimus-induced pneumonitis complicated by pentamidine-induced phospholipidosis in a renal transplant recipient: a case report. Transplant. Proc. 2011Sep.;43(7):2792–7.

[188] Pham P-TT, Pham P-CT, Danovitch GM, Ross DJ, Gritsch HA, Kendrick EA, et al. Sirolimus-Associated Pulmonary Toxicity. Transplantation. 2004Apr.27;77(8):1215.

[189] Lamming DW, Ye L, Katajisto P, Goncalves MD, Saitoh M, Stevens DM, et al. Rapamycin-induced insulin resistance is mediated by mTORC2 loss and uncoupled from longevity. Science. 2012Mar.30;335(6076):1638–43.

[190] Scaffidi P. Lamin A-Dependent Nuclear Defects in Human Aging. Science. 2006.

[191] Huang S, Chen L, Libina N, Janes J, Martin GM, Campisi J, et al. Correction of cellular phenotypes of Hutchinson-Gilford Progeria cells by RNA interference. Hum. Genet. 2005Dec.;118(3-4):444–50.

[192] Fong LG, Vickers TA, Farber EA, Choi C, Yun UJ, Hu Y, et al. Activating the synthesis of progerin, the mutant prelamin A in Hutchinson-Gilford progeria syndrome, with antisense oligonucleotides. Human Molecular Genetics. 2009Jun.10;18(13):2462–71.

[193] Flemming A. Regulatory watch: Pioneering gene therapy on brink of approval. Nat Rev Drug Discov. 2012Aug.31;11(9):664.

[194] Mazhari R, Hare JM. Mechanisms of action of mesenchymal stem cells in cardiac repair: potential influences on the cardiac stem cell niche. Nat Clin Pract Cardiovasc Med. 2007Feb.;4 Suppl 1:S21–6.

[195] Trollet C, Athanasopoulos T, Popplewell L, Malerba A, Dickson G. Gene therapy for muscular dystrophy: current progress and future prospects. Expert Opin. Biol. Ther. 2009Jul.;9(7):849–66.

[196] Merkulov S, Chen X, Chandler MP, Stelzer JE. In Vivo cMyBPC Gene Transfer Rescues Myofilament Contractile Dysfunction in cMyBPC Null Mice. Circ Heart Fail. 2012Aug.1.

Chapter 2

A Therapeutic Role for Hematopoietic Stem Cells in Osteogenesis Imperfecta

Meenal Mehrotra and Amanda C. LaRue

Additional information is available at the end of the chapter

1. Introduction

1.1. Osteogenesis Imperfecta (OI)

"Fragile bones" have been described in medical literature for centuries. Osteogenesis imperfecta (OI), whose name means "imperfect birth of bones", is one such fragile bone syndrome. A generalized disorder of the body's connective tissue, it is most obvious in its effects on the bone, but also involves the body's ligaments, tendons, fascia, eyes, skin, teeth and ears. It is a highly variable heritable disorder characterized by recurring bone fractures, low bone mass and bone fragility [1]. Bone fragility has led to the common name "brittle bone disease" for OI. Its overall incidence is approximately one in 10,000 births. The incidence of forms of OI recognizable at birth is 1/16-20,000, with about equal incidence of mild forms that are not recognizable until later in life. The clinical range of this condition is extremely broad, ranging from cases that are lethal in the perinatal period to cases that maybe difficult to detect and can present as early osteoporosis [2]. Individuals with OI may have varying combinations of growth deficiency, defective tooth formation (dentinogenesis imperfecta), hearing loss, macrocephaly, blue coloration of sclerae, scoliosis, barrel chest and ligamentous laxity. In more severe cases, people are susceptible to fracture from mild trauma and even from acts of daily living.

1.2. Classification and types of OI

Classical OI is an autosomal dominant condition caused by defects in type I collagen, the major structural component of the extracellular matrix of bone, skin and tendon. This deficiency arises from an amino acid substitution of glycine to bulkier amino acids in the collagen triple helix structure. The larger amino acid side-chains create steric hindrance that creates a bulge in the collagen complex, which in turn influences both the molecular nanomechanics as well as the interaction between molecules, which are both compromised [3]. As a result, the body may respond by hydrolyzing the improper collagen structure. If the body does not destroy the improper collagen, the relationship between the collagen fibrils and hydroxyapatite crystals to form bone is altered, causing brittleness. Another suggested disease mechanism is that the stress state within collagen fibrils is altered at the locations of mutations, where locally, larger shear forces lead to rapid failure of fibrils even at moderate loads as the homogeneous stress state found in healthy collagen fibrils is lost [3]. In the past several years, autosomal recessive forms of OI have been identified. Although recessive OI is not due to defects in collagen, its etiology in a collagen-modification complex is collagen-related. Hence, in ~10% of cases, genes encoding proteins involved in type I collagen's complex posttranslational modifications and intracellular trafficking can also be involved in the causation of OI [4]. Autosomal recessive OI is caused by defects in two of the components of the prolyl 3-hydroxylation complex, which modifies the $\alpha 1(I)$ chain of collagen in the endoplasmic reticulum, cartilage-associated protein (CRTAP) [5, 6] and prolyl 3-hydroxylase (P3H1) [7]. OI can also occur as a consequence of mutations in key osteoblast genes that code for proteins involved in matrix homeostasis [8, 9] and are not directly related to collagen metabolism and matrix structure. About 5% of OI cases are not caused by defects of type I collagen or the P3H1 hydroxylation complex and their etiology is presently unknown. Most people with OI receive it from a parent but in 35% of cases it is an individual (*de novo* or "sporadic") mutation.

1.3. Sillence classification

Classical OI is generally described using the Sillence classification, a nomenclature based on clinical and radiographic features, which was first proposed in 1979 [10]. This classification subdivides patients into four types based on disease severity and progression:

Type I OI, the most common and mildest form of the disease and is caused by a quantitative defect with synthesis of structurally normal type I procollagen at about half the normal amount [11]. Type I OI is non-deforming and results in patients attaining close to normal height, however vertebral fractures are common and can lead to mild scoliosis. Joint hyperextensibility is also a common feature. Growth deficiency and long bone deformities are generally mild. In these patients, fractures are rare at birth but begin with ambulation [1]. Patients also present with blue sclera and 50% may have hearing loss. Type I has been divided into A and B subtypes based on the absence or presence of dentinogenesis imperfecta, a genetic disorder of tooth development also known as hereditary opalescent dentin. This condition causes teeth to be discolored (most often a blue-gray or yellow-brown color) and translucent. Teeth are also weaker than normal, making them prone to rapid wear, breakage, and loss. These problems can affect both primary teeth and permanent teeth.

Type II OI is the most severe OI form, generally resulting in death in the perinatal period, although survival up to one year has been noted. These patients exhibit multiple intrauterine rib and long bone fractures and severe skeletal deformities, which eventually result in respiratory failure. Legs are usually held in a frog leg position with hips abducted and knees flexed. The skull is severely under mineralized with wide open fontanels. The bones of these infants are predominantly composed woven bone without haversian canals and organized lamellae. In 1984 a radiological sub classification of type II OI was proposed [12]: OI II A—broad ribs with multiple fractures, continuous beaded ribs, severe undermodeling of femur; OI II B—normal/thin ribs with some fractures, discontinuous beaded ribs, some undermodeling of femur; OI II C—varying thickness of ribs, discontinuous beading of ribs, malformed scapulae and ischiae, slender and twisted long bones.

Type III OI is a severe form of the disease, characterized by severe progressive skeletal deformities. This is due to the synthesis of mutated collagen. Fractures may be present *in utero* and are very common during the growth period as the bones are extremely fragile. The incidence of fracture remains high even in the adult life. The long bones are soft and deformed from normal muscle tension. Individuals are severely short statured and scoliosis can lead to respiratory problems. These patients also present with dentinogesisimperfecta. Radiographically, metphyseal flaring and "popcorn" formation at growth plate is seen. These patients require intensive physical rehabilitation to attain assisted ambulation.

Type IV OI is the most clinically diverse group of patients of OI. The phenotype can vary from mild to severe. Scleral hue is also variable. Typically, these patients suffer several fractures in a year and present with bowing of long bones. While fractures decrease after puberty, individuals have a short final stature. Radiographically, the patients have osteoporosis and mild modeling abnormalities. Like type I OI, this group can also be divided into two subgroups on the basis of the presence or absence of dentinogenesis imperfecta[13]. It is from this heterogeneous group that types V, VI and VII have been identified based on distinct clinical and histological features [14-16].

Although type V to VIII continues the Sillence classification, they are based on different criteria than other types. Type V and VI are defined using bone histology and have a phenotype that would be included in type IV. However, these individuals do not have defects in type I collagen. Type VII and VIII are recessive forms whose phenotype overlaps type II and III. These patients have deficiencies of components of collagen modification complex in endoplasmic reticulum.

Type V OI is moderately deforming and there are three distinctive features: the frequent development of hypertrophic calluses at the fracture site, the calcification of interosseous membranes between the bones of the forearm and the presence of radio-opaque metaphyseal band immediately adjacent to the growth plate on X-rays [14]. The calcified interosseous membrane severely limits the pronation/supination of the hand and may lead to secondary dislocation of the radial head. These patients have normal teeth and white sclerae. Patients with type V OI represent 4-5 % of the OI population seen the hospital.

Type VI OI also presents with moderate to severe deformities and do not have blue sclera and dentinogenesis imperfecta. Distinctive histiological features are the fish-scale like appearance of the bone lamellae and presence of excessive osteoid accumulation on bone forming surfaces. Inheritance is autosomal dominant and may represent approximately 4% of moderately to severely affected parents [15].

Type VII OI is an autosomal recessive form caused by defects in CRTAP, cartilage-associated protein [16]. Patients have moderate to severe skeletal deformities, bone fragility, lack of blue sclera and no dentinogenesis imperfecta. The distinctive clinical feature is the rhizomelic shortening of the humerous and femur. To date, this disorder has only been observed in a community of Native Americans in northern Quebec [16].

Type VIII OI is an autosomal recessive form caused by defects in prolyl 3-hydroxylase 1 (P3H1, encoded by LEPRE1). P3H1 forms a complex in the endoplasmic reticulum with CRTAP. This causes a phenotype which overlaps types II and III OI but has distinct features, including white sclera, extreme growth deficiency and under mineralization [7].

1.4. Dominantly inherited OI

Most patients with OI (~ 90%) have mutations in one of the type I collagen genes, COL1A1 or COL1A2. These mutations are dominantly inherited and the phenotype can vary from the very mild to lethal. There are two general cases of mutation in Type I collagen genes that result in OI: those that cause a quantitative defect with synthesis of structurally normal type I procollagen at about half the normal amount and those that result in synthesis of structurally abnormal collagen. The former is usually due to premature termination codons in one COL1A1 molecule that initiates decay of the mRNA from the affected allele. This generally results in mild nondeforming phenotype with blue sclera (Type I OI) [11]. The most prevalent mutation results in substitution of one of the invariant glycine residues that have a critical role in helix formation. A collagen type I molecule comprises a triple helix made up of two alpha 1 and one alpha 2 polypeptide chains. In the center of each helical turn, i.e. every third amino acid is a glycine residue, which is essential for the structure of the molecule. Any substitution of the residues can result in structural abnormalities and produce a mixture of normal and abnormal collagen strands. Depending on the substitution type and location, the phenotype can vary from mild to very severe. Usually, patients with the more severe type of the disease have a mutation at one essential glycine residue site [17]. Alterations in collagen type I molecules lead to structural changes in the bone and the abnormal collagen has lower tensile strength. This leads to the brittleness of the bones in OI. OI not only results in low trabecular bone mineral density and thin cortices, but also in small, slender bones. Together, these factors contribute to the fragility of the bones.

1.5. Recessively inherited OI

In the past decade, the genetic basis of 10 new OI variants has been discovered, seven of which result from mutations in genes encoding proteins involved in the post translational modifications of type I procollagen [6, 7, 18-22]. In 2007, mutations in *CRTAP* were identified in patients without mutations in COL1A1 and COL1A2 but with excess posttranslational modification of type I collagen indicative of delayed folding of the triple helix [6, 7]. Patients with similar phenotype with mutations in genes such as *LEPRE1* (proyl 3-hydroxylase, P3H) and *PPIB* (Peptidyl-prolylcis-trans isomerase B;cyclophilin B) have also been identified [19, 20]. FK binding protein 10 (FKBP10) mutations present as a milder phenotype in late childhood or adolescence with long bone fracture, acetabular protrusion and scoliosis

[22]. Among the most recent discoveries are the association of mutations in the gene *SERPINF1* (serpin peptidase inhibitor, clade F) with type VI OI [23]. The latter two are proteins responsible for chaperoning collagen through the endoplasmic reticulum. *SERPINF1* encodes pigment epithelium derived factor, a secreted glycoprotein with uncertain function in bone. Mutations in LRP5, a key regulator of osteoblast function, affects bone accrual during growth [8]. More recently, a child with moderate OI phenotype has been identified with homozygous mutation in SP7, which codes for osterix, a transcription factor specifically expressed in osteoblasts in the developing skeleton [9].

2. Animal models used for the study of OI

The many different types and subtypes of OI highlight the importance of developing animal models to study the disease. Canine, feline, bovine and ovine models of OI have been described (reviewed in [24]). However, the majority of animal studies have been conducted using engineered and spontaneously occurring murine models.

2.1. Mov-13 mouse: A model for OI type I

In Mov-13 mice, transcription of the proα1(I) gene was completely blocked as a result of Moloney leukemia virus integration at the 5′ end of the gene [25]. No functional α2(I) was detected in embryos [26], likely as a result of rapid degradation of proα2(I) procollagen chains which are unable to form stable triple helices. Mice homozygous for the null mutation produced no type I collagen and died at mid-gestation while heterozygotes survived to young adulthood [27]. Heterozygotes produced 50% less type I collagen which causes progressive hearing loss and alterations in the mechanical properties of long bones [28]. The heterozygous Mov-13 mouse therefore serves as a model for type I OI. As many as 5% of osteoblasts from long bones were shown to produce normal amounts of type I collagen, thus implying that a small set of osteoblasts did not express the mutant phenotype [29]. This bone tissue mosaicism for expression of the mutant allele may explain why Mov-13 heterozygotes do not display an obvious bone fragility phenotype.

2.2. Brittle II mouse: A model for type II OI

The cre/lox recombination system was used to develop a lethal murine knock in model of OI type II [30]. A 3.2 kbp transcription/translation stop cassette was introduced in intron 22 and flanked by directly repeating lox recombination sites. After homologous recombination in ES cells, two male chimeras were obtained. A knock in mouse carrying and intronic inclusion was generated by mating chimeras with wild-type females. Alternatively splicing involving the stop cassette resulted in retention of non-collagenous sequences. This mouse had the lethal phenotype of the similar human mutation and was designated BrtlII. Skeletal staining showed rib fractures, poor skeletal mineralization and shorter vertebral bodies. The mice die a few hours after birth from apparent respiratory distress.

2.3. Oim/Oim mouse: A model for type III OI

Chipman et al. [31] described a strain of mice with a nonlethal recessively inherited mutation that resulted in phenotypic and biochemical features that simulate moderate to severe human OI. This *oim* mutation arose spontaneously in 1985 in the Mutant Mouse Resource of The Jackson Laboratory. It has since been determined that the underlying defect in the *oim* mouse is a mutation in COL1A2 [32]. This mutation changes the reading frame at the 3′ end of the mRNA causing synthesis of an altered C-propeptide that ultimately inhibits the association of these molecules into heterotrimeric type I procollagen bundles in the bone matrix. Instead, homotrimers are formed which interferes with the integrity and quantity of the osteoid that accumulates in the bone. This mouse model has been shown to have a phenotype similar to that seen in human type III OI, including a decreased body size, abnormal bone mineralization (contributing to the brittleness of the bones), decreased bone density and a fragile skeleton susceptible to fractures. While the skeleton becomes progressively deformed with age, homozygous mice can live a normal life span. The heterozygous mice simulate the mild form of the disease in which the bones show abnormal cortical morphology and reduced bone mechanical strength even though no fractures are seen. Heterozygote oim/+ mice have subtle skeletal fragility whereas homozygous oim/oim mice have marked skeletal fragility. The dental phenotype in oim/oim is more severe in incisors than in molars and includes changes in pulp chamber size, tooth shape, and dentin ultrastructure. Teeth in oim/oim animals are clinically fragile. Although oim/+ teeth are grossly normal, ultrastructural abnormalities such as reduction in the number and regularity of spacing of the dentinal tubules, less mineralization, and blurring of the boundary between peritubular and intertubular dentin can be found in oim/+ teeth [33].

Breeding studies showed that the oim mutation was inherited in most crosses as a single recessive gene on chromosome 6, near the murine COL1A2 gene. Biochemical analyses of skin and bone, as well as isolated dermal fibroblast cultures, demonstrated that $\alpha1$(I) homotrimer collagen accumulated in these tissues. Short labeling studies in fibroblasts demonstrated an absence of pro$\alpha2$(I) collagen chains. Nucleotide sequencing of cDNA encoding the COOH-propeptide revealed a G deletion at pro$\alpha2$(I) nucleotide 3983; this results in an alteration of the sequence of the last 48 aminoacids. Normal-sized mRNA is transcribed, but no secreted protein has been identified in oim/oim fibroblasts and osteoblasts. Collagen from the oim/oim mouse showed reduced resistance to tensile stress [34]. Neutron activation analyses demonstrated that oim/oim femurs had significant differences in magnesium, fluoride, and sodium content compared to wild type mouse femurs [35]. These and other studies suggest that the known decreased biochemical properties of oim/oim bone reflect both altered mineral composition and decreased bone mineral density, which further suggests that the presence of $\alpha2$(I) chains plays an important role in bone mineralization [36].

2.4. Brittle IV mouse: A model for type IV OI

The cre/lox recombination system was used to develop a nonlethal knock-in murine model for OI [30]. A moderately severe OI phenotype was obtained from an$\alpha1$(I) 349 Gly→ Cys substitution in type I collagen, which is the same mutation in a type IV OI child. These mice, designated as Brittle IV (Brtl IV), have phenotypic variability ranging from perinatal lethality to long-term survival with reproductive success. The size of Brtl IV mice was about 50% that of normal littermates at 6 weeks of age, after which their size increased to about 80% of normal. Deformity of the rib cage was apparent and both forelegs and hindlegs were bowed and thinner than those of control littermates. The Brtl IV mouse has the molecular, biochemical, and radiographic features of human OI type IV. Heterozygous mutant mice have the undermineralization of the skeleton, the bone fragility, and the deformity characteristic of human patients. Their growth pattern, with normal size at birth followed by growth deficiency until 4–5 weeks of age, resembles the early childhood growth pattern reported for moderately severe OI patients. However, no significant deformities in long bones were evident in mutant mice after puberty and long bone fractures were also infrequent in adult mice.

3. Therapies for OI

At present, there is no cure for OI; however, some 'symptomatic' treatment options are available. The management of OI includes multidisciplinary input with experienced medical, orthopedic, physiotherapy and rehabilitation specialties. The current goals of therapy for OI are: to decrease the incidence of fractures; to increase growth velocity; to decrease pain; to have a positive effect on bone metabolic markers, bone histomorphometry and bone mineral density; and finally, to increase mobility and independence.

During past decades, various pharmacological agents have been administered to patients with OI and the majority of them initially claimed beneficial results, although none proved effective in controlled trials [37]. Among these were anabolic steroids, vitamin D, vitamin C, sodium fluoride, magnesium oxide, flavonoids (catechin) and calcitonin. Until 18 years ago, calcitonin was the most common therapy for OI, although its beneficial effects during the clinical course of the disease were disputed in the literature [38]; however it is no longer used. Thus, the search for effective treatments for OI remains ongoing.

3.1. Drug therapies

3.1.1. Bisphosphonates

In the last decade, the potential of bisphosphonate (BP) treatment has caused great excitement in the OI patient community and has generated new therapeutic options. BPs have been accepted as the standard of care for children with OI and in particular with moderate to severe forms of OI. The BP compounds are analogs of pyrophosphate which, when administered either orally or parentally, are characterized by a rapid and strong binding to hydroxyapatite crystals in the bone mineral. Once BPs are buried in the skeleton they are released only when bone is destroyed in the course of bone turnover. The success of BP appears to be related to the unremitting osteoclastic activity. These agents are potent inhibitors of bone resorption, decreasing osteoclast activity and number, although some effect on bone formation also occurs [39]. The potent anti-resorptive properties of BP inhibit the normal remodeling activity that acts to renew and repair bone. This activity results in improved vertebral shape and mass, higher cortical width, increased cancellous bone volume and suppressed bone turnover as shown by histomorphometric studies [40]. The net effect is to promote bone mineral accretion and at the same time to reduce bone turnover. Although the quality of the new bone that is formed remains unchanged, the bones benefit from greater mechanical strength due to overall increased bone mass [17].

A number of prospective studies have now shown that BPs can reduce fracture frequency, increase bone mineral content and improve the radiographic assessment of bone shape in growing children [41, 42]. In addition, linear growth is not impaired and fractures heal at their expected rate. Increase mobility was reported in the two largest studies conducted [42]. Muscle force measured by maximal isometric grip force of the non-dominant hand showed significant increases with BP therapy which was maintained for two years [43]. Patients with OI types I, II and IV showed significant improvement in height after four years of BP therapy [44]. It is difficult to assess the fracture rates as with increased mobility there might be a transient increase in fractures. However, overall decrease in fracture rate has been demonstrated after therapy when compared to historical controls [42]. Bone mineral density in the lumbar vertebrae also shows a rapid increase [45]. Radiographically, cycles of BP therapy leave dense sclerotic bands at the metaphysis of long bones which may contribute to the increased strength of the bones [46]. However, questions remain as to the selection of patients for treatment, which BPs to use, the minimum effective dose, the minimum effective treatment interval, appropriate duration of treatment and the role of oral BPs.

Concerns also remain regarding the potential buildup of microcracks and calcified cartilage which could lead to poor bone healing and increase fragility [47]. Osteonecrosis of the jaw is a complication of poor soft tissue and bone healing associated with BP therapy. While this is mainly reported in elderly patients with cancer who have been given very high doses of BP [48], there are concerns whether this complication could arise with long-term use of BP in children. However, the greatest concern in children with OI is over suppression of bone modeling and remodeling and worsening of bone quality. Long-term treatment, even at standard doses, interferes with bone remodeling and can be detected as metaphyseal undertubulation [49, 50]. Reports from surgeons describe treated bone as "rock-hard" and "crumbly", providing insight into paradoxical increases in fractures in some treated patients. Long-term suppression of bone turnover leads to accumulated micro-damage (microcracks) in bone [51] that may underlie the decrease in material strength. The equivocal improvement in fractures in children is illuminated by data from BP treatment of the Brtl mouse [52]. Treatment increases bone volume and load to fracture of murine femora, but concomitantly decreases material strength and elastic modulus. Femurs become, ironically, more brittle after prolonged treatment and bands of mineralized cartilage create matrix discontinuities that decrease bone quality. Prolonged treatment also alters osteoblast morphology. BP are also buried in the skeleton where they have a half-life of many years, so long term side effects may still surface. Thus, long-term use of BPs may not be beneficial as they decrease material properties and have detrimental effects on osteoblasts and bone formation.

3.1.2. Growth hormone

In mild forms of OI, agents increasing the production of type I collagen may have a therapeutic role. Growth hormone (GH) action positively affects bone growth and bone turnover by stimulating osteoblasts, collagen synthesis and longitudinal bone growth [53]. GH has a positive action on collagen metabolism, stimulating the expression in osteoblast cultures of insulin like-growth factor-1 (IGF-1) and IGF binding protein-3, which in turn regulate the synthesis of type I collagen [54, 55]. Osteoblasts from various species have IGF-I receptors and respond to both endogenous and exogenous IGF by accelerating the proliferation and increasing DNA and collagen synthesis [56, 57]. Animal studies in the *oim/oim* mouse model of OI, with bone phenotype comparable to a mild form of OI in humans, showed that systemic GH injections [58] or GH transgene expression in marrow [59] increased spine and femur length, produced significant changes in densitometric parameters and ameliorated biomechanical structural properties of bone. There is limited literature regarding GH in OI as only a few human studies have been performed using GH in patients with OI [60, 61]. One of the first attempts to treat OI with GH was more than 20 years ago by Kruse and Kuhlencordt[62], who treated two patients affected by OI with GH. The patients had an increase in periosteal new bone formation and in intracortical bone resorption with enhanced osteoblastic activity [62]. Following these results, no further study was reported in the literature until Marini and colleagues published their preliminary results from a limited number of patients treated with GH or clonidine (a pituitary GH secretagogue) [60]. In a further study by this group, the authors concluded that there is a group of type IV OI children who would benefit from GH treatment in terms of linear growth, bone matrix synthesis and bone histomorphometric parameters [63]. During GH therapy, patients have an improvement in general wellbeing, muscular performance and motor ability, which increases physical activity and, consequently, fracture risk in some cases [64]. In a study examining the efficacy of one year of GH treatment in patients affected by type I OI with an ascertained quantitative defect in type I collagen synthesis, GH treatment showed a positive effect on bone turnover, markers of bone apposition (i.e., osteocalcin and procollagen type I carboxy terminal propeptide levels) and bone mineral density, while the fracture risk did not change [65]. Thus, the results indicate that this is a useful therapy in patients with moderate forms of OI (the majority of type I and a good proportion of type IV). Patients with pre-existing scoliosis or bone deformities must be treated with particular caution because of the potential risk of worsening of these problems. Therefore, the selection of patients for GH treatment should be done carefully. It is possible that GH may be of benefit in combination with BP therapy [65, 66], but this has still to be adequately investigated [63].

3.1.3. Parathyroid hormone

Parathyroid hormone (PTH) also has anabolic effects on the bone and has been shown to have a positive effect for treatment of osteoporosis. Animal studies have shown that daily injection of recombinant human PTH results in increased bone mass, substantial new bone formation and altered bone architecture [67]. Based on this, daily injections of PTH should be beneficial in OI. However, these animal studies have demonstrated that sustained delivery in young rats resulted in development of bone lesions and tumors [67]. Due to this proposed increased risk for development of osteosarcoma, PTH is currently not recommended for children.

3.1.4. *RANKL inhibitors*

The potential therapeutic effects of receptor activator of nuclear factor kappa B ligand (RANKL) inhibitors in OI are currently under investigation. A recent study in a mouse model of OI (*oim/oim*) compared the effects of BP and RANKL inhibition. They found that although there were subtle differences between the two treatments, one was not superior to the other. There were similar decreases in fracture incidence with increases in metaphyseal bone volume via increase number of thinner trabeculae. BPs have the disadvantage of persisting in the bone for decades. Therefore RANKL inhibition is a newer, though more expensive treatment option, but may be preferred by some families and doctors as it is not deposited in the bone matrix. However, studies are needed to optimize the age of onset of therapy and the dose in children [68].

3.1.5. *Bortexomib*

The proteasome inhibitor Bortezomib is widely used in the treatment of multiple myeloma [69] and has been demonstrated to have an osteoblastogenic affect on adult murine and human mesenchymal stem cells by stabilizing RUNX-2 and acting directly on type I collagen [70]. It enhances osteoblast activity, differentiation [71] and also number [72]. Using the Brtl mouse model for OI, impairment in the differentiation of the progenitor cells towards osteoblasts has been demonstrated [73]. Treatment of the Brtl mice with Bortexomib rescued the osteoblastogenic capacity *in vitro* and ameliorated the bone properties *in vivo*, thus potentially identifying a new target for OI pharmacological treatment [73].

3.1.6. *Sclerostin*

A very recent study has investigated the potential of treating OI with antibodies to sclerostin, an anabolic bone agent produced by osteocytes that negatively regulated bone formation [74]. Antibodies to sclerostin are thought to stimulate osteoblasts and this agent is currently in clinical trials for treatment of osteoporosis [75]. Using the Brtl/+ mouse model, Sinder et al [74] demonstrated that treatment of OI mice for two weeks with antibodies to sclerostin stimulated bone formation, improved bone mass and increased bone load and stiffness to those of wildtype mice. These studies suggest short-term treatment of OI patients with sclerostin antibody may lead reduced fractures and improved bone quality.

3.2. Cell-based therapies

Normal bone responds to fracture or loading by increasing bone resorption and formation [76]. In a similar way, the OI bone initiates a cycle of bone remodeling in an attempt to form a stronger matrix. However, in OI, mutant collagen is synthesized, secreted from the cell and incorporated into matrix, where it actively participates in weakening the structure. Given the high turnover of bone seen in OI [77, 78], it is feasible that the deleterious effects in OI could be reduced or neutralized by the presence of normal osteoprogenitor cells. Thus, the potential to correct OI may lie in replicating the natural example of carriers, who have a substantial proportion of cells heterozygous for the collagen mutation, but are clinically normal. Studies of osteoblasts from carriers of type III and IV OI have shown that 40-75% of cells are mutant, setting the threshold for minimal symptoms at 30-40% normal cells [79]. Based on these findings, approaches that either target cells to suppress expression of mutant collagen or replace mutant cells with donated bone cell progenitors have potential to serve as long-term treatment for OI.

3.2.1. Gene-targeting therapy

While drug-based therapies may result in a more functional life for patients with moderate to severe OI, gene therapies aimed at correcting or replacing the defective gene may potentially provide long-term reversal of symptoms. Antisense technologies to inactivate mutant mRNA have been proposed as a method for mutation suppression [80]. In fibroblasts derived from a patient with type IV OI, antisense oligonucleotides were shown to suppress mutant protein $\alpha 2$(I) mRNA to 50% and mutant $\alpha 2$(I) mRNA to 40% [80]. While promising, these oligonucleotides also targeted the normal allele mRNA, suppressing it to 80% of its level in control cells, rendering this therapy ineffective. Similar studies have tested the ability of allele-specific suppression of mutant collagen expression by hammerhead ribozymes (short RNA molecules with catalytic potential) to biochemically transform the recipient from type II, III or IV OI into type I OI, in which individuals have a null allele, make half the normal amount of collagen and have mild disease [81]. These findings show that this suppression was complete and specific *in vitro* and substantial (50%) and highly selective (90%) in cells. However, the successful application to animal models is still to be tested.

Another approach involves gene targeting of mutant COL1A1 and COL1A2 using adeno-viral vectors in adult mesenchymal stem cells (MSCs). Two studies have shown successful production of normal collagen cells targeted with a COL1A1 or COL1A2 mutation [82, 83]. In a recent study by Deyle et al [84], MSCs were isolated from OI patients and mutant collagen genes were inactivated by adeno-virus-mediated gene targeting. Induced pluripotent stem cells (iPSC) were then derived from these gene-targeted cells with a floxed, polycistronic reprogramming vector, all vector-encoded transgenes were deleted with Cre recombinase. These iPSCs were then differentiated into mesenchymal and osteogenic cells *in vitro,* which produce bone *in vivo* after transplantation into the subrenal capsule of immunodeficient mice. These approaches could be potentially valuable for individuals with OI who are past early childhood. However, issues with low targeting success and random integration need to be solved before these approaches can be validated in humans.

3.2.2. Cellular replacement therapy

A number of reports in literature using animal models have suggested that bone marrow (BM) cells could be transplanted via the circulatory system and that the transplanted cells contribute to skeletal tissues including bone [85, 86]. Also encouraging have been transplantation studies of adult BM into Brtl pups *in utero* [87]. Despite low engraftment in bone (~ 2%), transplantation eliminated the perinatal lethality of Brtl mice and improved the biomechanical properties of femora in two-month old treated Brtl mice [87]. Current dogma suggests that BM contains two types of stem cells, mesenchymal stem cells (MSCs) and hematopoietic stem cells (HSCs), and that their repertoire of differentiation/reconstituting potentials are distinct and separate from each other. MSCs are defined by their adherence to plastic and potential to differentiate into mesenchymal tissue cells such as bone, fat, muscle, cartilage and fibroblasts [88-91]. The term "MSC" has been applied to define both mesenchymal stem cells and mesenchymal stromal cells [89]. HSCs are defined by their capability of hematopoietic reconstitution *in vivo* and have also been shown to give rise to a few tissue cell types including mast cells and osteoclasts. However, recent studies have begun to question the distinction between the potentials of MSCs and HSCs, particularly with regard to osteo-chondrogenic tissues.

4. MSC-based therapy

Transplantation studies using murine models have evaluated the potential of MSCs to directly differentiate into osteogenic cells to treat OI [92, 93]. Studies in a mouse model of OI showed that infusion of marrow stromal cells (MSCs) resulted in a significant increase in collagen production [85]. The data presented by Wang et al [92] demonstrated that murine MSCs migrate and incorporate into the developing neonatal heterozygous and homozygous OI mice, differentiate into osteoblasts and appear to participate in the bone formation of the recipient mouse *in vivo*. A recent study from the same group evaluated green fluorescent protein (GFP)-expressing single cell expanded, marrow-derived progenitors for engraftment in a neonatal model of OI following systemic transplantation [93]. Tissues from the recipient mice were examined at two and four weeks post transplantation. Their study shows that the progenitors infused in the neonatal OI mice engraft in the various tissues including bones, undergo differentiation, deposit matrix and form bone *in vivo*. The authors also state that the progenitor cell transplantation is more efficient in developing OI mice than adult mice [93].

Cell therapy protocols also involve direct delivery of cells into target tissues with the hope that the cells will differentiate into cells of the target tissues and repair or regenerate host tissues. Li et al (2010) have demonstrated that MSCs infused into femurs of the *oim/oim* mouse model contribute to bone formation *in vivo*. Improvement in mechanical properties of the recipient bones seen may be the result of bone deposition by both endogenous and donor cells or paracrine actions of donor cells. The recipient mice were followed for six weeks following cell infusion into femurs. It still remains to be investigated if this positive effect lasts beyond this time period.

Intrauterine transplantation of fetal human MSCs was shown to markedly reduced fracture rates and skeletal abnormalities in an *oim/oim* mouse model [94]. In a similar model, Vanleene et al [95] showed that human fetal MSCs isolated based on their adherence to plastic, transplanted *in utero* in *oim/oim* mice migrated to bone, differentiated into mature osteoblasts, and expressed the missing protein COL1a2, altering the apatite mineral structure and increasing bone matrix stiffness. The changes in microscopic material properties and micro-architecture contribute to the mechanical integrity of the bone, making the bone less brittle and resulting in a decreased incidence of fracture. However, further work needs to be done to investigate strategies to maximize donor cell homing to bone, differentiation, and collagen expression to maximize the therapeutic effects of transplantation.

While these studies suggest a role for MSCs in generation of osteogenic cells, the difficulty in defining and isolating MSCs as well as the sometimes complex history of manipulation before being tested for differentiation potentials *in vivo*, makes it difficult to determine the mechanism by which these cells have an effect [89, 96, 97].

5. HSC-based therapy

Recent studies have identified a population of circulating human osteoblastic cells which express osteocalcin or alkaline phosphatase and increase during pubertal growth and during fracture repair [98]. Studies showed that these osteocalcin positive cells were able to form mineralized nodules *in vitro* and bone *in vivo*. This population was subsequently shown to be $CD34^+$ [99], suggesting that it is derived from the HSC. In support of this, Chen et al [100] have shown that the frequency of osteoblast progenitor cells is higher in $CD34^+$ cells (approximately 1/5000) than in CD34- population (1/33,000) of human BM. Murine transplantation studies have demonstrated that transplantation of 3000 side population (SP) cells that are highly enriched for HSCs generated osteoblasts *in vivo* [101]. In another study, Dominici et al [102] transplanted marrow cells that had been transduced with GFP-expressing retroviral vector and observed a common retroviral integration site in clonogenic hematopoietic cells and osteoprogenitors from each of the recipient mice. This is consistent with observations that non-adherent BM cells, the fraction enriched for HSCs, give rise to bone in culture [101, 103]. A study of the kinetics and histological/anatomic pattern of osteopoietic engraftment after transplantation of ~ two million GFP-expressing non-adherent BM cells in 6-8 week old FVB/N OI mice revealed that osteopoietic engraftment was maximum two weeks after transplantation [104]. However, this osteogenic engraftment decreased to negligible levels after six months to one year while the hematopoietic reconstitution remained stable over the entire period of observation [104]. The authors explain the lack of durable donor derived osteopoiesis by the intrinsic genetic program or the external environmental signals that suppress the differentiation capacity of the donor stem cells. Studies in both an animal model and patients (CT NCT00187018) demonstrated that the non-adherent bone marrow population was able to significantly and robustly provide osteoprogenitors for treatment of OI [105]. Together, these studies provide compelling evidence for the existence of a common progenitor cell with both hematopoietic and osteocytic differentiation potentials in the non-adherent or CD34-expressing, HSC-enriched, fraction of BM cells.

In the last decade, many conflicting reports have been published regarding tissue-reconstituting ability of HSCs. To determine the tissue reconstituting potential of HSCs, we have carried out a series of studies based on BM reconstitution by a single HSC (reviewed in [106-108]). These studies have shown that transplantation of a clonal population derived from a single HSC expressing transgenic enhanced GFP (EGFP) results in efficient generation of mice exhibiting high-level, multi-lineage engraftment from a single HSC. In this model, putative HSCs are sorted based on surface marker expression and Hoechst dye efflux (side population, SP), identified by combining single cell deposition with short-term culture and functionally defined *in vivo* by the ability to reconstitute the BM when a single cell is transplanted into lethally irradiated mice [109-112]. It is important to note that there is no equivalent test for defining a MSC, making it difficult to isolate and characterize MSCs [96, 97]. Findings from studies using a single cell/clonal cell transplantation method have shown that HSCs can give rise to non-hematopoietic cells such as fibroblasts and fibrocytes [109], tumor-associated fibroblasts/myofibroblasts [110], valve interstitial cells [113], glomerular mesangial cells [111], brain microglial cells and perivascular cells [112], inner ear fibrocytes [114], retinal endothelial cells [115] and epithelial cells in multiple organs [116]. Most recently, our lab has demonstrated that HSCs give rise to adipocytes [117], a cell also thought to be of mesenchymal origin, and osteo-chondrogenic cells [118].

Based on these findings, we hypothesized that the primary defect in OI may lie in the HSC. As the bone turnover is high in OI, introduction of the normal progenitor cells would quickly populate the bone with cells making normal matrix and therefore ameliorate and/or prevent the occurrence of associated pathologies. To test this hypothesis, we conducted HSC transplantation in a mouse model of OI (*oim/oim*) [119]. In these studies, recipient *oim/oim* mice were first scanned by micro-computed tomography (micro-CT) before transplantation to obtain baseline images and information on bone histomorphometrics. The BM of lethally irradiated *oim/oim* mice was then reconstituted with $EGFP^+$ non-adherent mononuclear cells or purified HSCs from EGFP mice. Transgenic $EGFP^+$ mice (C57BL/6) [120] which ubiquitously express EGFP under the control of the actin promoter were used as BM donors for transplantation into homozygous OI mice (*oim/oim*; B6C3Fe a/a-Col1a2^{oim}/J; Jackson Labs). Either 2 x10^5 mononuclear cells or 50 Lin^- Sca-1^+ c-kit^+ $CD34^-$ SP cells (putative HSCs) prepared from the EGFP mice were injected via tail vein into irradiated *oim* mice. The mice transplanted with 50 Lin^- Sca-1^+ c-kit^+ $CD34^-$ SP cells also received injection of 2 x 10^5 un-manipulated BM cells from an *oim/oim* mouse which served as radio-protective cells during the post radiation pancytopenia period. *Oim/oim* mice with no engraftment and irradiated *oim/oim* mice transplanted with 2 x 10^5 MNCs from another *oim/oim* mouse were used as controls. Changes in bone parameters were analyzed using longitudinal micro-CT. To confirm participation of HSC-derived osteoblasts and osteocytes in *oim/oim* bones, the $EGFP^+$ cells were analyzed in paraffin sections.

Dramatic improvements in bone architecture were observed in the 3D micro-CT images of bones of HSC-engrafted oim mice at three, six and nine months post-transplantation which correlated with high levels of hematopoietic engraftment. These improvements corresponded to improvements in histomorphometric parameters including an increase in bone volume, trabecular number, thickness and density and a decrease in trabecular spacing. Decrease in trabecular pattern factor indicated an improvement in the connectivity and structure of the trabeculae.In addition to quantifiable improvements in the bone architecture, we also observed clinical improvements in the engrafted *oim/oim* mice. The weight of the mice increased over the course of the experiment, perhaps in part due to the dramatic improvements in the bone architecture and density. The mice also became more active and were less prone to fractures during routine bedding changes and animal husbandry. In contrast to the mice engrafted with normal HSCs, the bone architecture and clinical parameters in the control mice continued to deteriorate over the course of the experiment. Analysis of paraffin sections showed the presence of numerous $EGFP^+$ cells within the bone (unpublished data) that expressed Runx-2 and osteocalcin, demonstrating that they were osteoblasts and osteocytes as well as their origin from the HSCs. Studies are under way to determine the mechanisms by which HSCs affect structural and clinical improvements in the OI model.

6. Clinical bone marrow transplantations

Together, these preclinical studies suggest a potential for bone marrow transplantation in treating osteopoietic disorders. Findings from these studies are consistent with clinical transplantation of whole BM or fractionated MSCs in children with severe form of OI. In the first trial, three children with OI were transplanted with un-manipulated BM from a sibling donor [121]. Three months after osteoblast engraftment, specimens from trabecular bone show evidence of new dense bone formation. There was an increase in the total body bone mineral content associated with increase in growth velocity and reduced frequency of fracture [121]. Similar results were seen in an additional study with five children with severe OI [122]. With extended follow-up, the patients' growth rates either slowed down or plateaued, but bone mineral content continued to increase. These finding suggest a durable engraftment of osteogenic donor cells, which could potentially convert a severe clinical phenotype to a less severe one. Due to the promising results obtained with the previous trials, a study was conducted where gene marked, donor marrow derived mesenchymal cells were used to treat six children with severe OI. The cells engrafted in the bone, marrow stroma and skin and produced clinically measurable benefits in the form of increase growth velocities. But surprisingly, no increase was observed in the total body bone mineral content [123]. An additional study of a single human fetus receiving *in utero* transplantation of fetal MSCs reported that very low engraftment (0.3%) could still be demonstrated in bone at nine months of age, however evaluation of clinical outcome was complicated by treatment in infancy with bisphosphonate [124]. While statistical significance in these studies was often lacking because of the small number of patients in each study, these findings nonetheless suggest beneficial clinical effects of BM transplantation in OI.

7. Conclusions and future perspectives

There is significant interest in the use of BM transplantation to repair various tissues as illustrated by many ongoing clinical trials (reviewed in [89, 125]). Several preclinical studies have suggested that transplantation of BM cells may lead to improvements in other genetic diseases that involve collagen synthesis such as Alport syndrome [126, 127] and Epidermolysis bullosa [128]. As detailed above, preclinical studies and those in patients also demonstrate a therapeutic role for BM transplant for OI. Despite these studies, the mechanism by which marrow transplant ameliorates the genetic disorder remains unclear. Given that the BM is thought to contain two stem cell populations, MSCs and HSCs, elucidation of the stem cell with osteogenic potential would potentially drive therapies for OI. Our studies demonstrate that the HSC has this potential [118, 119] and can correct the osteogenic defect in an animal model of OI [119]. Our findings are supported by a recent study that compared the mechanisms of action for non-adherent mononuclear cells and MSCs in OI [105]. In this study, it was shown that both non-adherent BM cells enriched for HSCs and MSCs are clinically effective agents for cell therapy of bone, but that the two populations function by distinct mechanisms. Non-adherent BM cells were found to directly differentiate into osteoblasts and secrete normal collagen to the bone matrix. In contrast, MSCs did not engraft in the bone, but secreted soluble mediators that indirectly stimulated growth. Together, these studies demonstrate the potential for stem cell-based therapies for long-term treatment of OI. However, several issues remain to be elucidated including: what is the optimal delivery schedule, which type of cell to deliver for greatest efficacy (MSC, HSC or combination), and how to expand their potential with adjunct drug therapy.

Acknowledgements

This work was supported in part by the Biomedical Laboratory Research and Development Program of the Department of Veterans Affairs (Merit Award, ACL). The contents of this work do not represent the views of the Department of Veterans Affairs or the United States Government. This work was also supported by National Institutes of Health grants R01 CA148772 (ACL) and K01 AR059097-01 (MM).

Author details

Meenal Mehrotra[1] and Amanda C. LaRue[2*]

*Address all correspondence to: laruerc@musc.edu

1 Department of Pathology and Laboratory Medicine, Medical University of South Carolina, Charleston, SC, USA

2 Research Services, Department of Veterans Affairs Medical Center, Charleston, SC, USA and Department of Pathology and Laboratory Medicine, Medical University of South Carolina, Charleston, SC, USA

References

[1] Glorieux, F.H., *Osteogenesis imperfecta.* Best Pract Res Clin Rheumatol, 2008. 22(1): p. 85-100.

[2] Marini, J.C., *Osteogenesis Imperfecta,* in *Primer on the Metabolic Bone Diseases adn Disorders of Mineral Metabolism,* C.J. Rosen, Editor 2008, The American Society for Bone and Mineral Research: Washington. p. 446-450.

[3] Gautieri, A., S. Uzel, et al., *Molecular and mesoscale mechanisms of osteogenesis imperfecta disease in collagen fibrils.* Biophys J, 2009. 97(3): p. 857-65.

[4] Cundy, T., *Recent advances in osteogenesis imperfecta.* Calcif Tissue Int, 2012. 90(6): p. 439-49.

[5] Barnes, A.M., W. Chang, et al., *Deficiency of cartilage-associated protein in recessive lethal osteogenesis imperfecta.* N Engl J Med, 2006. 355(26): p. 2757-64.

[6] Morello, R., T.K. Bertin, et al., *CRTAP is required for prolyl 3- hydroxylation and mutations cause recessive osteogenesis imperfecta.* Cell, 2006. 127(2): p. 291-304.

[7] Cabral, W.A., W. Chang, et al., *Prolyl 3-hydroxylase 1 deficiency causes a recessive metabolic bone disorder resembling lethal/severe osteogenesis imperfecta.* Nat Genet, 2007. 39(3): p. 359-65.

[8] Ai, M., S. Heeger, et al., *Clinical and molecular findings in osteoporosis-pseudoglioma syndrome.* Am J Hum Genet, 2005. 77(5): p. 741-53.

[9] Lapunzina, P., M. Aglan, et al., *Identification of a frameshift mutation in Osterix in a patient with recessive osteogenesis imperfecta.* Am J Hum Genet, 2010. 87(1): p. 110-4.

[10] Sillence, D.O., A. Senn, and D.M. Danks, *Genetic heterogeneity in osteogenesis imperfecta.* J Med Genet, 1979. 16(2): p. 101-16.

[11] Marini, J.C., A. Forlino, et al., *Consortium for osteogenesis imperfecta mutations in the helical domain of type I collagen: regions rich in lethal mutations align with collagen binding sites for integrins and proteoglycans.* Hum Mutat, 2007. 28(3): p. 209-21.

[12] Sillence, D.O., K.K. Barlow, et al., *Osteogenesis imperfecta type II delineation of the phenotype with reference to genetic heterogeneity.* Am J Med Genet, 1984. 17(2): p. 407-23.

[13] Paterson, C.R., S. McAllion, and R. Miller, *Osteogenesis imperfecta with dominant inheritance and normal sclerae.* J Bone Joint Surg Br, 1983. 65(1): p. 35-9.

[14] Glorieux, F.H., F. Rauch, et al., *Type V osteogenesis imperfecta: a new form of brittle bone disease.* J Bone Miner Res, 2000. 15(9): p. 1650-8.

[15] Glorieux, F.H., L.M. Ward, et al., *Osteogenesis imperfecta type VI: a form of brittle bone disease with a mineralization defect.* J Bone Miner Res, 2002. 17(1): p. 30-8.

[16] Ward, L.M., F. Rauch, et al., *Osteogenesis imperfecta type VII: an autosomal recessive form of brittle bone disease.* Bone, 2002. 31(1): p. 12-8.

[17] Cheung, M.S. and F.H. Glorieux, *Osteogenesis Imperfecta: update on presentation and management.* Rev Endocr Metab Disord, 2008. 9(2): p. 153-60.

[18] Alanay, Y., H. Avaygan, et al., *Mutations in the gene encoding the RER protein FKBP65 cause autosomal-recessive osteogenesis imperfecta.* Am J Hum Genet, 2010. 86(4): p. 551-9.

[19] Baldridge, D., U. Schwarze, et al., *CRTAP and LEPRE1 mutations in recessive osteogenesis imperfecta.* Hum Mutat, 2008. 29(12): p. 1435-42.

[20] Barnes, A.M., E.M. Carter, et al., *Lack of cyclophilin B in osteogenesis imperfecta with normal collagen folding.* N Engl J Med, 2010. 362(6): p. 521-8.

[21] Christiansen, H.E., U. Schwarze, et al., *Homozygosity for a missense mutation in SERPINH1, which encodes the collagen chaperone protein HSP47, results in severe recessive osteogenesis imperfecta.* Am J Hum Genet, 2010. 86(3): p. 389-98.

[22] Kelley, B.P., F. Malfait, et al., *Mutations in FKBP10 cause recessive osteogenesis imperfecta and Bruck syndrome.* J Bone Miner Res, 2011. 26(3): p. 666-72.

[23] Becker, J., O. Semler, et al., *Exome sequencing identifies truncating mutations in human SERPINF1 in autosomal-recessive osteogenesis imperfecta.* Am J Hum Genet, 2011. 88(3): p. 362-71.

[24] Kamoun-Goldrat, A.S. and M.F. Le Merrer, *Animal models of osteogenesis imperfecta and related syndromes.* Journal of bone and mineral metabolism, 2007. 25(4): p. 211-8.

[25] Harbers, K., M. Kuehn, et al., *Insertion of retrovirus into the first intron of alpha 1(I) collagen gene to embryonic lethal mutation in mice.* Proc Natl Acad Sci U S A, 1984. 81(5): p. 1504-8.

[26] Lohler, J., R. Timpl, and R. Jaenisch, *Embryonic lethal mutation in mouse collagen I gene causes rupture of blood vessels and is associated with erythropoietic and mesenchymal cell death.* Cell, 1984. 38(2): p. 597-607.

[27] Jaenisch, R., K. Harbers, et al., *Germline integration of moloney murine leukemia virus at the Mov13 locus leads to recessive lethal mutation and early embryonic death.* Cell, 1983. 32(1): p. 209-16.

[28] Bonadio, J., T.L. Saunders, et al., *Transgenic mouse model of the mild dominant form of osteogenesis imperfecta.* Proc Natl Acad Sci U S A, 1990. 87(18): p. 7145-9.

[29] Kratochwil, K., K. von der Mark, et al., *Retrovirus-induced insertional mutation in Mov13 mice affects collagen I expression in a tissue-specific manner.* Cell, 1989. 57(5): p. 807-16.

[30] Forlino, A., F.D. Porter, et al., *Use of the Cre/lox recombination system to develop a non-lethal knock-in murine model for osteogenesis imperfecta with an alpha1(I) G349C substitution. Variability in phenotype in BrtlIV mice.* J Biol Chem, 1999. 274(53): p. 37923-31.

[31] Chipman, S.D., H.O. Sweet, et al., *Defective pro alpha 2(I) collagen synthesis in a recessive mutation in mice: a model of human osteogenesis imperfecta.* Proc Natl Acad Sci U S A, 1993. 90(5): p. 1701-5.

[32] McBride, D.J., Jr. and J.R. Shapiro, *Confirmation of a G nucleotide deletion in the Cola-2 gene of mice with the osteogenesis imperfecta mutation.* Genomics, 1994. 20(1): p. 135-7.

[33] Lopez Franco, G.E., A. Huang, et al., *Dental phenotype of the col1a2(oim) mutation: DI is present in both homozygotes and heterozygotes.* Bone, 2005. 36(6): p. 1039-46.

[34] Misof, K., W.J. Landis, et al., *Collagen from the osteogenesis imperfecta mouse model (oim) shows reduced resistance against tensile stress.* J Clin Invest, 1997. 100(1): p. 40-5.

[35] McBride, D.J., Jr., J.R. Shapiro, and M.G. Dunn, *Bone geometry and strength measurements in aging mice with the oim mutation.* Calcif Tissue Int, 1998. 62(2): p. 172-6.

[36] Camacho, N.P., L. Hou, et al., *The material basis for reduced mechanical properties in oim mice bones.* J Bone Miner Res, 1999. 14(2): p. 264-72.

[37] Albright, J.A., *Systemic treatment of osteogenesis imperfecta.* Clin Orthop Relat Res, 1981(159): p. 88-96.

[38] Pedersen, U., P. Charles, et al., *Lack of effects of human calcitonin in osteogenesis imperfecta.* Acta Orthop Scand, 1985. 56(3): p. 260-4.

[39] Russell, R.G., *Bisphosphonates: mode of action and pharmacology.* Pediatrics, 2007. 119 Suppl 2: p. S150-62.

[40] Munns, C.F., F. Rauch, et al., *Effects of intravenous pamidronate treatment in infants with osteogenesis imperfecta: clinical and histomorphometric outcome.* J Bone Miner Res, 2005. 20(7): p. 1235-43.

[41] Astrom, E. and S. Soderhall, *Beneficial effect of bisphosphonate during five years of treatment of severe osteogenesis imperfecta.* Acta Paediatr, 1998. 87(1): p. 64-8.

[42] Glorieux, F.H., N.J. Bishop, et al., *Cyclic administration of pamidronate in children with severe osteogenesis imperfecta.* N Engl J Med, 1998. 339(14): p. 947-52.

[43] Montpetit, K., H. Plotkin, et al., *Rapid increase in grip force after start of pamidronate therapy in children and adolescents with severe osteogenesis imperfecta.* Pediatrics, 2003. 111(5 Pt 1): p. e601-3.

[44] Zeitlin, L., F. Rauch, et al., *Height and weight development during four years of therapy with cyclical intravenous pamidronate in children and adolescents with osteogenesis imperfecta types I, III, and IV.* Pediatrics, 2003. 111(5 Pt 1): p. 1030-6.

[45] Land, C., F. Rauch, et al., *Osteogenesis imperfecta type VI in childhood and adolescence: effects of cyclical intravenous pamidronate treatment.* Bone, 2007. 40(3): p. 638-44.

[46] Rauch, F., R. Travers, et al., *Sclerotic metaphyseal lines in a child treated with pamidronate: histomorphometric analysis.* J Bone Miner Res, 2004. 19(7): p. 1191-3.

[47] Land, C., F. Rauch, and F.H. Glorieux, *Cyclical intravenous pamidronate treatment affects metaphyseal modeling in growing patients with osteogenesis imperfecta.* J Bone Miner Res, 2006. 21(3): p. 374-9.

[48] Migliorati, C.A., M.A. Siegel, and L.S. Elting, *Bisphosphonate-associated osteonecrosis: a long-term complication of bisphosphonate treatment.* Lancet Oncol, 2006. 7(6): p. 508-14.

[49] Whyte, M.P., W.H. McAlister, et al., *Bisphosphonate-induced osteopetrosis: novel bone modeling defects, metaphyseal osteopenia, and osteosclerosis fractures after drug exposure ceases.* J Bone Miner Res, 2008. 23(10): p. 1698-707.

[50] Whyte, M.P., D. Wenkert, et al., *Bisphosphonate-induced osteopetrosis.* N Engl J Med, 2003. 349(5): p. 457-63.

[51] Allen, M.R., K. Iwata, et al., *Alterations in canine vertebral bone turnover, microdamage accumulation, and biomechanical properties following 1-year treatment with clinical treatment doses of risedronate or alendronate.* Bone, 2006. 39(4): p. 872-9.

[52] Uveges, T.E., K.M. Kozloff, et al., *Alendronate treatment of the brtl osteogenesis imperfecta mouse improves femoral geometry and load response before fracture but decreases predicted material properties and has detrimental effects on osteoblasts and bone formation.* J Bone Miner Res, 2009. 24(5): p. 849-59.

[53] Antoniazzi, F., G. Zamboni, et al., *Bone development during GH and GnRH analog treatment.* Eur J Endocrinol, 2004. 151 Suppl 1: p. S47-54.

[54] Ernst, M. and G.A. Rodan, *Increased activity of insulin-like growth factor (IGF) in osteoblastic cells in the presence of growth hormone (GH): positive correlation with the presence of the GH-induced IGF-binding protein BP-3.* Endocrinology, 1990. 127(2): p. 807-14.

[55] McCarthy, T.L., M. Centrella, and E. Canalis, *Regulatory effects of insulin-like growth factors I and II on bone collagen synthesis in rat calvarial cultures.* Endocrinology, 1989. 124(1): p. 301-9.

[56] Hock, J.M., M. Centrella, and E. Canalis, *Insulin-like growth factor I has independent effects on bone matrix formation and cell replication.* Endocrinology, 1988. 122(1): p. 254-60.

[57] Wergedal, J.E., S. Mohan, et al., *Skeletal growth factor and other growth factors known to be present in bone matrix stimulate proliferation and protein synthesis in human bone cells.* J Bone Miner Res, 1990. 5(2): p. 179-86.

[58] King, D., D. Jarjoura, et al., *Growth hormone injections improve bone quality in a mouse model of osteogenesis imperfecta.* J Bone Miner Res, 2005. 20(6): p. 987-93.

[59] King, D., J. Chase, et al., *Effects of growth hormone transgene expression on vertebrae in a mouse model of osteogenesis imperfecta.* Spine (Phila Pa 1976), 2005. 30(13): p. 1491-5.

[60] Marini, J.C., S. Bordenick, et al., *Evaluation of growth hormone axis and responsiveness to growth stimulation of short children with osteogenesis imperfecta.* Am J Med Genet, 1993. 45(2): p. 261-4.

[61] Vieira, N.E., J.C. Marini, et al., *Effect of growth hormone treatment on calcium kinetics in patients with osteogenesis imperfecta type III and IV.* Bone, 1999. 25(4): p. 501-5.

[62] Kruse, H.P. and F. Kuhlencordt, *On an attempt to treat primary and secondary osteoporosis with human growth hormone.* Horm Metab Res, 1975. 7(6): p. 488-91.

[63] Marini, J.C., E. Hopkins, et al., *Positive linear growth and bone responses to growth hormone treatment in children with types III and IV osteogenesis imperfecta: high predictive value of the carboxyterminal propeptide of type I procollagen.* J Bone Miner Res, 2003. 18(2): p. 237-43.

[64] Kodama, H., K. Kubota, and T. Abe, *Osteogenesis imperfecta: Are fractures and growth hormone treatment linked?* J Pediatr, 1998. 132(3 Pt 1): p. 559-60.

[65] Antoniazzi, F., F. Bertoldo, et al., *Growth hormone treatment in osteogenesis imperfecta with quantitative defect of type I collagen synthesis.* J Pediatr, 1996. 129(3): p. 432-9.

[66] Antoniazzi, F., E. Monti, et al., *GH in combination with bisphosphonate treatment in osteogenesis imperfecta.* Eur J Endocrinol, 2010. 163(3): p. 479-87.

[67] Vahle, J.L., M. Sato, et al., *Skeletal changes in rats given daily subcutaneous injections of recombinant human parathyroid hormone (1-34) for 2 years and relevance to human safety.* Toxicol Pathol, 2002. 30(3): p. 312-21.

[68] Bargman, R., R. Posham, et al., *Comparable outcomes in fracture reduction and bone properties with RANKL inhibition and alendronate treatment in a mouse model of osteogenesis imperfecta.* Osteoporos Int, 2012. 23(3): p. 1141-50.

[69] Chen, R.A., Y. Tu, et al., *Bortezomib-dexamethasone or vincristine-doxorubicin-dexamethasone as induction therapy followed by thalidomide as maintenance therapy in untreated multiple myeloma patients.* J Int Med Res, 2011. 39(5): p. 1975-84.

[70] Mukherjee, S., N. Raje, et al., *Pharmacologic targeting of a stem/progenitor population in vivo is associated with enhanced bone regeneration in mice.* J Clin Invest, 2008. 118(2): p. 491-504.

[71] Zangari, M., E. Terpos, et al., *Impact of bortezomib on bone health in myeloma: A review of current evidence.* Cancer Treat Rev, 2012.

[72] Giuliani, N., F. Morandi, et al., *The proteasome inhibitor bortezomib affects osteoblast differentiation in vitro and in vivo in multiple myeloma patients.* Blood, 2007. 110(1): p. 334-8.

[73] Gioia, R., C. Panaroni, et al., *Impaired osteoblastogenesis in a murine model of dominant osteogenesis imperfecta: a new target for osteogenesis imperfecta pharmacological therapy.* Stem Cells, 2012. 30(7): p. 1465-76.

[74] Sinder, B.P., M.M. Eddy, et al., *Sclerostin antibody improves skeletal parameters in a Brtl/+ mouse model of osteogenesis imperfecta.* Journal of bone and mineral research : the official journal of the American Society for Bone and Mineral Research, 2012.

[75] Padhi, D., G. Jang, et al., *Single-dose, placebo-controlled, randomized study of AMG 785, a sclerostin monoclonal antibody.* Journal of bone and mineral research : the official journal of the American Society for Bone and Mineral Research, 2011. 26(1): p. 19-26.

[76] Raisz, L.G., *Physiology and pathophysiology of bone remodeling.* Clin Chem, 1999. 45(8 Pt 2): p. 1353-8.

[77] Baron, R., J.M. Gertner, et al., *Increased bone turnover with decreased bone formation by osteoblasts in children with osteogenesis imperfecta tarda.* Pediatr Res, 1983. 17(3): p. 204-7.

[78] Rauch, F., R. Travers, et al., *Static and dynamic bone histomorphometry in children with osteogenesis imperfecta.* Bone, 2000. 26(6): p. 581-9.

[79] Cabral, W.A. and J.C. Marini, *High proportion of mutant osteoblasts is compatible with normal skeletal function in mosaic carriers of osteogenesis imperfecta.* Am J Hum Genet, 2004. 74(4): p. 752-60.

[80] Wang, Q. and J.C. Marini, *Antisense oligodeoxynucleotides selectively suppress expression of the mutant alpha 2(I) collagen allele in type IV osteogenesis imperfecta fibroblasts. A molecular approach to therapeutics of dominant negative disorders.* The Journal of clinical investigation, 1996. 97(2): p. 448-54.

[81] Dawson, P.A. and J.C. Marini, *Hammerhead ribozymes selectively suppress mutant type I collagen mRNA in osteogenesis imperfecta fibroblasts.* Nucleic Acids Res, 2000. 28(20): p. 4013-20.

[82] Chamberlain, J.R., D.R. Deyle, et al., *Gene targeting of mutant COL1A2 alleles in mesenchymal stem cells from individuals with osteogenesis imperfecta.* Mol Ther, 2008. 16(1): p. 187-93.

[83] Chamberlain, J.R., U. Schwarze, et al., *Gene targeting in stem cells from individuals with osteogenesis imperfecta.* Science, 2004. 303(5661): p. 1198-201.

[84] Deyle, D.R., I.F. Khan, et al., *Normal collagen and bone production by gene-targeted human osteogenesis imperfecta iPSCs.* Mol Ther, 2012. 20(1): p. 204-13.

[85] Pereira, R.F., M.D. O'Hara, et al., *Marrow stromal cells as a source of progenitor cells for nonhematopoietic tissues in transgenic mice with a phenotype of osteogenesis imperfecta.* Proc Natl Acad Sci U S A, 1998. 95(3): p. 1142-7.

[86] Hou, Z., Q. Nguyen, et al., *Osteoblast-specific gene expression after transplantation of marrow cells: implications for skeletal gene therapy.* Proc Natl Acad Sci U S A, 1999. 96(13): p. 7294-9.

[87] Panaroni, C., R. Gioia, et al., *In utero transplantation of adult bone marrow decreases perinatal lethality and rescues the bone phenotype in the knockin murine model for classical, dominant osteogenesis imperfecta.* Blood, 2009. 114(2): p. 459-68.

[88] Pittenger, M.F., A.M. Mackay, et al., *Multilineage potential of adult human mesenchymal stem cells.* Science, 1999. 284(5411): p. 143-7.

[89] Prockop, D.J., *"Stemness" does not explain the repair of many tissues by mesenchymal stem/multipotent stromal cells (MSCs).* Clin Pharmacol Ther, 2007. 82(3): p. 241-3.

[90] Ziegelhoeffer, T., B. Fernandez, et al., *Bone marrow-derived cells do not incorporate into the adult growing vasculature.* Circulation research, 2004. 94(2): p. 230-8.

[91] Xing, F., J. Saidou, and K. Watabe, *Cancer associated fibroblasts (CAFs) in tumor micro-environment.* Frontiers in bioscience : a journal and virtual library, 2010. 15: p. 166-79.

[92] Wang, X., F. Li, and C. Niyibizi, *Progenitors systemically transplanted into neonatal mice localize to areas of active bone formation in vivo: implications of cell therapy for skeletal diseases.* Stem Cells, 2006. 24(8): p. 1869-78.

[93] Li, F., X. Wang, and C. Niyibizi, *Distribution of single-cell expanded marrow derived progenitors in a developing mouse model of osteogenesis imperfecta following systemic transplantation.* Stem Cells, 2007. 25(12): p. 3183-93.

[94] Guillot, P.V., O. Abass, et al., *Intrauterine transplantation of human fetal mesenchymal stem cells from first-trimester blood repairs bone and reduces fractures in osteogenesis imperfecta mice.* Blood, 2008. 111(3): p. 1717-25.

[95] Vanleene, M., Z. Saldanha, et al., *Transplantation of human fetal blood stem cells in the osteogenesis imperfecta mouse leads to improvement in multiscale tissue properties.* Blood, 2011. 117(3): p. 1053-60.

[96] Bianco, P., P.G. Robey, and P.J. Simmons, *Mesenchymal stem cells: revisiting history, concepts, and assays.* Cell Stem Cell, 2008. 2(4): p. 313-9.

[97] Javazon, E.H., K.J. Beggs, and A.W. Flake, *Mesenchymal stem cells: paradoxes of passaging.* Exp Hematol, 2004. 32(5): p. 414-25.

[98] Eghbali-Fatourechi, G.Z., J. Lamsam, et al., *Circulating osteoblast-lineage cells in humans.* N Engl J Med, 2005. 352(19): p. 1959-66.

[99] Eghbali-Fatourechi, G.Z., U.I. Modder, et al., *Characterization of circulating osteoblast lineage cells in humans.* Bone, 2007. 40(5): p. 1370-7.

[100] Chen, J.L., P. Hunt, et al., *Osteoblast precursor cells are found in CD34+ cells from human bone marrow.* Stem Cells, 1997. 15(5): p. 368-77.

[101] Olmsted-Davis, E.A., Z. Gugala, et al., *Primitive adult hematopoietic stem cells can function as osteoblast precursors.* Proc Natl Acad Sci U S A, 2003. 100(26): p. 15877-82.

[102] Dominici, M., C. Pritchard, et al., *Hematopoietic cells and osteoblasts are derived from a common marrow progenitor after bone marrow transplantation.* Proc Natl Acad Sci U S A, 2004. 101(32): p. 11761-6.

[103] Falla, N., V. Van, et al., *Characterization of a 5-fluorouracil-enriched osteoprogenitor population of the murine bone marrow.* Blood, 1993. 82(12): p. 3580-91.

[104] Dominici, M., R. Marino, et al., *Donor cell-derived osteopoiesis originates from a self-renewing stem cell with a limited regenerative contribution after transplantation.* Blood, 2008. 111(8): p. 4386-91.

[105] Otsuru, S., P.L. Gordon, et al., *Transplanted bone marrow mononuclear cells and MSCs impart clinical benefit to children with osteogenesis imperfecta through different mechanisms.* Blood, 2012.

[106] Ogawa, M., A.C. LaRue, and C.J. Drake, *Hematopoietic origin of fibroblasts/myofibroblasts: Its pathophysiologic implications.* Blood, 2006. 108(9): p. 2893-6.

[107] Ogawa, M., A.C. Larue, et al., *Hematopoietic stem cell origin of connective tissues.* Experimental hematology, 2010. 38(7): p. 540-7.

[108] Ogawa, M., A.C. Larue, et al., *Hematopoietic stem cell origin of mesenchymal cells: opportunity for novel therapeutic approaches.* International journal of hematology, 2010. 91(3): p. 353-9.

[109] Ebihara, Y., M. Masuya, et al., *Hematopoietic origins of fibroblasts: II. In vitro studies of fibroblasts, CFU-F, and fibrocytes.* Exp Hematol, 2006. 34(2): p. 219-29.

[110] LaRue, A.C., M. Masuya, et al., *Hematopoietic origins of fibroblasts: I. In vivo studies of fibroblasts associated with solid tumors.* Exp Hematol, 2006. 34(2): p. 208-18.

[111] Masuya, M., C.J. Drake, et al., *Hematopoietic origin of glomerular mesangial cells.* Blood, 2003. 101(6): p. 2215-8.

[112] Hess, D.C., T. Abe, et al., *Hematopoietic origin of microglial and perivascular cells in brain.* Exp Neurol, 2004. 186(2): p. 134-44.

[113] Visconti, R.P., Y. Ebihara, et al., *An in vivo analysis of hematopoietic stem cell potential: hematopoietic origin of cardiac valve interstitial cells.* Circ Res, 2006. 98(5): p. 690-6.

[114] Lang, H., Y. Ebihara, et al., *Contribution of bone marrow hematopoietic stem cells to adult mouse inner ear: mesenchymal cells and fibrocytes.* J Comp Neurol, 2006. 496(2): p. 187-201.

[115] Grant, M.B., W.S. May, et al., *Adult hematopoietic stem cells provide functional hemangioblast activity during retinal neovascularization.* Nat Med, 2002. 8(6): p. 607-12.

[116] Krause, D.S., N.D. Theise, et al., *Multi-organ, multi-lineage engraftment by a single bone marrow-derived stem cell.* Cell, 2001. 105(3): p. 369-77.

[117] Sera, Y., A.C. LaRue, et al., *Hematopoietic stem cell origin of adipocytes.* Exp Hematol, 2009. 37(9): p. 1108-20, 1120 e1-4.

[118] Mehrotra, M., C.R. Williams, et al., *Hematopoietic stem cells give rise to osteo-chondrogenic cells.* Blood Cells, Molecules & Diseases, 2012. *in press.*

[119] Mehrotra, M., M. Rosol, et al., *Amelioration of a mouse model of osteogenesis imperfecta with hematopoietic stem cell transplantation: microcomputed tomography studies.* Exp Hematol, 2010. 38(7): p. 593-602.

[120] Okabe, M., M. Ikawa, et al., *'Green mice' as a source of ubiquitous green cells.* FEBS Lett, 1997. 407(3): p. 313-9.

[121] Horwitz, E.M., D.J. Prockop, et al., *Transplantability and therapeutic effects of bone marrow-derived mesenchymal cells in children with osteogenesis imperfecta.* Nat Med, 1999. 5(3): p. 309-13.

[122] Horwitz, E.M., D.J. Prockop, et al., *Clinical responses to bone marrow transplantation in children with severe osteogenesis imperfecta.* Blood, 2001. 97(5): p. 1227-31.

[123] Horwitz, E.M., P.L. Gordon, et al., *Isolated allogeneic bone marrow-derived mesenchymal cells engraft and stimulate growth in children with osteogenesis imperfecta: Implications for cell therapy of bone.* Proc Natl Acad Sci U S A, 2002. 99(13): p. 8932-7.

[124] Le Blanc, K., C. Gotherstrom, et al., *Fetal mesenchymal stem-cell engraftment in bone after in utero transplantation in a patient with severe osteogenesis imperfecta.* Transplantation, 2005. 79(11): p. 1607-14.

[125] Dazzi, F. and N.J. Horwood, *Potential of mesenchymal stem cell therapy.* Curr Opin Oncol, 2007. 19(6): p. 650-5.

[126] Sugimoto, H., T.M. Mundel, et al., *Bone-marrow-derived stem cells repair basement membrane collagen defects and reverse genetic kidney disease.* Proc Natl Acad Sci U S A, 2006. 103(19): p. 7321-6.

[127] Prodromidi, E.I., R. Poulsom, et al., *Bone marrow-derived cells contribute to podocyte regeneration and amelioration of renal disease in a mouse model of Alport syndrome.* Stem Cells, 2006. 24(11): p. 2448-55.

[128] Tolar, J., A. Ishida-Yamamoto, et al., *Amelioration of epidermolysis bullosa by transfer of wild-type bone marrow cells.* Blood, 2009. 113(5): p. 1167-74.

Chapter 3

Genetic Determinants of Heart Rate Variation and Cardiovascular Diseases

Vyacheslav A. Korshunov, Igor A. Dyachenko and
Arkady N. Murashev

Additional information is available at the end of the chapter

1. Introduction

Heart rate (HR) is a variable parameter that rapidly adjusts to changing hemodynamic demands (Fig. 1). HR is determined by several mechanisms. First, chronotropic regulation of the heart occurs through spontaneous and periodic depolarization of sino-atrial (SA) pacemaker cells. The activity of the SA node is modulated by the autonomic nervous system, intrinsic cardiac nervous system, baroreflexes, and respiration. Second, the sympathetic nervous system (SNS) stimulates postganglionic sympathetic nerve fibers and triggers norepinephrine release in the SA node that results in an increase in HR. Third, the parasympathetic nervous system (PNS) also plays a significant role in regulation of HR. Parasympathetic vagal nerve endings release acetylcholine, which binds to muscarinic cholinergic receptors on pacemaker cells, causing opening of potassium channels, hyperpolarization of the membrane, and, consequently, a decrease in HR. Fourth, humoral and mechanical signals have an effect on HR and its variability. Mechanoreceptors in the atrium respond to stretch (occurs during respiration) and change HR without neural input [1]. Changes in blood pressure (BP) impact HR via baroreceptor reflexes. In response to high BP, stretch-sensitive receptors in the carotid sinus and aortic arch send action potentials via the vagus and glossopharyngeal nerves to the solitary tract nucleus (NTS) of the brainstem. The NTS affects the ventrolateral medulla is causing an inhibition of sympathetic drive and activates the PNS by triggering the nucleus ambiguous. The result is a decrease in HR and BP. In response to hypotension, the baroreceptor reflex works in the opposite direction, leading to an increase in sympathetic drive and decrease in vagal tone, which raises HR and BP. Mechanical signals also lead to respiratory sinus arrhythmia – increased in HR during inhalation and decreased HR during exhalation. This normal physiologic phenomenon involves an increase in intrathoracic volume during inspiration that results in an increase in HR by activation of SNS and a decrease in parasympathetic tone. The integrated spectral power of high frequency (HF, >0.15Hz) HR variability (HRV) is used as an index of the level of parasympathetic activity. Low frequency (LF, 0.04–0.15Hz) power of HRV reflects both sympathetic and parasympathetic activity and the LF/HF ratio is an indicator of sympatho-vagal balance [2]. Body temperature plays a relatively minor role in HRV. It has been shown that hypothermia is associated with bradycardia (decrease in HR) and fever associates with tachycardia (increase in HR) in neonates [3]. However, the contribution of baseline HR to HRV is relatively small. Very low and ultra low frequency ranges of HRV indicate alterations in body temperature.

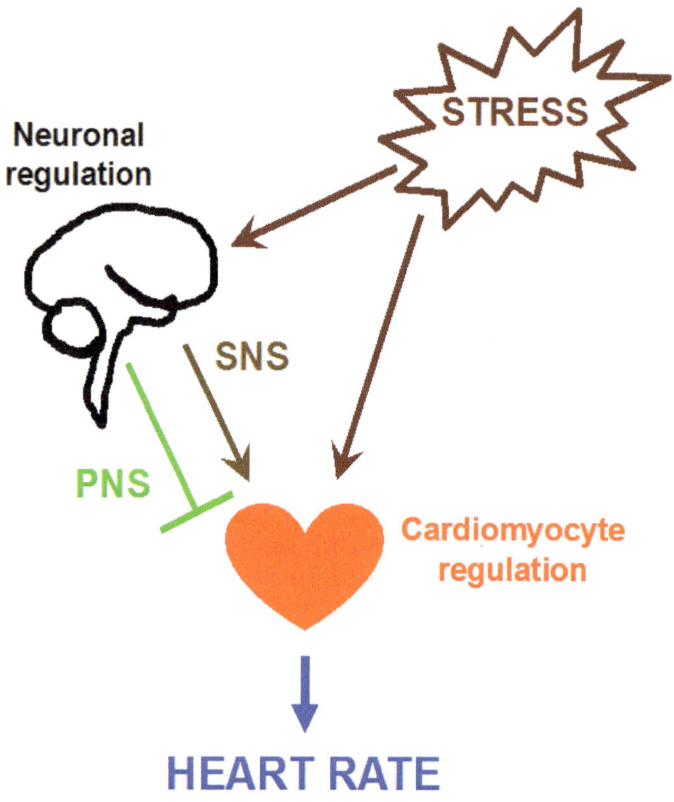

Figure 1. A scheme that shows regulation of heart rate. Heart rate (blue color) is determined by there major components. First, cardiomyocyte regulation (red color) is driven by depolarization of pacemaker cells. Second, neuronal regulation (black color) includes two components: sympathetic nervous system (SNS; brown color) and parasympathetic nervous system (PNS; green color). Third, stress factors (dark red color) are important for modulation of the heart rate. Please, see text for details.

Increased HR has been shown as a predictor of cardiovascular mortality in healthy people, myocardial infarction (MI) and heart failure patients [4]. The increased mortality observed with an increased HR may be a consequence of the SNS/PSN imbalance that can be characterized by SNS predominance, vagal depression, or the combined impact of this dysregulation of cardiovascular function [5]. Elevated HR increases short-term cardiac output and myocardial oxygen consumption, while simultaneously reducing time of diastole and myocardial blood supply that leads to development of myocardial ischemia and arrhythmias [6]. Analysis of HRV data has provided clinically useful information about the status of the cardiovascular system. For example, *Fourier* spectral analysis of HR data has shown that frequency profiles of HRV are altered in hypovolaemia, heart failure, hypertension, coronary artery disease, angina and MI [7-12]. Acute brain injury has been linked to decreased HRV as well [13]. Chronic pathological conditions like diabetes, hyperglycemia, hyperlipidemia, obesity, and kidney failure are shown to lead to autonomic dysregulation of HR and usually associates with low HRV values [14]. Inoue and colleagues [15] showed that for every 10 beats per minute (beats/min) increase in HR, the odds ratio of an increase in white blood cells is approximately 1.3 in both men and women. These findings indicate that resting HR is clinically important for chronic inflammation and future cardiovascular events. Numerous studies have demonstrated a strong association between decreased HRV and sepsis [16, 17]. HRV is also altered in psychiatric disorders like depression [18]. In some of these conditions abnormal HRV appears to be linked to an over-activation of the SNS and hypothalamic-pituitary-adrenal axis [19].

Given the complexity of HR regulation it is difficult to understand pathological mechanisms that alter HR. As shown in other complex traits, genetic factors play an important role in HR and HRV in humans. For example, Singh et al. [20] reported that heritability might explain a substantial proportion of the variance in HR and HRV based on twin study. Here, we summarize the current facts on the genetic mechanisms of HR regulation and discuss the potential impact of HR genes on progression of cardiovascular diseases.

2. Body

2.1. Genetics of HR trait in humans

The majority of clinical studies have focused on electrophysiological abnormalities in the heart (e.g., long QT syndrome) because of their importance in sudden death [21]. However, we still have an incomplete view on the genetic contribution to resting HR variation. For the past decade genetic studies in humans revealed a number of genomic loci that control HR variation (Table 1). A first linkage analysis for resting HR was performed in 962 Caucasians and 1,124 African-Americans in the Hypertension Genetic Epidemiology Network (HyperGEN) cohort [22]. A major locus was detected on chromosome 4 (195.06cM) with logarithm of odds ratio (LOD) score of 3.18 for both racial groups. This study also indicated that chromosome 10 may harbor a locus that contributes to HR [22]. Martin et al [23] investigated a population that contained 2,209 normotensive and hypertensive individuals. The authors reported ~26% heritability and found a significant locus on human chromosome 4 (128Mb; LOD=3.9). Ankyrin-B (ANK2) and myozenin 2 (MYOZ2) were proposed as candidate genes for variation in resting HR. ANK2 promotes targeting of ion channels to the membranes in cells. MYOZ2 may play a significant role in cardiac activity via excitation-contraction coupling. Thus, MYOZ2 may indirectly influence calcium signaling and pacemaker function in the heart. In a larger study of 3,282 Caucasian and African-American populations (Family Blood Pressure Program) two loci were found [24]. A significant locus on chromosome 10 (142.78cM; LOD=4.6) was linked to HR in the Caucasian group of HyperGEN. However, a common region on chromosome 5p13-14 (LOD=1.9) influenced HR in both races [24]. Genome-wide linkage for HR showed a peak on chromosome 18 (77cM; LOD = 2.03) in 73 Mongolian families [25]. Two genes SLC14A2 (solute carrier family 14 urea transporter) and LIPG (endothelial lipase precursor) are likely candidates in the chromosome 18 locus. The second peak (LOD=1.52) was identified on chromosome 5 (216cM). These findings further support the importance of the genes on human chromosome 5 for HR regulation (Table 1). The identified genomic region contains NSD1 (nuclear receptor SET domain-containing gene 1) gene that enhances transactivation of the androgen receptor. This region also contains F12 (coagulation factor XII) gene and is associated with cardiac risks [25]. The analyses of HR (measured as the RR interval) in 2,325 individuals from three isolated European populations revealed a significant locus on chromosome 12 [26]. In particular, two intronic single nucleotide polymorphisms (SNPs) (rs885389 and rs1725789) were located in a G-protein–coupled receptor 133 (GPR133) gene on chromosome 12 that exceeded the threshold of genome-wide significance ($P=3.9x10^{-8}$ and $1.5x10^{-7}$, respectively). For rs885389, each risk allele brings a decrease in 14ms in the length of the RR interval, and for rs1725789 – decrease in 16ms [26]. A significant quantitative trait locus (QTL) for HR (chromosome 9p21; LOD=4.8) was reported in the Strong Heart Family Study [27]. The linkage analyses were performed for HR, which was measured by electrocardiogram and echocardiograph Doppler recording in this population. Six significant SNPs were identified (rs7875153, rs7848524, rs4446809, rs10964759, rs1125488 and rs7853123) and the rs7875153 provided the strongest evidence for association and is located within a hypothetical protein with an undefined function (KIAA1797). However, KIAA1797 interacts with vinculin (VCL), which is involved in development of dilated cardiomypathy. Several genome-wide linkage studies assessed the involvement of the genetic factors in exercise HR response to training [28, 29]. In particular, the HERITAGE Family Study identified several genetic loci in 99 white and 127 black families [28]. Interestingly, there were differences in genetic loci between two races for baseline resting HR: for white families – chromosomes 4 and 11, for black – 2, 6, 7, 12, 14 and 15. For training HR response the following loci were identified: for white families – chromosomes 1 and 21, while loci on chromosomes 3, 20 and 21 were found in black families [28]. A follow up analysis of this cohort identified two SNPs that are located in the 5'-region of the cAMP-responsive element-binding protein 1 (CREB1) gene on chromosome 2 [29]. Most recently, the same group reported SNPs in nine genes (including CREB1) that explain heritability of training HR in the related to HERITAGE Family Study [30]. The proposed candidate genes might regulate cardiomyocyte and neuronal cell functions, as well as cardiac memory formation, fully accounting for the heritability of the submaximal HR training response.

Chromosome	Study	Reference
2	HERITAGE Family Study	An et al, 2006 Rankinen et al, 2010 Rankinen et al, 2012
4	Hypertension Genetic Epidemiology Network (HyperGEN) Metabolic Risk Complications of Genes Obesity Project HERITAGE Family Study	Wilk et al, 2002 Martin et al, 2004 An et al, 2006
5	Family Blood Pressure Program	Laramie et al, 2006
6	HERITAGE Family Study meta-analysis of 15 GWA studies	An et al, 2006 Eijgelsheim et al, 2010
7	HERITAGE Family Study meta-analysis of 15 GWA studies	An et al, 2006 Eijgelsheim et al, 2010
9	Strong Heart Family Study in American Indians	Melton et al, 2010
10	Hypertension Genetic Epidemiology Network (HyperGEN) Family Blood Pressure Program	Wilk et al, 2002 Laramie et al, 2006
11	HERITAGE Family Study meta-analysis of 15 GWA studies	An et al, 2006 Eijgelsheim et al, 2010
12	HERITAGE Family Study 3 isolated European populations meta-analysis of 15 GWA studies	An et al, 2006 Marroni et al, 2009 Eijgelsheim et al, 2010
14	HERITAGE Family Study meta-analysis of 15 GWA studies	An et al, 2006 Eijgelsheim et al, 2010
15	HERITAGE Family Study	An et al, 2006
18	Mongolian Family Study	Gombojav et al, 2008

Table 1. Heart rate controlling genetic loci in humans

Genome-wide association (GWA) studies became a powerful approach to identify common variants associated with cardiovascular diseases. A recent meta-analysis of 15 GWA studies for HR variation included 38,991 subjects of European ancestry [31]. Authors used an adjusted RR interval for association analyses in approximately 2.5 million genomic markers. Six novel associations with resting HR were found: 6q22; 14q12; 12p12; 6q22; 7q22; and 11q12. Locus 6q22 is near a gap junction protein, alpha 1 (GJA1) gene that encodes connexin-43 protein and is crucial in electrical coupling of the myocytes. Mutations in GJA1 cause an inherited hypoplastic left heart syndrome. The second locus on 6q22 is located near SLC35F1 that encodes hospholamban. The 14q12 locus is near myosin heavy chain-6 protein (MYH6), which is related to hypertrophic cardiomyopathy, atrial-septal defects and dilated cardiomyopathy. The locus on chromosome 12p12 includes several genes (SOX5, c12orf67, BCAT1,

LRMP and CASC1) without any pathophysiological association with cardiac diseases. In the 7q22 locus a candidate gene, SLC12A9, encodes a cation-chloride co-transporter-interacting protein was found. Finally, the 11q12 locus is near FADS1 (arachidonyl-CoA) gene, which has been shown to release Ca^{2+} from the sarcoplasmic reticulum. Previously published associations were confirmed for GJA1, MYH6 and CD34. These variants explain approximately 0.7% of RR interval variance. Only 1.6% of resting HR variance can be explained by 20 polymorphisms in this study [31]. The latter suggest a substantial polygenic nature of the resting HR trait. Despite great progress in our understanding of the genetics of HR variation we have a limited knowledge of the genetic causes.

2.2. Genetic studies of HR trait in rodents

Utilization of laboratory animals has been successful in uncovering genetic causes of cardiovascular diseases. One of the major advantages of animal studies is that they have minimal environmental and methodological effects as compared to human studies. Historically, genetic crosses between two inbred lines with a robust cardiovascular variation are widely used to identify QTLs in rodents (Table 2). Studies in rats have been aimed at understanding the genetics of BP variation by using spontaneously hypertensive rats (SHR), stroke-prone spontaneously hypertensive rats (SHRSP) and Dahl rats (salt-sensitive hypertension). However, several genetic crosses uncovered QTLs that control HR trait independently from BP (Table 2). For example, HR variation after 12 days of salt-load was tested in the cross between SHRSP and Wistar-Kyoto rats (WKY), and identified a significant locus (LOD=5.9) on rat chromosome 3 [32]. In the center of the locus is SNC2α1 gene that encodes a brain isoform of α1 polypeptide of the type 2 voltage-gated sodium channel. In a cross between SHR and normotensive Brown-Norway (BN) rats a significant locus that controls elevated HR was found on rat chromosome 8 (6.8cM; LOD= 8.7) [33]. This segment of rat chromosome 8 harbors over 200 genes. The more likely candidates for HR are subtypes of nicotinic acetylcholine receptor α3 (CHRNA3), α5 (CHRNA5), and β (CHRNB4); hyperpolarization-activated channel (HCN4); 5-hydroxytryptamine (serotonin) receptor 3A (HTR3A) and 3B (HTR3B); and sodium channel (SCN2). Studies on congenic strains with varying segments of chromosome 2 between SHR and WKY rats identified a new HR locus [34]. Another congenic strain of chromosome 10 from Dahl rat revealed increased HR and short QT interval loci [35]. Authors found that overexpression of a candidate gene, rififylin (RFFL), increased cardiomyocyte beating in congenic rats. In addition to resting HR, one genetic study examined a stress-related HR variation in WKY and SHR cross progeny with 23 recombinant inbred rat strains (HXB-BXH) [36]. Specifically, genetic loci that are involved in HR responses to stress (an airpuff startle test) are located on rat chromosomes 1, 2 and 10. BN allele on rat chromosome 2 (D2Rat62-D2Rat247, LOD=2.9) enhanced the bradycardia in early response to the stress. Two significant QTLs for tachycardia responses were identified on rat chromosome 1 (D1Rat287-D1Rat292, LOD=3.1) and chromosome 10 (D10Rat26- D10Rat267, LOD=2.4). Thus, seven loci were identified in hypertensive rat models that are specific to HR variation with minimal effect from BP.

Chromosome	Study	Reference
Rat		
1	WKY x SHR cross and 23 HXB-BXH strains	Jaworski et al, 2002
2	WKY x SHR cross and 23 HXB-BXH strains Congenic SHR	Jaworski et al, 2002 Alemayehu et al, 2002
3	SHRSP x WKY cross	Kreutz et al, 1997
8	BN x SHR	Silva et al, 2007
10	WKY x SHR cross and 23 HXB-BXH strains Congenic Dahl	Jaworski et al, 2002 Gopalakrishnan et al, 2011
Mouse		
1	BALB x CBA cross C57BL/6 x DBA/2 cross	Sugiyama et al, 2002 Blizard et al, 2009
2	BALB x CBA cross	Sugiyama et al, 2002
4	FVB/NJ x 129P2 sensitized mutants cross	Scicluna et al, 2011
5	30 Inbred strains and 29 AXB-BXA strains C57BL/6 x DBA/2 cross	Howden et al, 2008 Blizard et al, 2009
6	30 Inbred strains and 29 AXB-BXA strains	Howden et al, 2008
7	C3HeB x SJL cross, 30 Inbred strains and 28 AXB-BXA strains	Smolock et al, 2012
15	BALB x CBA cross C57BL/6 x DBA/2 cross	Sugiyama et al, 2002 Blizard et al, 2009

Table 2. Heart rate controlling genetic loci in rodents

Mouse studies identified HR genetic loci that independent of BP variation (Table 2). Three significant QTLs were identified on mouse chromosomes 1, 2, and 15 in the BALB/CJxCBA/J backcross [37]. The HR quantitative trait 1 (Hrq1) locus was found on mouse chromosome 2 (72cM; LOD=4.0) and Hrq2 on chromosome 15 (25cM; LOD=3.1). The chromosome 2 locus contains a cholinergic receptor, nicotinic, polypeptide alpha 1 (CHRNA1) gene. Two of the muscarinic receptors are also the Hrq1 locus, CHRM4 (cholinergic receptor, muscarinic 4) and CHRM5. The authors also found the Hrq3 locus on chromosome 1 that significantly interacts with the Hrq1 locus [37]. Electrocardiographic evaluation of 26 AXA/BXA recombinant mouse inbred strains and linkage analyses revealed HR and HRV loci [38]. The most significant QTL for HR was found on mouse chromosome 6 (54Mb, LOD=3.8). This locus contains several candidate genes associated with HR regulation, including corticotropin-releasing factor receptor 2 (CRHR2) and neuropeptide Y (NPY). This study also uncovered a HF-HRV locus that was identified on mouse chromosome 5 (54Mb, LOD=3.1). Candidate genes for HF-HRV included D5 dopamine receptor (DRD5), peroxisome proliferative-activated receptor-coactivator-1 (PCG1), and endothelial nitric oxide synthase (ENOS). Two significant QTLs were reported in a cross between C57BL/6J and DBA/2J strains [39]. In particular, a female-specific locus was found on mouse chromosome 1 (72cM, LOD=7.9) and gender-uniform locus on mouse chromosome 5 (54cM, LOD=8.5). A repeaded HR measurements showed a locus for HR on chromosome 15 (2cM, LOD=3.1). Importantly, two significant QTLs for HR were confirmed in BXD recombinant inbred strains. L-type calcium channel (CAV1.1) and regulator of G protein signaling (RGS2) are the two candidate genes within the HR locus [39]. A linkage analysis for HR variation in a sensitized mouse mutant (SCN5A-1798$^{insD/+}$) was studied in F2 progeny from the FVB/NJx129P2 cross [40]. Interval mapping found a HR locus on chromosome 4 (136-151Mb, LOD=4.2). Finally, we reported a highly significant QTL for elevated HR on chromosome 7 (41 cM, LOD = 6.7) in the C3HeB/FeJxSJL/J backcross [41]. We mapped this locus using a GWA analyses in the Hybrid Mouse Diversity Panel (HMDP) that included 30 inbred and 28 AXB/BXA recombinant inbred strains. We detected seventeen significant SNPs within a 0.9Mb interval on mouse chromosome 7. This locus contains a cluster of three gamma-Aminobutyric acid (GABA) A receptor subunit genes: GABRβ3, GABRα5, and GABRγ3. These receptor subunits are responsible for inhibitory effects of neurotransmitter $GABA_A$ in the brain. Taken together, animal studies yielded a similar number of the genetic loci as reported in humans for HR variation.

2.3. Challenges and future directions in the genetic studies on HR variation

Despite the progress in technology of the high throughput wide-genome screens in human populations, the methodological challenges are attributed to variability of HR. In addition, BP levels and/or responses to therapy may further limit our abilities to dissect the genetic basis of HR variation in humans. For example, retrospective analyses of several anti-hypertensive trials revealed potential methodological differences [42]. Specifically, clinical, ambulatory and home monitoring methods might introduce inter-individual variability that could complicate genetic analyses. One approach is to increase the number of the assessments of hemodynamics per individual. For example, repeated measurements have improved reproducibility between the measurements taken on the same day and between days in heart failure patients [43]. Therefore, more uniform methods of evaluation of HR trait should be considered in large genetic studies in humans. Animal experiments are proven as better-controlled genetic models for complex traits. However, there are similar genetic loci identified on the HR trait between human and animal studies (Tables 1-2). The latter suggests a clear need for more genetic experiments in animal models. GWA and traditional genetic approaches (genetic intercrossed and congenic lines) should improve mapping results. We recently combined two approaches and mapped a novel genetic locus on mouse chromosome 7 that contains three candidate genes [41]. Overview of the current candidate genes suggests involvement of three major components in HR regulation: 1) cardiomyocyte cell function; 2) neuronal cell functions; and, 3) stress-related pathways (Fig. 1). So far only a limited number of HR candidates were validated in genetically targeted animal models. In particular, mice heterozygous for ANK2 that phenocopy human sinus node dysfunction, displayed severe bradycardia and HRV [44]. Several mouse mutants were made to target a class of hyperpolarization-activated cyclic nucleotidegated (HCN) cation channels [45]. It was concluded that the HCN4, HCN1 and HCN2 subunits are important for generation of the pacemaker current in the SA cells [45]. RGS2 knockout mice exhibited autonomic abnormalities in regulation of hemodynamic parameters [46]. Authors found that RGS2 knockout mice had an increased sympathetic tone and exhibited baroreceptor-HR reflex resetting. In addition, two HR candidates were implicated in stress-dependent responses [47, 48]. First, studies in CRHR2 knockout mice suggest its involvement in stress-responses in the brain and periphery [47]. Second, mice that overexpressed NPY showed enhanced sympatho-adrenal activity and adaptive responses to various stresses [48]. Although gene targeting is widely used in mice, transgenic rats can be generated by zinc-finger nucleases [49]. A recent report showed successful generation of a renin knockout rat on the Dahl salt-sensitive background [50]. However, development of systems genetics approaches would dramatically elevate our understanding of the contribution of the each regulatory component of HR variation. We think that utilization of systems biology approaches will provide significantly more insights into HR variation [51]. Ultimately, validation of the HR candidate genes and pathways in animals will validate HR studies in humans. These research efforts may lead to personalized diagnostic and treatment strategies for cardiovascular patients.

3. Conclusions

HR is regulated by very complex mechanisms (Fig. 1). Abnormal HR is a strong predictor for cardiovascular diseases. However, pathophysiology of HR regulation is not well understood. It is also well established that genetic factors play an important role in HR variation. Genetic studies in humans identified over 20 loci that are linked to the HR trait. Despite the recent progress we can explain only a small portion of the genetic contribution to HR variation. Inter-individual variability in hemodynamic parameters remains one of the key challenges in large population studies. In fact, identification of the stress-related genes may suggest that the methods of evaluation of HR might affect the stress-response in humans. Genetic experiments in animals significantly reduce effects of the environmental/methodological factors. However, only a similar number of the HR loci were identified in rodents compared to humans (Tables 1-2). Overview of the candidates revealed that they contribute to the HR variation via three major mechanisms: cardiomyocyte, neuronal cell functions and stress-responses. In general, there is a lack of validation of both, human and animal studies. We think that generation of transgenic animal models of HR candidate genes should also be coupled with systems genetics approaches. Experimental studies will lead to translational applications for preventing cardiovascular diseases related to HR pathophysiology.

Acknowledgments

We would like to thank Dr. Elaine Smolock for critical reading of the manuscript. This study was supported in part by funds from University of Rochester, Russian Program "Scientific and scientific-pedagogical personnel of innovative Russia" for 2009-2013 GK №14.740.11.0923 and HL105623 (VAK).

Abbreviations

HR, heart rate

SA, sino-atrial (cells/node)

SNS, sympathetic nervous system

PNS, parasympathetic nervous system

BP, blood pressure

NTS, solitary tract nucleus

HF, high frequency

HRV, heart rate variation

LF, low frequency

MI, myocardial infarction

LOD, logarithm of odds ratio

SNP, single nucleotide polymorphism

QTL, quantitative trait locus

GWA, Genome-wide association

SHR, spontaneously hypertensive rats

SHRSP, stroke-prone spontaneously hypertensive rats

Dahl, salt-sensitive rats

WKY, Wistar-Kyoto rats

BN, Brown-Norway rats

HMDP, hybrid mouse diversity panel

Author details

Vyacheslav A. Korshunov[1*], Igor A. Dyachenko[2,3] and Arkady N. Murashev[2,3]

*Address all correspondence to: Slava_Korshunov@URMC.rochester.edu

1 Department of Medicine, Aab Cardiovascular Research Institute, University of Rochester School of Medicine and Dentistry, Rochester, NY, USA

2 Pushchino State Natural-Science Institute, Pushchino, Russia

3 Pushchino Branch, Shemyakin-Ovchinnikov Institute of Bioorganic Chemistry, Pushchino, Russia

References

[1] Saul JP, Berger RD, Albrecht P, Stein SP, Chen MH, Cohen RJ. Transfer function analysis of the circulation: Unique insights into cardiovascular regulation. *The American journal of physiology*. 1991;261:H1231-1245

[2] Togo F, Takahashi M. Heart rate variability in occupational health - a systematic review. *Industrial health*. 2009;47:589-602

[3] Fairchild KD, O'Shea TM. Heart rate characteristics: Physiomarkers for detection of late-onset neonatal sepsis. *Clinics in perinatology*. 2010;37:581-598

[4] Lanza GA, Fox K, Crea F. Heart rate: A risk factor for cardiac diseases and outcomes? Pathophysiology of cardiac diseases and the potential role of heart rate slowing. *Advances in cardiology*. 2006;43:1-16

[5] Lurje L, Wennerblom B, Tygesen H, Karlsson T, Hjalmarson A. Heart rate variability after acute myocardial infarction in patients treated with atenolol and metoprolol. *International journal of cardiology*. 1997;60:157-164

[6] Feldman D, Elton TS, Menachemi DM, Wexler RK. Heart rate control with adrenergic blockade: Clinical outcomes in cardiovascular medicine. *Vascular health and risk management*. 2010;6:387-397

[7] Triedman JK, Cohen RJ, Saul JP. Mild hypovolemic stress alters autonomic modulation of heart rate. *Hypertension*. 1993;21:236-247

[8] Pal GK, Pal P, Nanda N, Amudharaj D, Karthik S. Spectral analysis of heart rate variability (hrv) may predict the future development of essential hypertension. *Medical hypotheses*. 2009;72:183-185

[9] Maule S, Rabbia F, Perni V, Tosello F, Bisbocci D, Mulatero P, Veglio F. Prolonged qt interval and reduced heart rate variability in patients with uncomplicated essential hypertension. *Hypertension research*. 2008;31:2003-2010

[10] Bailon R, Serrano P, Laguna P. Influence of time-varying mean heart rate in coronary artery disease diagnostic performance of heart rate variability indices from exercise stress testing. *Journal of electrocardiology*. 2011;44:445-452

[11] Buccelletti E, Gilardi E, Scaini E, Galiuto L, Persiani R, Biondi A, Basile F, Silveri NG. Heart rate variability and myocardial infarction: Systematic literature review and metanalysis. *European review for medical and pharmacological sciences*. 2009;13:299-307

[12] Garan H. Heart rate variability in acute myocardial infarction. *Cardiology*. 2009;114:273-274

[13] Goldstein B, Toweill D, Lai S, Sonnenthal K, Kimberly B. Uncoupling of the autonomic and cardiovascular systems in acute brain injury. *The American journal of physiology*. 1998;275:R1287-1292

[14] Thayer JF, Sternberg E. Beyond heart rate variability: Vagal regulation of allostatic systems. *Annals of the New York Academy of Sciences*. 2006;1088:361-372

[15] Inoue T, Iseki K, Iseki C, Kinjo K. Elevated resting heart rate is associated with white blood cell count in middle- aged and elderly individuals without apparent cardiovascular disease. *Angiology*. 2012;67:541-546

[16] Ahmad S, Ramsay T, Huebsch L, Flanagan S, McDiarmid S, Batkin I, McIntyre L, Sundaresan SR, Maziak DE, Shamji FM, Hebert P, Fergusson D, Tinmouth A, Seely AJ. Continuous multi-parameter heart rate variability analysis heralds onset of sepsis in adults. *PloS one*. 2009;4:e6642

[17] Papaioannou VE, Dragoumanis C, Theodorou V, Gargaretas C, Pneumatikos I. Relation of heart rate variability to serum levels of c-reactive protein, interleukin 6, and 10 in patients with sepsis and septic shock. *Journal of critical care*. 2009;24:625 e621-627

[18] Brown AD, Barton DA, Lambert GW. Cardiovascular abnormalities in patients with major depressive disorder: Autonomic mechanisms and implications for treatment. *CNS drugs*. 2009;23:583-602

[19] Dunser MW, Hasibeder WR. Sympathetic overstimulation during critical illness: Adverse effects of adrenergic stress. *Journal of intensive care medicine*. 2009;24:293-316

[20] Singh JP, Larson MG, O'Donnell CJ, Tsuji H, Evans JC, Levy D. Heritability of heart rate variability: The framingham heart study. *Circulation*. 1999;99:2251-2254

[21] Chopra N, Knollmann BC. Genetics of sudden cardiac death syndromes. *Current opinion in cardiology*. 2011;26:196-203

[22] Wilk JB, Myers RH, Zhang Y, Lewis CE, Atwood L, Hopkins PN, Ellison RC. Evidence for a gene influencing heart rate on chromosome 4 among hypertensives. *Human genetics*. 2002;111:207-213

[23] Martin LJ, Comuzzie AG, Sonnenberg GE, Myklebust J, James R, Marks J, Blangero J, Kissebah AH. Major quantitative trait locus for resting heart rate maps to a region on chromosome 4. *Hypertension*. 2004;43:1146-1151

[24] Laramie JM, Wilk JB, Hunt SC, Ellison RC, Chakravarti A, Boerwinkle E, Myers RH. Evidence for a gene influencing heart rate on chromosome 5p13-14 in a meta-analysis

of genome-wide scans from the nhlbi family blood pressure program. *BMC medical genetics*. 2006;7:17

[25] Gombojav B, Park H, Kim JI, Ju YS, Sung J, Cho SI, Lee MK, Ohrr H, Radnaabazar J, Seo JS. Heritability and linkage study on heart rates in a mongolian population. *Experimental & molecular medicine*. 2008;40:558-564

[26] Marroni F, Pfeufer A, Aulchenko YS, Franklin CS, Isaacs A, Pichler I, Wild SH, Oostra BA, Wright AF, Campbell H, Witteman JC, Kaab S, Hicks AA, Gyllensten U, Rudan I, Meitinger T, Pattaro C, van Duijn CM, Wilson JF, Pramstaller PP. A genome-wide association scan of rr and qt interval duration in 3 european genetically isolated populations: The eurospan project. *Circulation. Cardiovascular genetics*. 2009;2:322-328

[27] Melton PE, Rutherford S, Voruganti VS, Goring HH, Laston S, Haack K, Comuzzie AG, Dyer TD, Johnson MP, Kent JW, Jr., Curran JE, Moses EK, Blangero J, Barac A, Lee ET, Best LG, Fabsitz RR, Devereux RB, Okin PM, Bella JN, Broeckel U, Howard BV, MacCluer JW, Cole SA, Almasy L. Bivariate genetic association of kiaa1797 with heart rate in american indians: The strong heart family study. *Human molecular genetics*. 2010;19:3662-3671

[28] An P, Rice T, Rankinen T, Leon AS, Skinner JS, Wilmore JH, Bouchard C, Rao DC. Genome-wide scan to identify quantitative trait loci for baseline resting heart rate and its response to endurance exercise training: The heritage family study. *International journal of sports medicine*. 2006;27:31-36

[29] Rankinen T, Argyropoulos G, Rice T, Rao DC, Bouchard C. Creb1 is a strong genetic predictor of the variation in exercise heart rate response to regular exercise: The heritage family study. *Circulation. Cardiovascular genetics*. 2010;3:294-299

[30] Rankinen T, Sung YJ, Sarzynski MA, Rice TK, Rao DC, Bouchard C. Heritability of submaximal exercise heart rate response to exercise training is accounted for by nine snps. *J Appl Physiol*. 2012;112:892-897

[31] Eijgelsheim M, Newton-Cheh C, Sotoodehnia N, de Bakker PI, Muller M, Morrison AC, Smith AV, Isaacs A, Sanna S, Dorr M, Navarro P, Fuchsberger C, Nolte IM, de Geus EJ, Estrada K, Hwang SJ, Bis JC, Ruckert IM, Alonso A, Launer LJ, Hottenga JJ, Rivadeneira F, Noseworthy PA, Rice KM, Perz S, Arking DE, Spector TD, Kors JA, Aulchenko YS, Tarasov KV, Homuth G, Wild SH, Marroni F, Gieger C, Licht CM, Prineas RJ, Hofman A, Rotter JI, Hicks AA, Ernst F, Najjar SS, Wright AF, Peters A, Fox ER, Oostra BA, Kroemer HK, Couper D, Volzke H, Campbell H, Meitinger T, Uda M, Witteman JC, Psaty BM, Wichmann HE, Harris TB, Kaab S, Siscovick DS, Jamshidi Y, Uitterlinden AG, Folsom AR, Larson MG, Wilson JF, Penninx BW, Snieder H, Pramstaller PP, van Duijn CM, Lakatta EG, Felix SB, Gudnason V, Pfeufer A, Heckbert SR, Stricker BH, Boerwinkle E, O'Donnell CJ. Genome-wide association analysis identifies multiple loci related to resting heart rate. *Human molecular genetics*. 2010;19:3885-3894

[32] Kreutz R, Struk B, Stock P, Hubner N, Ganten D, Lindpaintner K. Evidence for primary genetic determination of heart rate regulation: Chromosomal mapping of a genetic locus in the rat. *Circulation*. 1997;96:1078-1081

[33] Silva GJ, Pereira AC, Krieger EM, Krieger JE. Genetic mapping of a new heart rate qtl on chromosome 8 of spontaneously hypertensive rats. *BMC medical genetics*. 2007;8:17

[34] Alemayehu A, Breen L, Krenova D, Printz MP. Reciprocal rat chromosome 2 congenic strains reveal contrasting blood pressure and heart rate qtl. *Physiological genomics*. 2002;10:199-210

[35] Gopalakrishnan K, Morgan EE, Yerga-Woolwine S, Farms P, Kumarasamy S, Kalinoski A, Liu X, Wu J, Liu L, Joe B. Augmented rififylin is a risk factor linked to aberrant cardiomyocyte function, short-qt interval and hypertension. *Hypertension*. 2011;57:764-771

[36] Jaworski RL, Jirout M, Closson S, Breen L, Flodman PL, Spence MA, Kren V, Krenova D, Pravenec M, Printz MP. Heart rate and blood pressure quantitative trait loci for the airpuff startle reaction. *Hypertension*. 2002;39:348-352

[37] Sugiyama F, Churchill GA, Li R, Libby LJ, Carver T, Yagami K, John SW, Paigen B. Qtl associated with blood pressure, heart rate, and heart weight in cba/caj and balb/cj mice. *Physiological genomics*. 2002;10:5-12

[38] Howden R, Liu E, Miller-DeGraff L, Keener HL, Walker C, Clark JA, Myers PH, Rouse DC, Wiltshire T, Kleeberger SR. The genetic contribution to heart rate and heart rate variability in quiescent mice. *American journal of physiology. Heart and circulatory physiology*. 2008;295:H59-68

[39] Blizard DA, Lionikas A, Vandenbergh DJ, Vasilopoulos T, Gerhard GS, Griffith JW, Klein LC, Stout JT, Mack HA, Lakoski JM, Larsson L, Spicer JM, Vogler GP, McClearn GE. Blood pressure and heart rate qtl in mice of the b6/d2 lineage: Sex differences and environmental influences. *Physiological genomics*. 2009;36:158-166

[40] Scicluna BP, Tanck MW, Remme CA, Beekman L, Coronel R, Wilde AA, Bezzina CR. Quantitative trait loci for electrocardiographic parameters and arrhythmia in the mouse. *Journal of molecular and cellular cardiology*. 2011;50:380-389

[41] Smolock EM, Ilyushkina IA, Ghazalpour A, Gerloff J, Murashev AN, Lusis AJ, Korshunov VA. A genetic locus on mouse chromosome 7 controls elevated heart rate. *Physiological genomics*. 2012;44:689-698

[42] Krakoff LR. Fluctuation: Does blood pressure variability matter? *Circulation*. 2012;126:525-527

[43] Greenberg BH, Hermann DD, Pranulis MF, Lazio L, Cloutier D. Reproducibility of impedance cardiography hemodynamic measures in clinically stable heart failure patients. *Congest Heart Fail*. 2000;6:74-80

[44] Le Scouarnec S, Bhasin N, Vieyres C, Hund TJ, Cunha SR, Koval O, Marionneau C, Chen B, Wu Y, Demolombe S, Song LS, Le Marec H, Probst V, Schott JJ, Anderson

ME, Mohler PJ. Dysfunction in ankyrin-b-dependent ion channel and transporter targeting causes human sinus node disease. *Proceedings of the National Academy of Sciences of the United States of America*. 2008;105:15617-15622

[45] Herrmann S, Hofmann F, Stieber J, Ludwig A. Hcn channels in the heart: Lessons from mouse mutants. *British journal of pharmacology*. 2012;166:501-509

[46] Gross V, Tank J, Obst M, Plehm R, Blumer KJ, Diedrich A, Jordan J, Luft FC. Autonomic nervous system and blood pressure regulation in rgs2-deficient mice. *American journal of physiology. Regulatory, integrative and comparative physiology*. 2005;288:R1134-1142

[47] Coste SC, Kesterson RA, Heldwein KA, Stevens SL, Heard AD, Hollis JH, Murray SE, Hill JK, Pantely GA, Hohimer AR, Hatton DC, Phillips TJ, Finn DA, Low MJ, Rittenberg MB, Stenzel P, Stenzel-Poore MP. Abnormal adaptations to stress and impaired cardiovascular function in mice lacking corticotropin-releasing hormone receptor-2. *Nature genetics*. 2000;24:403-409

[48] Ruohonen ST, Savontaus E, Rinne P, Rosmaninho-Salgado J, Cavadas C, Ruskoaho H, Koulu M, Pesonen U. Stress-induced hypertension and increased sympathetic activity in mice overexpressing neuropeptide y in noradrenergic neurons. *Neuroendocrinology*. 2009;89:351-360

[49] Geurts AM, Cost GJ, Freyvert Y, Zeitler B, Miller JC, Choi VM, Jenkins SS, Wood A, Cui X, Meng X, Vincent A, Lam S, Michalkiewicz M, Schilling R, Foeckler J, Kalloway S, Weiler H, Menoret S, Anegon I, Davis GD, Zhang L, Rebar EJ, Gregory PD, Urnov FD, Jacob HJ, Buelow R. Knockout rats via embryo microinjection of zinc-finger nucleases. *Science*. 2009;325:433

[50] Moreno C, Hoffman M, Stodola TJ, Didier DN, Lazar J, Geurts AM, North PE, Jacob HJ, Greene AS. Creation and characterization of a renin knockout rat. *Hypertension*. 2011;57:614-619

[51] Ghazalpour A, Rau CD, Farber CR, Bennett BJ, Orozco LD, van Nas A, Pan C, Allayee H, Beaven SW, Civelek M, Davis RC, Drake TA, Friedman RA, Furlotte N, Hui ST, Jentsch JD, Kostem E, Kang HM, Kang EY, Joo JW, Korshunov VA, Laughlin RE, Martin LJ, Ohmen JD, Parks BW, Pellegrini M, Reue K, Smith DJ, Tetradis S, Wang J, Wang Y, Weiss JN, Kirchgessner T, Gargalovic PS, Eskin E, Lusis AJ, Leboeuf RC. Hybrid mouse diversity panel: A panel of inbred mouse strains suitable for analysis of complex genetic traits. *Mammalian genome*. 2012; 23:680-92

Chapter 4

Hutchinson-Gilford Progeria Syndrome

Jean-Ha Baek, Tomás McKenna and Maria Eriksson

Additional information is available at the end of the chapter

1. Introduction

Hutchinson-Gilford Progeria Syndrome (HGPS) is a lethal congenital disorder, characterised by premature appearance of accelerated ageing in children. Although HGPS was first described by Jonathan Hutchinson [1] and then by Hastings Gilford [2] more than a century ago, it was not until 2003 that the genetic basis of HGPS was uncovered [3, 4]. Approximately 90% of HGPS patients have an identical mutation in paternal allele of the *LMNA* gene – a substitution of cytosine to thymine at nucleotide 1824, c.1824C>T. Although apparently a silent mutation (that is, no change in the amino acid, G608G), it causes aberrant mRNA splicing, which leads to the production of a truncated and partially processed pre-lamin A protein called "progerin" [3, 4]. Accumulation of progerin is thought to underlie the pathophysiology of HGPS. Individuals with HGPS appear to show ageing-related phenotypes at a much faster rate than normal, consequently leaving young children with the appearance and health conditions of an aged individual. The reported incidence of HGPS is 1 in 4 to 8 million newborns and 89 patients are currently known to be alive with HGPS worldwide [5]. The observed male to female ratio of incidence of HGPS is 1.2:1 and there has been no report on ethnic-specific recurrence. HGPS affect diverse body systems including growth, skeleton, body fat, skin, hair, and cardiovascular system. However, patients show no defects in their mental and intellectual abilities [6-8]. Surprisingly, progerin has also been found in normal unaffected individuals and its level increases with age, suggesting a similar genetic mechanism in progeria as in normal physiological ageing. Thus, numerous animal models have been developed to better understand the mechanism(s) of HGPS and to develop cure for this devastating disease.

In this chapter, the main aspects of HGPS such as signs and symptoms, genetic basis, animal models, and treatments will be discussed.

2. Signs and symptoms

The median age at diagnosis of HGPS is 2.9 years [6]. The diagnosis is generally straightforward as affected patients show classical symptoms and strongly resembles one another. The affected individuals display no signs of disease at birth, but within their first years of life they gradually develop an appearance often referred to as aged-like [9, 10]. Some of the typical physical characteristics of HGPS include alopecia (loss of hair including scalp and eyebrows), prominent scalp veins and forehead, classical facial features including frontal bossing, protruding ears with absent lobes, a glyphic (broad, mildly concave nasal ridge) nose, prominent eyes, thin lips and micrognathia (small jaw) with a vertical midline groove in the chin [7, 11, 12] (Figure 1). Abnormal and delayed dentition is also common, and thin and often tight skin results from significant loss of subcutaneous fat [7, 10] (Figure 1). HGPS patients have high-pitched voices, a horse-riding stance, limited joint mobility and have short stature (median final height of 100-110 cm; median final weight of 10-15 kg). As they mature, they develop osteolysis, particularly involving the distal phalanges and clavicles [6-8, 11, 13]. On average, death occurs at the age of 13, with at least 90% of HGPS subjects dying from progressive atherosclerosis of the coronary and cerebrovascular arteries [7].

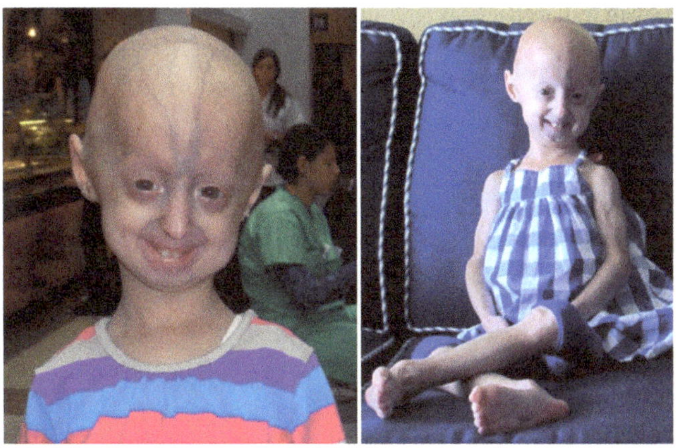

Figure 1. Photographs of a 7 year-old girl with HGPS (*LMNA* c.1824C>T, p.G608G). This patient has typical phenotypes, including alopecia, thin and tight skin, loss of subcutaneous fat, prominent scalp veins and forehead, prominent eyes, protruding ears, thin lips, and small jaw. Photos were from courtesy of The Progeria Research Foundation.

Recently, Olive *et al.* reported similarities between many aspects of cardiovascular disease in HGPS patients and normal adult individuals with atherosclerosis and suggested that progerin may be a contributor to the risk of atherosclerosis in the general population [14]. HGPS patients exhibited features that are classically associated with the atherosclerosis of ageing, including presence of plaques in the coronary arteries, arterial lesions showing calcification, inflammation, and evidence of plaque erosion or rupture. Authors speculated that progerin accumulation in vascular cells causes nuclear defects and increases susceptibility to mechanical strain that in turn triggers cell death and inflammatory response, giving rise to atherosclerosis [14].

Interestingly, despite the presence of multiple premature ageing symptoms, many other organs, such as liver, kidney, lung, brain, gastrointestinal tract, and bone marrow, appear to be unaffected. Furthermore, not all of the ageing processes are advanced in affected children. For example, the prevalence of mental deterioration, cancer, and cataract, is not higher in HGPS patients [7]. To date, there are scarce explanations as to why only certain organs are affected in HGPS. Nevertheless, researchers have been trying to clarify some of these puzzling observations. Recently, Jung and colleagues suggested that the absence of cognitive deficits in HGPS patients may be explained by the down regulation of pre-lamin A expression in the brain [15]. Furthermore, authors hypothesised that low level of pre-lamin A in the brain may be regulated by a brain-specific microRNA (miRNA), miRNA-9. In support of the result from this study, Nissan *et al.* lately published a promising result showing that miRNA-9 inversely regulates lamin A and progerin expression in neural cells and proposed that protection of neural cells from toxic accumulation of progerin in HGPS may be due to expression of miRNA-9 [16]. Further studies, possibly using animal models, are required to investigate changes in the expression of miRNA-9 and its effects on the level of progerin in the brain.

The clinical features seen in HGPS strongly resemble several aspects of natural ageing. For this reason, HGPS has served as a useful model for deciphering some of the mechanisms underlying physiological ageing. The first evidence for changes of nuclear architecture during the normal ageing process came from work in *C. elegans* [17]. In this study, the authors demonstrated that nuclear defects accumulate during ageing and suggested that HGPS may be a result of increased rate of the normal ageing process [17]. Scaffidi and Misteli showed that cells from HGPS patients and normally aged individuals share several common nuclear defects [18]. In addition, a small amount of progerin protein was detected in protein extracts derived from elderly individuals which was absent in young samples [19]. Rodriguez *et al.* quantified the levels of progerin transcripts using real time quantitative RT-PCR and showed that the progerin transcript is present in unaffected old individuals, though at a very low level compared to HGPS patients, and this level increased with *in vitro* ageing, similarly to HGPS cells [20]. Recently, Olive and others have also reported that although the level of progerin is much higher in HGPS patients, progerin is also present in the coronary arteries of non-HGPS ageing individuals and significantly increases with advancing age [14]. On the whole, accumulation of progerin, which is formed sparsely over time as a result of the ageing process, appears to be a possible candidate and partially responsible for cellular senescence and genomic instability that is observed in ageing cells. In HGPS, this occurs at a substantially faster rate compared to normally-aged cells due to enhanced use of the cryptic splice donor site, producing higher level of progerin. The relationship between this disease of accelerating ageing and the onset of analogous symptoms during the lifespan of a normal individual is unclear. Nevertheless, the idea that progerin may play a role in general human ageing is supported by the numerous studies mentioned above.

3. Genetic basis

The *LMNA* gene is known to be a hotspot for disease-causing mutations and has gained much attention due to its association with a variety of human diseases. To date, more than 400 mutations spreading across the protein-coding region of the *LMNA* gene have been discovered (see review [21]). The *LMNA* gene is found at chromosome 1q21.2-q21.3 and is composed of 12 exons. Through alternative splicing, the *LMNA* gene encodes the A-type lamins, lamins A and C (lamin A, AΔ10, C, and C2), of which lamin A (encoded by exons 1-12) and lamin C (encoded by exons 1-10) are the major isoforms expressed in all differentiated cells in vertebrates [22, 23]. The B-type lamins, lamins B1 and B2, are another type of lamins, which are encoded by the *LMNB1* and *LMNB2* genes, respectively. The B-type lamins are found in all cells and are expressed during development. Lamin A, C, B1 and B2 are key structural components of the nuclear lamina, an intermediate filament structure that lies on the inner surface of the inner nuclear membrane and is responsible for maintaining structural stability and organising chromatin (see review [24]). The nuclear lamina determines the shape and size of the cell nucleus, and is involved in DNA replication and transcription. In addition, nuclear lamina has been shown to interact with several nuclear membrane-associated proteins, transcription factors, as well as heterochromatin itself. The nuclear lamina is required for most nuclear activities, such as chromatin organisation, DNA replication, cell cycle regulation, nuclear positioning within the cell, assembly/disassembly of the nucleus during cell division, as well as for modulating master regulatory genes and signalling pathways [25-27]. There are more than 10 different disorders that are caused by mutations in the *LMNA* gene and these disorders are collectively called laminopathies and include neuropathies, muscular dystrophies, cardiomyopathies, lipodystrophies, in addition to progeroid syndromes (see Chapter on Laminopathies).

The genetic basis for HGPS was unknown until it was found to be a single nucleotide mutation on the paternal allele with autosomal-dominant expression [3, 4]. Although numerous mutations have been reported to cause HGPS [4, 28-33], approximately 90% of cases are caused by a recurrent, dominant, *de novo* heterozygous silent amino acid substitution at c. 1824C>T, G608G (a change from glycine GGC to glycine GGT, referred to as G608G) of the *LMNA* gene [4] (Figure 2). This mutation is located in exon 11 of *LMNA* gene and results in increased activation of the cryptic splice donor site, splicing the *LMNA* gene at 5 nucleotides upstream of the mutation, leading to accumulation of aberrant mRNA transcript, missing 150 nucleotides from normal pre-lamin A. This mutated mRNA is then translated into a protein termed 'progerin', which is missing 50 amino-acid residues from its C-terminal region. It has been suggested that different mutations cause activation of the same cryptic splice site in exon 11 of *LMNA* gene, and disease severity is correlated with the usage of this splice site (Figure 2). For instance, Moulson and others described two patients with particularly severe progeroid symptoms, clearly more severe than a typical case of HGPS [30]. In both cases, the amount of progerin relative to properly processed pre-lamin A was significantly greater than that of in typical HGPS, suggesting that the severity of the disease appears to be dependent on the amount of progerin in cells [30]. Very recently, another more severe case was reported by Reunert *et al* [31]. This patient had the heterozygous *LMNA* mutation c.

1821G>A, which lead to neonatal progeria with death in the first year of life [31]. Authors showed that the ratio of progerin protein to mature lamin A was higher in this patient compared to classical HGPS and also proposed that this ratio determines the disease severity in progeria [31]. Opposite cases were also shown by Hisama and colleagues. In this study, mutations at the junction of exon 11 and intron 11 of the *LMNA* gene resulted in a considerably lower level of progerin compared to HGPS, giving rise to an adult-onset progeroid syndrome closely resembling Werner syndrome [33].

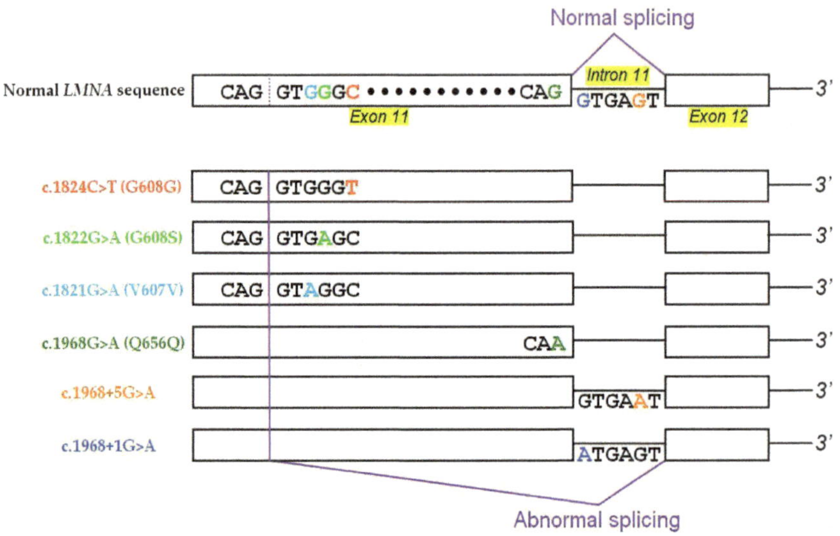

Figure 2. A schematic diagram showing point mutations leading to increased activation of a cryptic splice site within exon 11 of the *LMNA* gene [4, 30, 31, 33]. All of these mutations results in an internal deletion of 150 nucleotides of exon 11, ultimately leading to the production of an abnormally processed protein called 'progerin'. It is interesting to note that the normal *LMNA* sequence can also be spliced abnormally, removing 150 nucleotides of exon 11, in healthy individuals and this incidence may increase with age, leading to cellular senescence [18, 20].

Under the normal condition, mature lamin A protein is produced from a precursor, pre-lamin A, via a series of post-translational processing steps, which begins at the C-terminal end. The *CaaX* motif at the C-terminal tail (where the *C* is a cysteine, the *a* residues are aliphatic amino acids, and the *X* can be any amino acids) signals for 4 sequential modifications (Figure 3A). Firstly, the cysteine of the *CaaX* motif is farnesylated by a farnesyltransferase (FTase), then the last three amino acids (*aaX*) are cleaved by a zinc metalloprotease, ZMPSTE24 (mouse) or FACE-1 (human). Following this cleavage, farnesylated C-terminal cysteine is methylated by isoprenylcysteine carboxy-methyl transferase (ICMT). Finally, the last 15 amino acids of the protein are cleaved again by ZMPSTE24, producing mature lamin A.

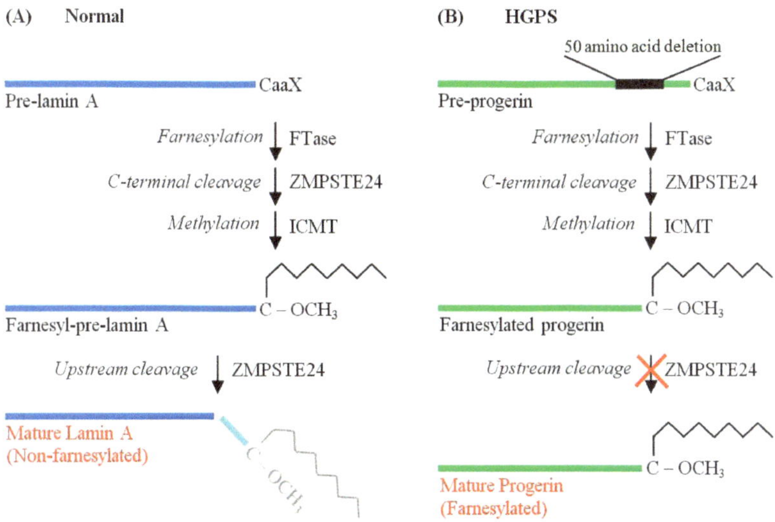

Figure 3. Post-translational processing of pre-lamin A in (A) normal condition and of truncated pre-lamin A ("pre-progerin") in (B) HGPS. The proteolytic cleavage site (RSYLLG motif) lies within the 50 amino acid region that is lost due to HGPS mutation, and as a result, the ZMPSTE24 endoprotease cannot recognise and perform subsequent upstream cleavage. Consequently, a truncated lamin A protein (that is, progerin) remains farnesylated, which is believed to have a dominant negative effect in HGPS.

In HGPS, the first 3 steps of post-translational maturation can be performed (that is, farnesylation, cleavage, and methylation), while the fourth processing step cannot be completed as the G608G mutation eliminates the second cleavage site recognised by ZMPSTE24 of pre-lamin A resulting a permanently farnesylated form of progerin (Figure 3B) [34]. This improperly processed protein in HGPS is thought to underlie the progression of the disease phenotype [35]. Because progerin, unlike mature lamin A, remains farnesylated, it gains a high affinity for the nuclear membrane, consequently causing a disruption in the integrity of the nuclear lamina. Indeed, HGPS patient cells show a number of abnormalities in nuclear structure and function. Upon indirect immunofluorescence labelling with antibodies directed against lamins A/C, fibroblasts from individuals with HGPS were characterised by the presence of dysmorphic nuclei with altered size and shape, presence of lobules, wrinkles, herniations of the nuclear envelope, thickening of the nuclear lamina, loss of peripheral heterochromatin, and clustering of nuclear pores [4, 36, 37]. These features worsen with passages in cell culture and are correlated with an apparent intranuclear accumulation of progerin (Figure 4) [36, 38]. In addition to permanent farnesylation of the progerin, it has been hypothesised that the deletion of the phosphorylation site (Ser 625) found in the 50 amino acid-deleted region may also account for some of the HGPS phenotypes as cell cycle dependent phosphorylation of lamin A is important for its normal function [4, 39].

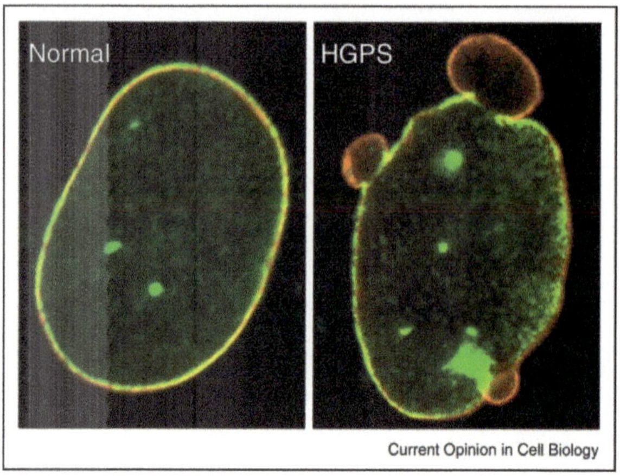

Figure 4. Immunostaining of skin fibroblasts taken from a normal individual (left) and a HGPS patient (right) showing nuclear blebbing. Lamin A/C is labelled red and lamin B1 in green. Note that the expression of lamin B1 is lost in the blebbed region. The figure has been adapted from Shimi *et al.* (2012) [40], with permission from Elsevier.

Numerous studies have addressed the senescent characteristics of HGPS cells, which intriguingly parallel with properties of fibroblasts from aged individuals. Cellular senescence is a hallmark characteristic of the ageing process, and cell nuclei from old individuals have similar defects to those of HGPS patient cells, including increased DNA damage [18, 41, 42], down-regulation of several nuclear proteins, such as the heterochromatin protein HP1 and the LAP2 group of lamin A-associated proteins [18, 37], and changes in histone modifications [18]. Heterochromatin becomes more disorganised with increased ageing in patients [43], and deregulation of chromatin organisation is a common phenomenon in HGPS, where progerin is known to alter histone methylation [44, 45]. Interestingly, the cryptic splice site that is constitutively activated in HGPS is seldom used in "normal" pre-lamin A processing in healthy aged individuals (Figure 2). To directly demonstrate that the production of progerin by sporadic use of the cryptic splice donor site in *LMNA* exon 11 is responsible for the observed changes in nuclear architecture in cells from aged individuals, Scaffidi and Mistelli used a morpholino oligonucleotide to inhibit this cryptic splice site and consequently the production of progerin and showed that the nuclear defects were reversed [18].

Although the amount of progerin in cells is considerably lower than the amount of lamin A and lamin C [46], it is obvious that this small amount of progerin is very potent in terms of causing disease phenotypes in humans and in causing misshaped nuclei in cultured cells. Supporting the hypothesis that progerin exerts dominant negative effect in HGPS, Goldman and colleagues introduced progerin into normal cells via transfection and showed that progerin is targeted to the nuclear envelope and is entirely responsible for the misshapen nuclei. Same changes were observed when progerin protein was microinjected into cytoplasm of the normal cells [36]. It was hypothesised that retention of the farnesyl group on progerin may be the key factor in the development of the HGPS phenotype. Indeed, several different research groups showed that the nuclear abnormalities were alleviated or reversed by the inhibition of farnesylation [47-49]. Briefly, Yang and colleagues used mouse embryonic fibroblasts from a transgenic mouse expressing progerin ($Lmna^{HG/+}$) and showed that the treatment with a protein farnesyltransferase inhibitor (FTI) reduced nuclear blebbing to a baseline level observed in untreated wild-type cells [47]. Capell's group used transfection technique to demonstrate that the percentage of blebbed nuclei in HeLa cells that are transfected with progerin vector, decreased with FTI treatment in a dose-dependent manner [48]. Finally, Glynn and Glover showed a significant improvement in the nuclear morphology of HGPS cells or cells expressing mutant lamin A following FTI treatment [49].

There are several other *de novo* dominant *LMNA* mutations that are found less frequently and are known to cause atypical HGPS (see review [50]). Clinically, atypical HGPS patients exhibit additional signs and symptoms of classical HGPS or lack some of phenotypes observed in classical form. These overlapping and distinct clinical features of atypical HGPS are well described by Garg and colleagues [51].

4. Animal models

Animal models of HGPS have been a valuable tool in the study of the pathological processes implicated in the origin of this disease as well as finding a cure. Some of these mouse models are designed to express the exact mutation that is observed in human HGPS patients, or have defect in the lamin A processing. These mouse models are summarised in Table 1.

In 2006, Varga and colleagues generated a transgenic mouse model for HGPS by introducing a human bacterial artificial chromosome (BAC) c.1824C>T mutated *LMNA* gene. These animals over-expressed human lamin A/C and progerin in all tissues. Although this animal model did not display any external phenotypes seen in HGPS patients, such as growth retardation, alopecia, micrognathia and abnormal dentition, it progressively lost vascular smooth muscle cells in the medial layer of large arteries that closely resembled the most deadly aspect of the HGPS patients. Surprisingly, these animals showed no differences in their life expectancy compared to their wild-type littermates [52].

The $Zmpste24^{-/-}$ model was first developed by Leung and co-workers [53]. This model is a complete knock-out model, in which animals do not have any *ZMPSTE24* enzyme. Disruption of the gene encoding *ZMPSTE24* in mice causes defective lamin A processing, which results in the accumulation of farnesylated pre-lamin A at the nuclear envelope [54, 55]. Since these *ZMPSTE24*-deficient mice have shown to have many features that resemble HGPS and other laminopathies (diseases that are caused by mutations in the nuclear lamina), this model has served as a crucial tool to explore the mechanisms underlying these diseases and to design therapies for the treatment [55, 56]. In addition to being a model for HGPS, $Zmpste24^{-/-}$ mice also showed numerous characteristics of mandibuloacral dysplasia (MAD) [54], which promoted researchers to search for *ZMPSTE24* mutations in MAD patients [57]. Furthermore, loss of *ZMPSTE24* in humans has been shown to cause restrictive dermopathy, a lethal perinatal progeroid syndrome characterised by tight and rigid skin with erosions, loss of fat and prominent superficial vasculature, thin hair, micrognathia, joint contractures, and thin dysplastic clavicles [58]. The *Zmpste24*$^{-/-}$ mice look normal at birth, but develop skeletal abnormalities with spontaneous bone fractures. Furthermore, they show progressive hair loss, abnormal teething, muscle weakness, which ultimately lead to premature death at the age of 20-30 weeks [54, 55].

As an additional proof of the toxic effects of pre-lamin A accumulation, Fong and others compared the phenotypes of *Zmpste24*$^{-/-}$ mice and littermate *Zmpste24*$^{-/-}$ mice bearing one *Lmna* knock-out allele (*Zmpste24*$^{-/-}$*Lmna*$^{+/-}$) [59]. In this study, the authors showed that double knock-out mice carrying the *Zmpste24*$^{-/-}$*Lmna*$^{+/-}$ genotype, expressing half the pre-lamin A of *Zmpste24*$^{-/-}$*Lmna*$^{+/+}$ mice were completely protected from all disease phenotypes, including reduced growth rate, muscle strength and impaired bone and soft tissue development, and shortened lifespan. Furthermore, the frequency of misshapen nuclei in *Zmpste24*$^{-/-}$*Lmna*$^{+/-}$ fibroblasts was significantly lower than fibroblasts from *Zmpste24*$^{-/-}$*Lmna*$^{+/+}$ mice. The results from this study not only suggest that the accumulation of the farnesylated pre-lamin A is toxic, but also show that lowering the level of pre-lamin A have a beneficial effect on disease phenotypes in mice and on nuclear shape in cultured cells [59].

The *Lmna*$^{HG/+}$ model is a progerin knock-in mouse model, in which one of the *LMNA* alleles only expresses progerin, while the other expresses lamin A/C. These animals show several HGPS-related phenotypes, including bone alterations, reduction in subcutaneous fat and premature death at around 28 weeks of age [47, 60]. Although *Lmna*$^{HG/+}$ mice clearly show many of the early symptoms of HGPS, they do not display any signs of atherosclerosis in the intima or media of the aorta. This was surprising as most of HGPS patients die from cardiovascular complications and authors speculated that absence of these cardiovascular-related phenotypes in *Lmna*$^{HG/+}$ mice is simply because these mice do not live long enough to develop these deficits [60]. In the homozygous *Lmna*$^{HG/HG}$ animals, both *LMNA* alleles express progerin and therefore, lamin A/C is not produced. These animals exhibit severe growth retardation with complete absence of adipose tissue and numerous spontaneous bone fractures. They die at 3-4 weeks of age with poorly mineralised bones, micrognathia, craniofacial abnormalities [60].

In all of the mouse models described above, both pre-lamin A and progerin are farnesylated. Since the disease phenotypes in *Lmna*$^{HG/+}$ mice were alleviated with a FTI, it was logical to suppose that the protein prenylation is important for disease pathogenesis [60-62]. To further elucidate this subject, Yang *et al.* created a knock-in mice expressing non-farnesylated progerin (*Lmna*$^{nHG/+}$), in which progerin's C-terminal –CSIM motif was changed to –SSIM. This single amino acid substitution eliminated protein prenylation and two following processing steps (cleavage of the last 3 amino acids and methylation, Figure 3) [63]. Yang and colleagues expected that *Lmna*$^{nHG/+}$ mice would be free of disease, but surprisingly these animals developed all of the same disease phenotypes found in *Lmna*$^{HG/+}$ mice and invariably succumbed to the disease [63]. Persistence of disease phenotype in *Lmna*$^{nHG/+}$ mice, though milder than *Lmna*$^{HG/+}$ mice, raised doubts about the primacy of the protein prenylation in disease pathogenesis suggesting that features of progerin other than the accumulation of farnesylated progerin may underlie the severity of the disease [63]. In order to investigate the toxicity of the non-farnesylated progerin produced by the $Lmna^{nHG}$ allele, Yang *et al.* generated another non-fanesylated progerin allele ($Lmna^{csmHG}$), in which the progerin's C-terminal ends with the –CSM compared to the –SSIM ending in $Lmna^{nHG}$ allele [64]. CSM progerin cannot be prenylated, but it retains a C-terminal cysteine similar to the CSIM progerin that accumulates in FTI-treated $Lmna^{HG/+}$ mice. Astonishingly, mice containing the $Lmna^{csmHG}$ allele were free of HGPS-like disease phenotypes. Even the homozygous mice ($Lmna^{csmHG/csmHG}$), which produce exclusively progerin and no lamin A/C, were absent of all the characteristics of HGPS [64]. Furthermore, nuclear abnormalities were also milder in both types of mice. This study demonstrated that the toxicity of non-farnesylated progerin depends on the mutation used to abolish protein farnesylation [64]. The absence of HGPS-like phenotypes in mice expressing $Lmna^{csmHG}$ allele is consistent in mice expressing farnesylated and non-farnesylated forms of pre-lamin A. While expression of farnesylated pre-lamin A in $Zmpste24^{-/-}$ mice results in a severe HGPS-like symptoms [54, 59, 65, 66], mice expressing non-farnesylated pre-lamin A ($Lmna^{nPLAO/nPLAO}$) exhibited no HGPS-like phenotypes [67].

Although all differentiated cells express lamin A [22], there is still no clear explanation as to why the HGPS-related symptoms are limited to particular tissues and organs. Due to this segmental nature of HGPS with clinical features only present in restricted tissues, developing an ideal representative mouse model for HGPS has been a challenge. However, by using tissue-specific promoters, researchers have succeeded in designing transgenic mouse models expressing progerin in specific tissues. Unlike general knock-out or knock-in mouse models, transgenic mouse models using tissue-specific promoters provide a wealth of information about the function of specific genes, the *LMNA*, in case of HGPS. For example, Wang and others created a transgenic mouse line that expresses progerin in the epidermis by using the keratin 14 promoter [68]. Although keratinocytes of these mice showed abnormalities in nuclear morphology, their hair growth and wound healing were normal [68]. Although the advantages in using tissue-specific promoters to directly control the expression of target genes in specified tissues in transgenic animals have been acknowledged, the limitations of this system had become clear. This constitutive system had no control over the timing of the target gene expression, which depend entirely on the properties of the promoters used. The promoters in this setting is constitutively active, many starting early in the embryonic stage. In order to overcome this drawback, numerous researchers have invested time and effort in establishing conditional or inducible transgenic modelling system, one of which is regulated by tetracycline. The tetracycline-controlled transcriptional regulation system (tet-on/off) is a binary transgenic system that enables spatial and temporal regulation of gene expression [69]. By adding/removing doxycycline (a tetracycline derivative) to/from the system, it is possible to switch on/off the expression of the target gene in *in vivo*, which in turn is under the control of the tissue specific promoter. Using this system, Eriksson's group has generated a number of transgenic mouse models that express the HGPS mutation in isolated organ systems [70, 71], which served as a useful tool to study mechanism of disease progress. Briefly, transgenic mice carrying a human minigene of lamin A with the most common HGPS mutation, c.1824C>T; p.G608G, under the control of the tetracycline-regulated (tet-off) keratin 5 promoter (K5tTA) expressed the mutation in the skin, ameloblasts layer of the teeth, salivary glands, oesophagus, stomach, tongue, nose cavity and trachea [70]. These animals showed growth retardation, hair thinning, tooth fractures and premature death, all of which are similar clinical features observed in HGPS patients [70]. In order to study skeletal abnormalities of HGPS, the osterix (Sp7-tTA) promoter was used to create a bone-specific expression model of the HGPS mutation with expression of the HGPS mutation during osteoblast development (tetop-LA^{G608G}; Sp7-tTA mice). These mice showed growth retardation, gait imbalance and abnormalities in bone structure [71]. Recently, Osorio and colleagues have designed another mouse model expressing the HGPS mutation [72]. In this knock-in mouse model, the wild-type mouse *LMNA* gene was replaced with a mutant allele that carried the c.1827C>T; p.G609G mutation, which is equivalent to the HGPS c.1824C>T; p.G608G mutation in the human *LMNA* gene (*Lmna*$^{G609G/G609G}$). These mice accumulate progerin and exhibit key clinical features of HGPS, such as shortened life span and bone and cardiovascular abnormalities [72].

Mouse Model	*Description*	*References*
BAC transgenic G608G	Over expression of human lamin A/C and progerin	[51]
Zmpste24$^{-/-}$	Knockout of the gene encoding *Zmpste24*	[53, 54]
Zmpste24$^{-/-}$ ***Lmna***$^{+/-}$	Intercross between *Zmpste24*$^{-/-}$ mice and *Lmna*$^{+/-}$ mice No expression of *Zmpste24* with only one allele expressing lamin A/C	[58]
Lmna$^{HG/+}$	One allele expresses progerin, while the other expresses lamin A/C	[46, 59]
Lmna$^{nHG/+}$	One allele expresses non-farnesylated progerin, while the other expresses lamin A/C	[62]
Lmna$^{csmHG/csmHG}$	Both alleles express non-fanesylated progerin allele (*Lmna*^{csmHG}), in which the progerin's C-terminal ends with the –CSM compared to the –SSIM ending in *Lmna*^{nHG} allele	[63]
K14 promoter – FLAG - progerin	Tissue specific over expression of progerin with FLAG tag	[67]
tetop-LA^{G608G}; K5-tTA	Tissue specific over expression of human lamin A and progerin by using a Keratin 5 promoter	[69]
tetop-LA^{G608G}; Sp7-tTA	Bone specific over expression of human lamin A and progerin by using a osterix promoter	[70]
Lmna$^{G609G/G609G}$	*Lmna* gene replaced with a mutant allele that carries the c. 1827C>T; p.G609G mutation, which is equivalent to the HGPS c. 1824C>T; p.G608G mutation in the human *LMNA* gene	[71]

Table 1. A summary table of the most relevant mouse models for HGPS.

5. Treatments

Although the cause of HGPS has been discovered nearly 10 years ago, HGPS remains incurable, with no therapy other than symptomatic treatment. Nevertheless, not long after the discovery of a mutation in *LMNA* gene as the cause of HGPS, a number of potential therapeutic strategies have emerged. A great deal of evidence suggests that the accumulation of progerin may be the key to the pathogenesis of HGPS [18, 20, 30, 31, 36, 72]. As progerin is permanently farnesylated, researchers initially turned to farnesyltransferase inhibitors (FTIs) in the search for a pathogenic treatment. FTIs were initially developed for the treatment of cancer [73]. The theory to this invention was simple: to abolish the farnesyl lipid from mutationally activated Ras proteins, thus mislocalising these signalling proteins away from the plasma membrane, where they stimulate uncontrolled cell division. Analogous concept was applied to HGPS: to mislocalise farnesylated progerin away from the nuclear envelope, with the hope that the mislocalisation would reduce the ability of the molecule to cause disease. However, potential shortcomings to the FTI treatment were recognised from the start. For example, these drugs would be expected to interfere with the farnesylation of lamin B1 and B2, possibly causing more damage to the nuclear lamina. Moreover, these molecules would be expected to disturb farnesylation of other cellular proteins, possibly loading a second insult on already compromised cells. Finally, there was a concern that pre-lamin A might be geranylgeranylated in the presence of FTI, in which case would forbid the overall strategy. Indeed, negative effects of FTI treatment were reported both *in vitro* and *in vivo* by Verstraeten and colleagues. They showed that FTI treatment caused defects in centrosome separation leading to donut-shaped nuclei [74]. However, despite these concerns, investigators cautiously raised their hopes about the possibility of testing FTIs in HGPS.

In 2004, it was first hypothesised that farnesylated progerin might be a key player in the pathogenesis of HGPS [59]. Within a year, Yang *et al.* generated a mice carrying a "progerin-only" *Lmna* allele ($Lmna^{HG/+}$) and showed that the number of $Lmna^{HG/+}$ fibroblasts with misshapen nuclei was significantly decreased following the treatment of a FTI [47]. Shortly thereafter, several groups reported similar observations and demonstrated the possibility of farnesyltransferase inhibition as a therapeutic strategy for HGPS [48, 49, 75]. The finding that FTIs improve nuclear abnormalities led to testing the efficacy of FTIs in mouse models of HGPS. Fong *et al.* showed that administration of FTI restored disease phenotypes in *Zmpste24* deficient ($Zmpste24^{-/-}$) mice [76], and Yang *et al.* found that FTI significantly alleviated HGPS-related disease phenotypes (e.g. rib fractures, body weight curves, reduced bone density) and increased the survival of mice with a HGPS mutation ($Lmna^{HG/+}$) [60, 62]. Furthermore, Capell and colleagues demonstrated that treatment with FTI to HGPS mouse (BAC transgenic G608G; [52]) significantly prevented both the onset and late progression of cardiovascular disease, which is one of the most prevalent cause of death in HGPS patients [77]. However, some of enthusiasm about FTI treatment was dampened by unexpected emergence of HGPS-related disease phenotypes in mice expressing non-farnesylated progerin ($Lmna^{nHG/+}$) [63]. In order to further elucidate the fact that protein farnesylation is relevant to the pathogenesis and treatment of disease, Yang and others compared the effects of an FTI on disease phenotypes in both $Lmna^{HG/+}$ and $Lmna^{nHG/+}$ mice [61]. In this study, authors showed that the FTI reduced disease phenotypes only in *Lmna*$^{HG/+}$ mice, and had no effect in *Lmna*$^{nHG/+}$ mice, which supported the idea that the beneficial effects of FTI in *Lmna*$^{HG/+}$ mice are due to the inhibition of progerin farnesylation [61].

The encouraging results from both cell and animal studies led to the initiation of the clinical trial with FTI for HGPS patients. In 2007, 28 patients with classical HGPS were enrolled for the first clinical trial, in which children were treated with Lonafarnib (an FTI) for 2 years. Although the trial ended in December 2009, no report has been published on how effective the drug was in treating HGPS. While this first trial was in progress, the statins and aminobisphosphonates gained attention as potential therapies for the treatment of HGPS. Varela and others reported that combined treatment with statins and aminobisphosphonates effectively inhibit the farnesylation and gernaylgeranylation (an alternative prenylation) of progerin and pre-lamin A, which was accompanied by an alleviation in the disease phenotype of the *Zmpste24*$^{-/-}$ knockout mice [78]. Statins and aminobisphosphonates, both inhibit protein prenylation at different points than FTIs in the isoprenoids and cholesterol biosynthetic pathway, and are already in clinical use (Figure 5). Statins are renowned inhibitors of cholesterol synthetic pathway and are widely used in the clinic to lower cholesterol level and prescribed for cholesterol associated diseases, such as atherosclerosis. Statins inhibit the production of isoprenoid precursors involved in protein modification, thereby inhibiting lamin A maturation [79-81]. The aminobisphosphonates are currently used to treat osteoporosis. It inhibits farnesylpyrophosphate synthase, thus reducing the production of both geranyl-geranyl and farnesyl group [82, 83]. In addition to results from Varela *et al.* [78], Wang and colleagues also showed that treatment of transgenic mice that express progerin in epidermis with a FTI or a combination of a statin plus an aminobisphosphonate significantly improved nuclear morphological abnormalities in intact tissue [84]. Based on these hopeful animal studies, the Triple Drug Trial to test the therapeutic effect of a combination of a statin (Pravastatin), a biosphosphonate (Zoledronic Acid), and a FTI (Lonafarnib) was initiated in August 2009, including 45 HGPS patients [5]. This trial was planned to last for 2 years, but announcement about its outcome is yet to be made.

Besides interfering the post-translational processing of mutated pre-lamin A, another major path for HGPS treatment is to reduce the expression of progerin in cells and tissue [37, 72, 85, 86]. This was first shown by Scaffidi and Misteli [37]. They used antisense morpholino oligonucleotides specifically directed against the aberrant exon 11 and exon 12 junction contained in mutated pre-mRNAs to target the splicing defect observed in HGPS, and consequently decrease the production of progerin. Authors showed that once splicing defect is corrected and the level of progerin is decreased, morphological abnormalities of HGPS fibroblasts were ameliorated [37]. More recently, Osorio *et al.* designed a 25-nucleotide morpholino that bound to the exon 10-lamin A splice donor site, and showed that its administration reduced the percentage of cells with nuclear abnormalities to wild-type levels in a dose-dependent manner [72]. It remains to be seen, however, whether these oligonucleotides can be effectively and safely administered to patients. Another approach to reduce progerin expression at mRNA level is to use a short hairpin RNA (shRNA). Huang and colleagues showed that the reduced expression of mutated *LMNA* mRNA level was associated with amelioration of abnormal nuclear morphology [86]. However, the efficacy of shRNA in whole organism is yet to be confirmed.

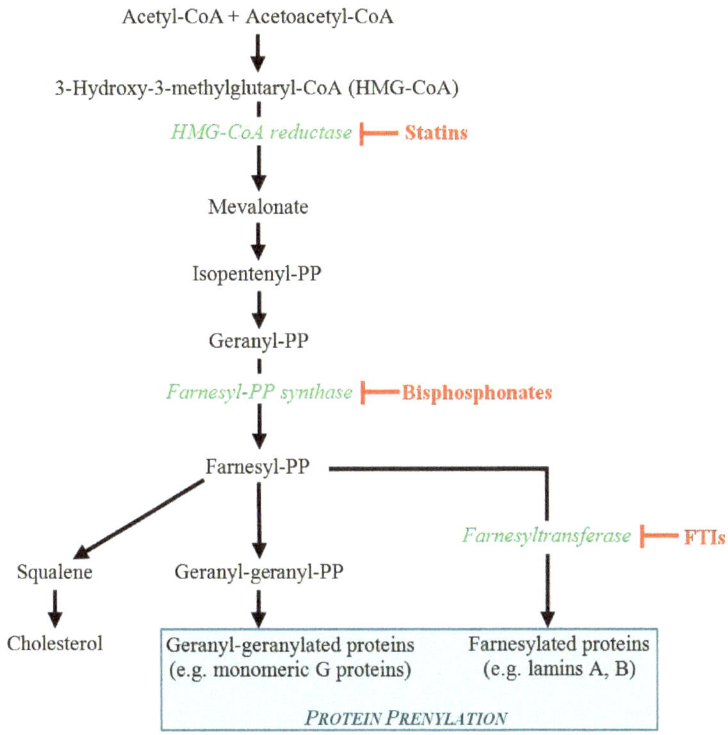

Figure 5. Isoprenoids and cholesterol biosynthetic pathway and its inhibitors for the treatment possibilities of HGPS. PP stands for pyrophosphate.

More recently, rapamycin has been gaining much attention as a new candidate for the treatment of HGPS. Rapamycin (also known as Sirolimus) is an FDA-approved drug that has been used for a long time in transplant patients as an anti-rejection drug. In addition to its historical use as an immunosuppressant, pre-clinical studies demonstrated life-span extending effect of rapamycin or rapamycin derivatives in mice [87, 88]. The effect of rapamycin is due to the inhibition of mammalian target of rapamycin (mTOR) pathway by rapamycin and is at least partly dependant on autophagy [89, 90]. Cao and colleagues have recently demonstrated that HGPS cells treated with rapamycin showed enhanced progerin degradation, slowed senescence, and reduced nuclear blebbing compared to untreated cells [91, 92]. Furthermore, similar results were reported by Cenni and others [93]. Since rapamycin is already an approved drug, its effect should be further examined in mouse models of HGPS and considered as a potential therapy for HGPS patients.

6. Conclusion

Since the discovery of the genetic basis for HGPS almost a decade ago, there has been progress in understanding the mechanism(s) of this premature ageing syndrome and its possible implications for physiological ageing. Results from numerous studies have uniformly suggested that the accumulation of an abnormally processed lamin A protein, progerin, mediates dominant-negative effects in cells from HGPS patients. Notably, over the last few years, many achievements in basic research have driven the development of potential therapies which have resulted in several clinical trials for patients with HGPS. It was inevitable to have hopes that these compounds targeting the isoprenoids and cholesterol biosynthetic pathway would alleviate the clinical course of HGPS. Nevertheless, drugs that are currently in clinical trials do not have the ability to target the cryptic splice site; therefore, additional approaches may still need to be considered.

In summary, by better understanding the mechanisms of HGPS, it may be possible to minimise the pathological process observed in HGPS, and to develop potential treatments for age-related diseases.

Acknowledgements

Our work is supported by a VINNMER fellow grant from VINNOVA, and an Innovator grant from The Progeria Research Foundation. We thank the patients and their families, and The Progeria Research Foundation for contributing the HGPS patient photos.

Author details

Jean-Ha Baek*, Tomás McKenna and Maria Eriksson

*Address all correspondence to: jean-ha.baek@ki.se

Department of Biosciences and Nutrition, Center for Biosciences, Karolinska Institutet, Huddinge, Sweden

References

[1] Hutchinson, J. (1886). Congenital Absence of Hair and Mammary Glands with Atrophic Condition of the Skin and its Appendages, in a Boy whose Mother had been almost wholly Bald from Alopecia Areata from the age of Six. *Medico-chirurgical transactions.*, 69, 473-7, Epub 1886/01/01.

[2] Gilford, H. (1897). On a Condition of Mixed Premature and Immature Development. *Medico-chirurgical transactions.*, 80, 17-46, Epub 1897/01/01.

[3] De Sandre-Giovannoli, A., Bernard, R., Cau, P., Navarro, C., Amiel, J., Boccaccio, I., et al. (2003). Lamin a truncation in Hutchinson-Gilford progeria. *Science.*, 300(5628), 2055 EOF, Epub 2003/04/19.

[4] Eriksson, M., Brown, W. T., Gordon, L. B., Glynn, M. W., Singer, J., Scott, L., et al. (2003). Recurrent de novo point mutations in lamin A cause Hutchinson-Gilford progeria syndrome. *Nature*, 423(6937), 293-8, Epub 2003/04/26.

[5] Progeria Research Foundation. (2012). www.progeriaresearch.org].

[6] Hennekam, R. C. (2006). Hutchinson-Gilford progeria syndrome: review of the phenotype. *American journal of medical genetics Part A.*, 140(23), 2603-24, Epub 2006/07/14.

[7] Merideth, M. A., Gordon, L. B., Clauss, S., Sachdev, V., Smith, A. C., Perry, M. B., et al. (2008). Phenotype and course of Hutchinson-Gilford progeria syndrome. *New England journal of medicine*, 358(6), 592-604, Epub 2008/02/08.

[8] Gordon, C. M., Gordon, L. B., Snyder, Nazarian. A., Quinn, N., Huh, S., et al. (2011). Hutchinson-Gilford progeria is a skeletal dysplasia. *Journal of bone and mineral research : the official journal of the American Society for Bone and Mineral Research*, 26(7), 1670-9, Epub 2011/03/30.

[9] Kieran, M. W., Gordon, L., & Kleinman, M. (2007). New approaches to progeria. *Pediatrics*, 120(4), 834-41, Epub 2007/10/03.

[10] Gordon, L. B., Mc Carten, K. M., Giobbie-Hurder, A., Machan, J. T., Campbell, S. E., Berns, S. D., et al. (2007). Disease progression in Hutchinson-Gilford progeria syndrome: impact on growth and development. *Pediatrics*, 120(4), 824-33, Epub 2007/10/03.

[11] Domingo, D. L., Trujillo, M. I., Council, S. E., Merideth, Gordon. L. B., Wu, T., et al. (2009). Hutchinson-Gilford progeria syndrome: oral and craniofacial phenotypes. *Oral diseases*, 15(3), 187-95, Epub 2009/02/25.

[12] De Busk, F. L. (1972). The Hutchinson-Gilford progeria syndrome Report of 4 cases and review of the literature. *The Journal of pediatrics.*, 80(4), 697-724, Epub 1972/04/01.

[13] Cleveland, R. H., Gordon, L. B., Kleinman, Miller. D. T., Gordon, C. M., Snyder, et., & al, . (2012). A prospective study of radiographic manifestations in Hutchinson-Gilford progeria syndrome. *Pediatric radiology*, 42(9), 1089-98, Epub 2012/07/04.

[14] Olive, M., Harten, I., Mitchell, R., Beers, J. K., Djabali, K., Cao, K., et al. (2010). Cardiovascular pathology in Hutchinson-Gilford progeria: correlation with the vascular pathology of aging. *Arteriosclerosis thrombosis, and vascular biology.*, 30(11), 2301-9, Epub 2010/08/28.

[15] Jung, H. J., Coffinier, C., Choe, Y., Beigneux, A. P., Davies, Yang. S. H., et al. (2012). Regulation of prelamin A but not lamin C by miR-9, a brain-specific microRNA. *Pro-*

ceedings of the National Academy of Sciences of the United States of America., 109(7), 423-31, Epub 2012/02/07.

[16] Nissan, X., Blondel, S., Navarro, C., Maury, Y., Denis, C., Girard, M., et al. (2012). Unique Preservation of Neural Cells in Hutchinson- Gilford Progeria Syndrome Is Due to the Expression of the Neural-Specific miR-9 MicroRNA. *Cell reports,* 2(1), 1-9, Epub 2012/07/31.

[17] Haithcock, E., Dayani, Y., Neufeld, E., Zahand, A. J., Feinstein, N., Mattout, A., et al. (2005). Age-related changes of nuclear architecture in Caenorhabditis elegans. *Proc Natl Acad Sci U S A.,* 102(46), 16690-5, Epub 2005/11/05.

[18] Scaffidi, P., & Misteli, T. (2006). Lamin A-dependent nuclear defects in human aging. *Science.,* 312(5776), 1059-63, Epub 2006/04/29.

[19] Mc Clintock, D., Ratner, D., Lokuge, M., Owens, D. M., Gordon, L. B., Collins, F. S., et al. (2007). The mutant form of lamin A that causes Hutchinson-Gilford progeria is a biomarker of cellular aging in human skin. *PloS one,* e1269 EOF, Epub 2007/12/07.

[20] Rodriguez, S., Coppede, F., Sagelius, H., & Eriksson, M. (2009). Increased expression of the Hutchinson-Gilford progeria syndrome truncated lamin A transcript during cell aging. *European journal of human genetics,* 17(7), 928-37, Epub 2009/01/29.

[21] Bertrand, A. T., Chikhaoui, K., Yaou, R. B., & Bonne, G. (2011). Clinical and genetic heterogeneity in laminopathies. *Biochemical Society transactions,* 39(6), 1687-92, Epub 2011/11/23.

[22] Dechat, T., Pfleghaar, K., Sengupta, K., Shimi, T., Shumaker, D. K., Solimando, L., et al. (2008). Nuclear lamins: major factors in the structural organization and function of the nucleus and chromatin. *Genes & development.,* 22(7), 832-53, Epub 2008/04/03.

[23] Rober, R. A., Weber, K., & Osborn, M. (1989). Differential timing of nuclear lamin A/C expression in the various organs of the mouse embryo and the young animal: a developmental study. *Development.,* 105(2), 365-78, Epub 1989/02/01.

[24] Capell, B. C., & Collins, F. S. (2006). Human laminopathies: nuclei gone genetically awry. *Nature reviews Genetics.,* 7(12), 940-52, Epub 2006/12/02.

[25] Goldman, R. D., Gruenbaum, Y., Moir, R. D., Shumaker, D. K., & Spann, T. P. (2002). Nuclear lamins: building blocks of nuclear architecture. *Genes & development,* 16(5), 533-47, Epub 2002/03/06.

[26] Gruenbaum, Y., Margalit, A., Goldman, R. D., Shumaker, D. K., & Wilson, K. L. (2005). The nuclear lamina comes of age. *Nature reviews Molecular cell biology.,* 6(1), 21-31, Epub 2005/02/03.

[27] Boban, M., Braun, J., & Foisner, R. (2010). Lamins:'structure goes cycling'. *Biochemical Society transactions Pt 1,* 301 EOF-306 EOF, Epub 2010/01/16.

[28] Cao, H., & Hegele, R. A. (2003). LMNA is mutated in Hutchinson-Gilford progeria (MIM 176670) but not in Wiedemann-Rautenstrauch progeroid syndrome (MIM 264090). *Journal of human genetics*, 48(5), 271-4, Epub 2003/05/28.

[29] Verstraeten, V. L., Broers, J. L., van Steensel-Justin, Zinn., Ramaekers, S., Steijlen, F. C., et, P. M., & al, . (2006). Compound heterozygosity for mutations in LMNA causes a progeria syndrome without prelamin A accumulation. *Human molecular genetics.*, 15(16), 2509-22, Epub 2006/07/11.

[30] Moulson, C. L., Fong, L. G., Gardner, J. M., Farber, E. A., Go, G., Passariello, A., et al. (2007). Increased progerin expression associated with unusual LMNA mutations causes severe progeroid syndromes. *Human mutation*, 28(9), 882-9, Epub 2007/05/01.

[31] Reunert, J., Wentzell, R., Walter, M., Jakubiczka, S., Zenker, M., Brune, T., et al. (2012). Neonatal progeria: increased ratio of progerin to lamin A leads to progeria of the newborn. *European journal of human genetics*, Epub 2012/03/16.

[32] Fukuchi, K., Katsuya, T., Sugimoto, K., Kuremura, M., Kim, H. D., Li, L., et al. (2004). LMNA mutation in a 45 year old Japanese subject with Hutchinson-Gilford progeria syndrome. *Journal of medical genetics*, e67 EOF, Epub 2004/05/04.

[33] Hisama, F. M., Lessel, D., Leistritz, D., Friedrich, K., Mc Bride, K. L., Pastore, M. T., et al. (2011). Coronary artery disease in a Werner syndrome-like form of progeria characterized by low levels of progerin, a splice variant of lamin A. *American journal of medical genetics Part A.*, 155(12), 3002 EOF-6 EOF, Epub 2011/11/09.

[34] Dechat, T., Shimi, T., Adam, S. A., Rusinol, A. E., Andres, D. A., Spielmann, H. P., et al. (2007). Alterations in mitosis and cell cycle progression caused by a mutant lamin A known to accelerate human aging. *Proceedings of the National Academy of Sciences of the United States of America.*, 104(12), 4955-60, Epub 2007/03/16.

[35] Young, S. G., Fong, L. G., Michaelis, S., & Prelamin, A. (2005). Zmpste24, misshapen cell nuclei, and progeria--new evidence suggesting that protein farnesylation could be important for disease pathogenesis. *Journal of lipid research.*, 46(12), 2531-58, Epub 2005/10/07.

[36] Goldman, R. D., Shumaker, D. K., Erdos, M. R., Eriksson, M., Goldman, A. E., Gordon, L. B., et al. (2004). Accumulation of mutant lamin A causes progressive changes in nuclear architecture in Hutchinson-Gilford progeria syndrome. *Proceedings of the National Academy of Sciences of the United States of America*, 101(24), 8963-8, Epub 2004/06/09.

[37] Scaffidi, P., & Misteli, T. (2005). Reversal of the cellular phenotype in the premature aging disease Hutchinson-Gilford progeria syndrome. *Nature medicine*, 11(4), 440-5, Epub 2005/03/08.

[38] Bridger, J. M., & Kill, I. R. (2004). Aging of Hutchinson-Gilford progeria syndrome fibroblasts is characterised by hyperproliferation and increased apoptosis. *Experimental gerontology*, 39(5), 717-24, Epub 2004/05/08.

[39] Eggert, M., Radomski, N., Linder, D., Tripier, D., Traub, P., & Jost, E. (1993). Identification of novel phosphorylation sites in murine A-type lamins. *European journal of biochemistry / FEBS*, 213(2), 659-71, Epub 1993/04/15.

[40] Shimi, T., Butin-Israeli, V., & Goldman, R. D. (2012). The functions of the nuclear envelope in mediating the molecular crosstalk between the nucleus and the cytoplasm. *Current opinion in cell biology*, 24(1), 71-8, Epub 2011/12/24.

[41] Liu, B., Wang, J., Chan, K. M., Tjia, W. M., Deng, W., Guan, X., et al. (2005). Genomic instability in laminopathy-based premature aging. *Nature medicine*, 11(7), 780-5, Epub 2005/06/28.

[42] Musich, P. R., & Zou, Y. (2011). DNA-damage accumulation and replicative arrest in Hutchinson-Gilford progeria syndrome. *Biochemical Society transactions*, 39(6), 1764-9, Epub 2011/11/23.

[43] Dimauro, T., & David, G. (2009). Chromatin modifications: the driving force of senescence and aging? *Aging.*, 1(2), 182-90, Epub 2010/02/17.

[44] Brown, W. T. (1992). Progeria: a human-disease model of accelerated aging. *The American journal of clinical nutrition.*, 55(6), 1222S-4S, Epub 1992/06/01.

[45] Columbaro, M., Capanni, C., Mattioli, E., Novelli, G., Parnaik, V. K., Squarzoni, S., et al. (2005). Rescue of heterochromatin organization in Hutchinson-Gilford progeria by drug treatment. *Cellular and molecular life sciences : CMLS*, 62(22), 2669-78, Epub 2005/11/02.

[46] Reddel, C. J., & Weiss, . (2004). Lamin A expression levels are unperturbed at the normal and mutant alleles but display partial splice site selection in Hutchinson-Gilford progeria syndrome. *Journal of medical genetics*, 41(9), 715-7, Epub 2004/09/03.

[47] Yang, S. H., Bergo, M. O., Toth, J. I., Qiao, X., Hu, Y., Sandoval, S., et al. (2005). Blocking protein farnesyltransferase improves nuclear blebbing in mouse fibroblasts with a targeted Hutchinson-Gilford progeria syndrome mutation. *Proceedings of the National Academy of Sciences of the United States of America*, 102(29), 10291-6, Epub 2005/07/15.

[48] Capell, B. C., Erdos, M. R., Madigan, J. P., Fiordalisi, J. J., Varga, R., Conneely, K. N., et al. (2005). Inhibiting farnesylation of progerin prevents the characteristic nuclear blebbing of Hutchinson-Gilford progeria syndrome. *Proceedings of the National Academy of Sciences of the United States of America*, 102(36), 12879-84, Epub 2005/09/01.

[49] Glynn, M. W., & Glover, T. W. (2005). Incomplete processing of mutant lamin A in Hutchinson-Gilford progeria leads to nuclear abnormalities, which are reversed by farnesyltransferase inhibition. *Human molecular genetics*, 14(20), 2959-69, Epub 2005/08/30.

[50] Rodriguez, S., & Eriksson, M. (2010). Evidence for the involvement of lamins in aging. *Current aging science*, 3(2), 81-9, Epub 2010/01/05.

[51] Garg, A., Subramanyam, L., Agarwal, A. K., Simha, V., Levine, B., D'Apice, M. R., et al. (2009). Atypical progeroid syndrome due to heterozygous missense LMNA muta-

tions. *The Journal of clinical endocrinology and metabolism.*, 94(12), 4971-83, Epub 2009/10/31.

[52] Varga, R., Eriksson, M., Erdos, M. R., Olive, M., Harten, I., Kolodgie, F., et al. (2006). Progressive vascular smooth muscle cell defects in a mouse model of Hutchinson-Gilford progeria syndrome. *Proceedings of the National Academy of Sciences of the United States of America*, 103(9), 3250-5, Epub 2006/02/24.

[53] Leung, G. K., Schmidt, W. K., Bergo, M. O., Gavino, B., Wong, D. H., Tam, A., et al. (2001). Biochemical studies of Zmpste24-deficient mice. *The Journal of biological chemistry*, 276(31), 29051-8, Epub 2001/06/16.

[54] Bergo, M. O., Gavino, B., Ross, J., Schmidt, W. K., Hong, C., Kendall, L. V., et al. (2002). Zmpste24 deficiency in mice causes spontaneous bone fractures, muscle weakness, and a prelamin A processing defect. *Proceedings of the National Academy of Sciences of the United States of America.*, 99(20), 13049-54, Epub 2002/09/18.

[55] Pendas, A. M., Zhou, Z., Cadinanos, J., Freije, J. M., Wang, J., Hultenby, K., et al. (2002). Defective prelamin A processing and muscular and adipocyte alterations in Zmpste24 metalloproteinase-deficient mice. *Nature genetics*, 31(1), 94-9, Epub 2002/03/30.

[56] Osorio, F. G., Obaya, A. J., Lopez-Otin, C., & Freije, J. M. (2009). Accelerated ageing: from mechanism to therapy through animal models. *Transgenic research*, 18(1), 7-15, Epub 2008/11/19.

[57] Agarwal, A. K., Fryns, J. P., Auchus, R. J., & Garg, A. (2003). Zinc metalloproteinase, ZMPSTE24, is mutated in mandibuloacral dysplasia. *Human molecular genetics*, 12(16), 1995-2001, Epub 2003/08/13.

[58] Navarro, C. L., De Sandre-Giovannoli, A., Bernard, R., Boccaccio, I., Boyer, A., Genevieve, D., et al. (2004). Lamin A and ZMPSTE24 (FACE-1) defects cause nuclear disorganization and identify restrictive dermopathy as a lethal neonatal laminopathy. *Human molecular genetics*, 13(20), 2493-503, Epub 2004/08/20.

[59] Fong, L. G., Ng, J. K., Meta, M., Cote, N., Yang, S. H., Stewart, C. L., et al. (2004). Heterozygosity for Lmna deficiency eliminates the progeria-like phenotypes in Zmpste24-deficient mice. *Proc Natl Acad Sci U S A.*, 101(52), 18111-6, Epub 2004/12/21.

[60] Yang, S. H., Meta, M., Qiao, X., Frost, D., Bauch, J., Coffinier, C., et al. (2006). A farnesyltransferase inhibitor improves disease phenotypes in mice with a Hutchinson-Gilford progeria syndrome mutation. *The Journal of clinical investigation*, 116(8), 2115-21, Epub 2006/07/25.

[61] Yang, S. H., Chang, S. Y., Andres, D. A., Spielmann, H. P., Young, S. G., & Fong, L. G. (2010). Assessing the efficacy of protein farnesyltransferase inhibitors in mouse models of progeria. *Journal of lipid research.*, 51(2), 400-5, Epub 2009/12/08.

[62] Yang, S. H., Qiao, X., Fong, L. G., & Young, S. G. (2008). Treatment with a farnesyltransferase inhibitor improves survival in mice with a Hutchinson-Gilford progeria

syndrome mutation. *Biochimica et biophysica acta.*, 1781(1-2), 36 EOF-39 EOF, Epub 2007/12/18.

[63] Yang, S. H., Andres, D. A., Spielmann, H. P., Young, S. G., & Fong, L. G. (2008). Progerin elicits disease phenotypes of progeria in mice whether or not it is farnesylated. *The Journal of clinical investigation.*, 118(10), 3291-300, Epub 2008/09/05.

[64] Yang, S. H., Chang, S. Y., Ren, S., Wang, Y., Andres, D. A., Spielmann, H. P., et al. (2011). Absence of progeria-like disease phenotypes in knock-in mice expressing a non-farnesylated version of progerin. *Human molecular genetics*, 20(3), 436-44, Epub 2010/11/23.

[65] Denecke, J., Brune, T., Feldhaus, T., Robenek, H., Kranz, C., Auchus, R. J., et al. (2006). A homozygous ZMPSTE24 null mutation in combination with a heterozygous mutation in the LMNA gene causes Hutchinson-Gilford progeria syndrome (HGPS): insights into the pathophysiology of HGPS. *Human mutation*, 27(6), 524-31, Epub 2006/05/04.

[66] Shackleton, S., Smallwood, D. T., Clayton, P., Wilson, L. C., Agarwal, A. K., Garg, A., et al. (2005). Compound heterozygous ZMPSTE24 mutations reduce prelamin A processing and result in a severe progeroid phenotype. *Journal of medical genetics.*, 42(6), e36, Epub 2005/06/07.

[67] Davies, B. S., Barnes, R. H., 2nd, Tu. Y., Ren, S., Andres, D. A., Spielmann, H. P., et al. (2010). An accumulation of non-farnesylated prelamin A causes cardiomyopathy but not progeria. *Human molecular genetics*, 19(13), 2682-94, Epub 2010/04/28.

[68] Wang, Y., Panteleyev, Owens. D. M., Djabali, K., Stewart, C. L., & Worman, H. J. (2008). Epidermal expression of the truncated prelamin A causing Hutchinson-Gilford progeria syndrome: effects on keratinocytes, hair and skin. *Human molecular genetics*, 17(15), 2357-69, Epub 2008/04/30.

[69] Zhu, Z., Zheng, T., Lee, C. G., Homer, R. J., & Elias, J. A. (2002). Tetracycline-controlled transcriptional regulation systems: advances and application in transgenic animal modeling. *Seminars in cell & developmental biology.*, 13(2), 121-8, Epub 2002/07/20.

[70] Sagelius, H., Rosengardten, Y., Hanif, M., Erdos, M. R., Rozell, B., Collins, F. S., et al. (2008). Targeted transgenic expression of the mutation causing Hutchinson-Gilford progeria syndrome leads to proliferative and degenerative epidermal disease. *Journal of cell science Pt 7*, 969 EOF-78 EOF, Epub 2008/03/13.

[71] Schmidt, E., Nilsson, O., Koskela, A., Tuukkanen, J., Ohlsson, C., Rozell, B., et al. (2012). Expression of the Hutchinson-Gilford progeria mutation during osteoblast development results in loss of osteocytes, irregular mineralization, and poor biomechanical properties. *The Journal of biological chemistry*, Epub 2012/08/16.

[72] Osorio, F. G., Navarro, C. L., Cadinanos, J., Lopez-Mejia, I. C., Quiros, P. M., Bartoli, C., et al. (2011). Splicing-directed therapy in a new mouse model of human accelerated aging. *Science translational medicine*, ra7. Epub 2011/10/28.

[73] Reiss, Y., Goldstein, J. L., Seabra, M. C., Casey, P. J., & Brown, MS. (1990). Inhibition of purified p21ras farnesyl:protein transferase by Cys-AAX tetrapeptides. *Cell*, Epub 1990/07/13.

[74] Verstraeten, V. L., Peckham, L. A., Olive, M., Capell, B. C., Collins, F. S., Nabel, E. G., et al. (2011). Protein farnesylation inhibitors cause donut-shaped cell nuclei attributable to a centrosome separation defect. *Proceedings of the National Academy of Sciences of the United States of America.*, 108(12), 4997-5002, Epub 2011/03/09.

[75] Mallampalli, M. P., Huyer, G., Bendale, P., Gelb, M. H., & Michaelis, S. (2005). Inhibiting farnesylation reverses the nuclear morphology defect in a HeLa cell model for Hutchinson-Gilford progeria syndrome. *Proceedings of the National Academy of Sciences of the United States of America*, 102(40), 14416-21, Epub 2005/09/28.

[76] Fong, L. G., Frost, D., Meta, M., Qiao, X., Yang, S. H., Coffinier, C., et al. (2006). A protein farnesyltransferase inhibitor ameliorates disease in a mouse model of progeria. *Science.*, 311(5767), 1621-3, Epub 2006/02/18.

[77] Capell, B. C., Olive, M., Erdos, M. R., Cao, K., Faddah, D. A., Tavarez, U. L., et al. (2008). A farnesyltransferase inhibitor prevents both the onset and late progression of cardiovascular disease in a progeria mouse model. *Proceedings of the National Academy of Sciences of the United States of America.*, 105(41), 15902-7, Epub 2008/10/08.

[78] Varela, I., Pereira, S., Ugalde, A. P., Navarro, C. L., Suarez, M. F., Cau, P., et al. (2008). Combined treatment with statins and aminobisphosphonates extends longevity in a mouse model of human premature aging. *Nature medicine.*, 14(7), 767-72, Epub 2008/07/01.

[79] Sinensky, M., Beck, L. A., Leonard, S., & Evans, R. (1990). Differential inhibitory effects of lovastatin on protein isoprenylation and sterol synthesis. *The Journal of biological chemistry*, 265(32), 19937-41, Epub 1990/11/15.

[80] Lutz, R. J., Trujillo, Denham. K. S., Wenger, L., & Sinensky, M. (1992). Nucleoplasmic localization of prelamin A: implications for prenylation-dependent lamin A assembly into the nuclear lamina. *Proceedings of the National Academy of Sciences of the United States of America*, 89(7), 3000-4, Epub 1992/04/01.

[81] Baker, S. K. (2005). Molecular clues into the pathogenesis of statin-mediated muscle toxicity. *Muscle & nerve*, 31(5), 572-80, Epub 2005/02/16.

[82] Amin, D., Cornell, S. A., Gustafson, S. K., Needle, S. J., Ullrich, J. W., Bilder, G. E., et al. (1992). Bisphosphonates used for the treatment of bone disorders inhibit squalene synthase and cholesterol biosynthesis. *Journal of lipid research*, 33(11), 1657-63, Epub 1992/11/01.

[83] Keller, R. K., & Fliesler, S. J. (1999). Mechanism of aminobisphosphonate action: characterization of alendronate inhibition of the isoprenoid pathway. *Biochemical and biophysical research communications*, 266(2), 560-3, Epub 1999/12/22.

[84] Wang, Y., Ostlund, C., & Worman, H. J. (2010). Blocking protein farnesylation improves nuclear shape abnormalities in keratinocytes of mice expressing the prelamin A variant in Hutchinson-Gilford progeria syndrome. *Nucleus*, 1(5), 432-9, Epub 2011/02/18.

[85] Fong, L. G., Ng, J. K., Lammerding, J., Vickers, T. A., Meta, M., Cote, N., et al. (2006). Prelamin A and lamin A appear to be dispensable in the nuclear lamina. *The Journal of clinical investigation.*, 116(3), 743-52, Epub 2006/03/03.

[86] Huang, S., Chen, L., Libina, N., Janes, J., Martin, G. M., Campisi, J., et al. (2005). Correction of cellular phenotypes of Hutchinson-Gilford Progeria cells by RNA interference. *Hum Genet.*, 118(3-4), 444 EOF-450 EOF, Epub 2005/10/07.

[87] Harrison, D. E., Strong, R., Sharp, Z. D., Nelson, J. F., Astle, C. M., Flurkey, K., et al. (2009). Rapamycin fed late in life extends lifespan in genetically heterogeneous mice. *Nature*, 460(7253), 392-5, Epub 2009/07/10.

[88] Miller, R. A., Harrison, D. E., Astle, C. M., Baur, J. A., Boyd, A. R., de Cabo, R., et al. (2011). Rapamycin, but not resveratrol or simvastatin, extends life span of genetically heterogeneous mice. The journals of gerontology Series A,. *Biological sciences and medical sciences.*, 66(2), 191-201, Epub 2010/10/27.

[89] Mendelsohn, A. R., & Larrick, J. W. (2011). Rapamycin as an antiaging therapeutic?: targeting mammalian target of rapamycin to treat Hutchinson-Gilford progeria and neurodegenerative diseases. *Rejuvenation research*, 14(4), 437-41, Epub 2011/08/20.

[90] Graziotto, J. J., Cao, K., Collins, F. S., & Krainc, D. (2012). Rapamycin activates autophagy in Hutchinson-Gilford progeria syndrome: implications for normal aging and age-dependent neurodegenerative disorders. *Autophagy*, 8(1), 147-51, Epub 2011/12/16.

[91] Cao, K., Graziotto, J. J., Blair, C. D., Mazzulli, J. R., Erdos, M. R., Krainc, D., et al. (2011). Rapamycin reverses cellular phenotypes and enhances mutant protein clearance in Hutchinson-Gilford progeria syndrome cells. *Science translational medicine*, 89ra58 EOF, Epub 2011/07/01.

[92] Driscoll, M. K., Albanese, J. L., Xiong, Z. M., Mailman, M., Losert, W., & Cao, K. (2012). Automated image analysis of nuclear shape: what can we learn from a prematurely aged cell? *Aging.*, 4(2), 119-32, Epub 2012/02/23.

[93] Cenni, V., Capanni, C., Columbaro, M., Ortolani, M., D'Apice, M. R., Novelli, G., et al. (2011). Autophagic degradation of farnesylated prelamin A as a therapeutic approach to lamin-linked progeria. *European journal of histochemistry*, 55(4), e36., Epub 2012/02/03.

Chapter 5

Structural Insights Into Disease Mutations of the Ryanodine Receptor

Zhiguang Yuchi, Lynn Kimlicka and
Filip Van Petegem

Additional information is available at the end of the chapter

1. Introduction

Ca^{2+} ions form important intracellular messenger molecules in nearly every cell type of the human body. Under so-called "resting" states of the cell, the concentration of Ca^{2+} in the cytoplasm is extremely low (~10^{-7}M), but this can rapidly rise ~2 orders of magnitude when an appropriate signal is generated. Ca^{2+} ions can enter the cytoplasm either from the extracellular space or from intracellular compartments, through specialized membrane proteins. These "calcium channels" are complex proteins, often consisting of multiple subunits, and are targets for multiple regulatory events.

A major intracellular Ca^{2+} store is the endoplasmic reticulum (ER), or its specialized form, the sarcoplasmic reticulum (SR) in muscle tissue. The mobilization of Ca^{2+} from these organelles can trigger many Ca^{2+}-dependent events, such as the contraction of muscle tissue. The coupling between electrical excitation of a muscle cell and its subsequent contraction (excitation-contraction coupling, E-C coupling) is a finely orchestrated process that requires a functional cross-talk between proteins embedded in the plasma membrane and in the SR membrane (Figure 1). An electrical signal, a depolarization of the plasma membrane, can lead to opening of L-type voltage-gated calcium channels (Ca_V), which results in the influx of Ca^{2+} into the cytoplasm. In the SR membrane, large calcium release channels called Ryanodine Receptors (RyRs) can detect this initial influx, and release more Ca^{2+} in a process known as Ca^{2+}-induced Ca^{2+} release (CICR). The latter event provides the bulk of the Ca^{2+} required for contraction to occur. In this scenario, the RyRs form signal amplifiers, which both detect and augment the Ca^{2+} signal [1, 2]. This scenario likely predominates in cardiac tissue, but Ca^{2+} is not always required to open RyRs. In skeletal muscle, for example, various pieces of evidence suggest a direct interaction between the L-type calcium channel ($Ca_V1.1$) and the RyR [3-6]. In this case, the depolarization of the plasma membrane causes distinct conformational changes in $Ca_V1.1$, which are then transmitted directly to the RyR, causing them to open.

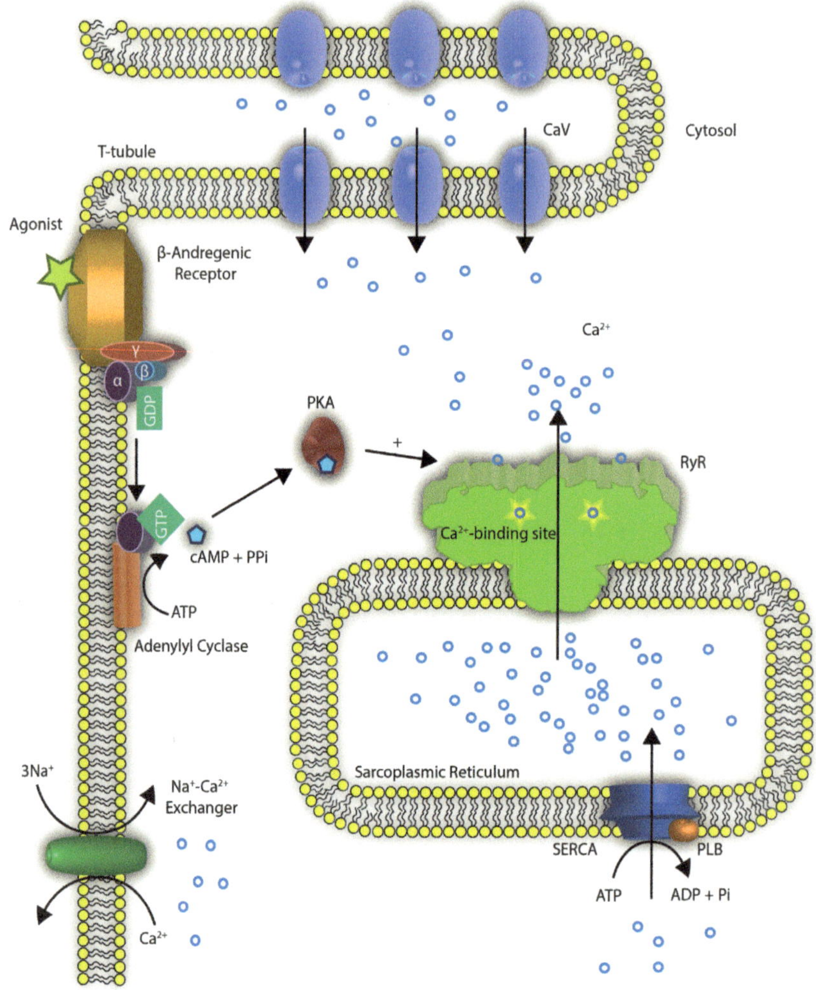

Figure 1. Schematic diagram of components in E-C coupling. Depolarization of plasma membrane (PM) activates the embedded voltage-gated calcium channel (CaV) which conducts Ca^{2+} influx into the cytoplasm. RyRs in SR membrane sense this Ca^{2+} signal and amplify it by releasing more Ca^{2+} from SR store (Ca^{2+} -induced Ca^{2+} release, CICR). This will provide enough Ca^{2+} for the muscle contraction to occur. SERCA pump in the SR and Na^+-Ca^{2+} exchanger in the PM pump out the Ca^{2+} from cytoplasm and restore the resting [Ca^{2+}]. The activity of RyR can be upregulated by the PKA phosphoryaltion upon the activation of β-adrenergic receptor on the PM.

RyRs owe their name to the binding of ryanodine, a toxic compound from the South American plant *Ryania speciosa* [7]. RyRs are currently the largest known ion channels, with a massive size of >2.2MDa. They form homotetrameric assemblies [8, 9], and each monomer contains ~5000 amino acid residues. In humans and all other mammalian organisms investigated so far, three different isoforms (RyR1-3) have been found to date. RyR1 is widely expressed in skeletal muscle, and was the first one to be cloned [10, 11]. RyR2 is primarily found in the heart [12, 13] and RyR3 was originally identified in the brain [14], although each isoform is found in many different cell types [15].

Since Ca^{2+} ions form very potent intracellular messenger molecules, it is not surprising that their entry into the cytoplasm is under intense regulation. RyRs therefore form the targets for a plethora of auxiliary proteins and small molecules that are known to regulate their ability to open or close [15-17]. The primary regulatory molecule is cytoplasmic Ca^{2+}, which triggers the channel to open. However, higher Ca^{2+} levels can trigger closing, indicating that there is more than one Ca^{2+} binding site. Under conditions whereby the SR is overloaded with Ca^{2+}, RyRs can also open spontaneously in a process known as store-overload-induced calcium release (SOICR) [18, 19].

An overview of several positive and negative RyR modulators is shown in Figure 2. Well-known regulators include FK506 binding proteins (FKBPs), small proteins that stabilize the closed state of the channels and can prevent the formation of subconductance states [20, 21]. Calmodulin (CaM) is a ~17kDa protein that can bind 4 Ca^{2+} ions in separate EF hands, well-known Ca^{2+}-binding motifs. CaM binds RyR in a 4:1 stoichiometry and can either inhibit or stimulate RyRs depending on the isoform and Ca^{2+} levels [22-25]. RyRs are also the target for several kinases (PKA, PKG, CaMKII) and phosphatases (PP1, PP2A, PDE4D3), and the degree of phosphorylation seems to affect RyR activity [26]. In this chapter, we discuss the involvement of RyRs in several genetic diseases, summarize the outcome of several years of functional studies on disease variants of the RyR, and describe the insights into disease mechanisms through low- and high-resolution structural studies.

2. Ryanodine receptors and genetic disease

2.1. Malignant hyperthermia

Malignant hyperthermia (MH) is a pharmacogenetic disorder, requiring both a genetic mutation and an external trigger to cause a disease phenotype. The condition is mostly linked to mutations in the RyR skeletal muscle isoform (RyR1), but some mutations in the skeletal muscle L-type calcium channel ($Ca_V1.1$) can also cause MH [27]. It is typically triggered by the use of inhalational anesthetics or succinylcholine, a muscle relaxant [28]. The condition is considered rare, with an incidence of 1:60,000 for adults or 1:15,000 for children [29]. An MH episode is characterized by an abnormal rise in the core body temperature, skeletal muscle rigidity, acidosis, and tachycardia. Most modern surgery rooms monitor for these signs, and will make use of dantrolene, which can rapidly reverse the symptoms. Dantrolene acts by decreasing the intracellular Ca^{2+} concentration [30]. Several studies suggest a direct interaction between dantrolene and RyR1, and it is thought that dantrolene directly prevents Ca^{2+} release through RyR1 [31, 32].

The first link between MH and RyR1 came through a related disorder in pigs, known as porcine stress syndrome (PSS). It was found that the pig RyR1 mutation R615C underlies PSS [33], and soon after the corresponding mutation in humans was linked to MH [34].

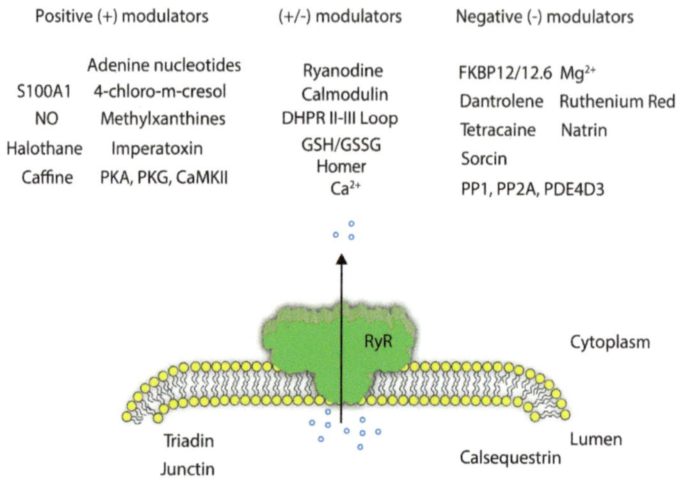

Figure 2. Regulation of RyRs. RyRs are regulated by a number of postive and negative modulators from both the cytoplasmic and SR luminal sides. S100A1: S100 calcium-binding protein A1; NO: nitric oxide; PKA: cAMP-dependent protein kinase; PKG: cGMP-dependent protein kinase; CaMKII: Ca^{2+}/calmodulin-dependent protein kinase II; DHPR: dihydropyridine receptor/L-type voltage-dependent calcium channel; GSH: glutathione; GSSG: glutathione disulfide; FKBP12/12.6: FK506 binding protein 12/12.6; PP1: protein phosphatase 1; PP2A: protein phosphatase 2; PDE4D3: cAMP-specific 3',5'-cyclic phosphodiesterase 4D3.

2.2. Core myopathies

Central core disease (CCD) is a congenital myopathy, characterized by progressive muscle weakness and the presence of metabolically inactive tissue (cores) in the center of muscle fibers. These cores lack mitochondria and the myofibrillar organization is disrupted. The common phenotype of CCD includes muscle atrophy, floppy infant syndrome and skeletal muscle deformities [35, 36]. It was found early on that there is a connection between CCD and MH susceptibility [37], and some RyR1 mutations have been found to cause both. Multi-mini core disease (MmD) is another inherited congenital myopathy. Different from CCD, whose inheritance is autosomal dominant, MmD is usually considered recessive [35]. As its name suggests, MmD is characterized by the presence of multiple not-well-defined cores in muscle fibers. MmD can cause axial muscle weakness that can lead to severe scoliosis [35]. Although MmD is mainly associated with mutations in RyR1 [38], mutations in selenoprotein N 1 [39], a protein required for RyR1 calcium release [40], and α-actin (ACTA1) [41] have also been found to underlie MmD.

2.3. Catecholaminergic polymorphic ventricular tachycardia

Also known as CPVT, this disorder manifests itself in young individuals, with either syncope or sudden cardiac death as the first symptom. Many affected individuals will develop cardiac arrhythmias that are triggered by exercise or emotional stress. CPVT is mostly detected through stress tests, which indicate bidirectional ventricular tachycardia. Typically no morphological abnormalities of the myocardium are detected. The disease is mostly due to mutations in the cardiac RyR2 isoform [42], but mutations in the associated proteins calsequestrin [43] and triadin [44] can also be the cause. As CPVT is triggered by β-adrenergic stimulation, it can be treated by β-blockers [45]. Flecainide, a sodium channel blocker, has also been found to be beneficial for CPVT patients [46].

Now more than 20 years since the initial identification of the first RyR disease mutations, nearly 500 mutations have been found in RyR1 and RyR2 combined. In RyR1, most disease mutations seem to be spread across the gene, with some clustering in distinct areas, whereas in RyR2, most mutations are found in one of 3 or 4 different disease hot spots (Figure 3). The appearance of clusters may be due to bias in sequencing, as historically only the areas that had already shown to be involved in disease were being considered for sequence analysis.

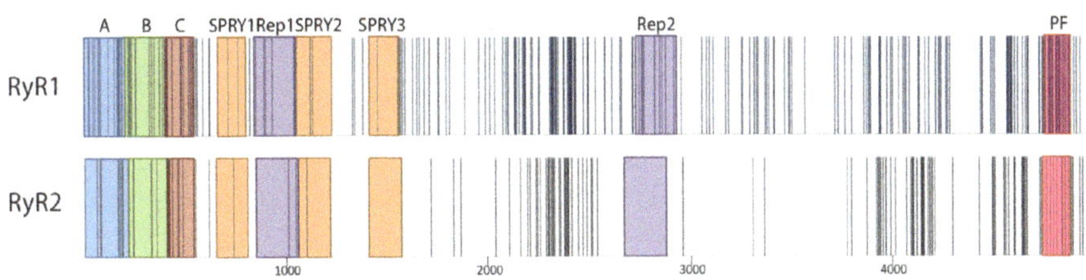

Figure 3. Disease hot spots. Linear view of the RyR1 and RyR2 sequences with each vertical line representing a disease mutation. The areas of solid colors correspond to domains A(blue), B (green), C (red), SPRY (orange), Tandem Repeat domains (Rep) (purple) and Pore-forming domain (PF) (pink).

3. Functional studies

Although increasing numbers of RyR mutations are identified in patients and their family members, only a handful of them have been validated as causative disease mutations [29]. Functional studies are necessary to prove the molecular basis of the mutations as pathogenic. Without functional characterizations, the possibility that the mutations are the result of polymorphism cannot be ruled out. In this section, different methods of performing functional studies and their results are highlighted.

3.1. Model systems

There are a variety of ways to prepare model systems to study functional effects of mutations in RyRs: endogenous or recombinant expression systems and *in vivo* models.

In the early days, before and shortly after the discovery of RyR mutations in MH-susceptible pigs and individuals, SR vesicles were prepared from muscle biopsies [47-55]. SR vesicles from non-MH-susceptible animals or individuals were also obtained to serve as controls. These are endogenous expression systems since SR vesicles contain RyRs, and therefore, can be used as a whole or can be further purified to obtain single RyR channels. These approaches can be invasive, as they involve acquisition of native RyRs expressed in patients or knock-in mice carrying mutations. For example, skeletal myotubes have been isolated from MH-susceptible and/or CCD patients [56-59]. Both RyR1 and RyR2 can be studied by isolating skeletal myotubes and cardiomyocytes from knock-in mice, respectively [60-73]. Flexor digitorum brevis fibers, present in the feet, have also been derived from knock-in mice for the study of RyR1 mutations [67, 74-76]. In some cases, measures have been taken to alleviate some of the affliction on obtaining native RyRs from patients by using less invasive approaches. In one study of a CCD-associated RyR1 mutation, fibroblasts from a CCD patient were differentiated into muscle by myoD conversion with adenovirus [77]. In other cases, immortalized lymphoblastoid cells were generated using B-lymphocytes isolated from blood samples [78-83].

A more commonly used model is a recombinant expression system. By using cells that lack the native expression of RyRs, all results will arise only from the mutant RyR. One of the most commonly used systems are dyspedic myotubes, which are derived from mice that lack RyR1, called "RyR1-null mice" [80, 84-90]. Also commonly used are human embryonic kidney (HEK)-293 cells. HEK-293 cells not only lack native RyR expression but also lack other complexes involved in E-C coupling and yet have been demonstrated to express functional RyR when its cDNA is transfected [19, 79, 80, 89-115]. Other cell lines used in functional studies include COS-7 [116], myoblastic C_2C_{12} [117], HL-1 cardiomyocytes [108, 110, 115, 118], and CHO cells [119].

Finally, knock-in mice have served as valuable models for the study of mutations in RyR1 and RyR2 [60-64, 66-76, 120-128]. The comparison between mice that are homozygous or heterozygous for the mutation in question has provided clues about the gene dosage effects. Studying the effect of mutations on the body as a whole provides insights that are more relevant to clinical phenotypes.

3.2. Methods

Multiple techniques have been implemented to study mutant RyRs from different expression systems. Five major methods are introduced here.

One way to measure Ca^{2+} release through RyR channels is through [$^{45}Ca^{2+}$]-uptake and -release assays [50, 52, 98]. Microsomal vesicles expressing recombinant RyR and SERCA1a are prepared. The vesicles are then incubated with $^{45}Ca^{2+}$, during which SERCA1a pumps $^{45}Ca^{2+}$ into the vesicles. By comparing the amount of $^{45}Ca^{2+}$ accumulation in the presence or absence of the potent RyR inhibitor Ruthenium Red, the amount of Ca^{2+} release through RyR can be determined.

A more widely used technique is a Ca^{2+} fluorescence assay involving whole cell samples (Figure 4A,B) [19, 57-59, 70, 71, 73, 77, 79, 89, 91-93, 95, 102, 104-106, 108, 109, 112, 113, 115-118]. Cells with either endogenous or recombinant expression of RyR are loaded with a fluorescent Ca^{2+} indicator, such as fura-2, which diffuses throughout the cytoplasm. By measuring fluorescence with confocal microscopy, resting [Ca^{2+}] levels in the cytoplasm, as well as frequency, duration, and extent of Ca^{2+} release from RyR can be calculated.

Commonly used is a [^{3}H]ryanodine binding assay (Figure 4C) [19, 51, 54, 60, 67, 77, 79, 86, 90, 92, 93, 95, 96, 103, 105, 108, 113, 129]. SR vesicles containing endogenous or recombinant RyR are incubated with radioactive [^{3}H]ryanodine. Since ryanodine binds to the channels in the open state, binding of [^{3}H]ryanodine is indicative of the measure of open channels. The extent of RyR activation is then measured by radioactive counting.

As opposed to whole-cell measurements, activities of a single channel can be recorded using planar lipid bilayer electrophysiology (Figure 4D) [19, 53, 54, 67, 69, 77, 79, 99-101, 105, 107, 108, 111, 112, 114]. Recombinant or endogenous RyR from crude SR vesicle preparations or from purified material are fused into an artificial lipid bilayer formed across two chambers. The current generated by ions passing through the channel is recorded. This method allows various properties of the single channel to be determined, including the open probability, duration of the open and closed time, and conductance. The two chambers can resemble cytoplasmic and luminal sides of the channel, allowing the studies of Ca^{2+}-induced Ca^{2+} release (CICR) from the cytoplasmic side or store-overload-induced Ca^{2+} release (SOICR) from the luminal side. The planar lipid bilayer technique also allows for additional control because purified auxiliary proteins or pharmacological modulators can be added to either side.

3.3. Highlight of the results

Functional studies of mutant RyR channels have generated multitudes of insights into the molecular basis of the RyR channelopathies. Accordingly, complex sets of results have been generated that require careful interpretation and have resulted in a lot of debate. For example, many mutations seem to make the RyR channels more active, but the exact nature of this change is still under scrutiny. In some cases, mutations seem to be more sensitive to cytosolic activators, while other evidence suggests they are more sensitive to luminal Ca^{2+} levels. Others suggest that altered phosphorylation states of the channel or affinity to auxiliary proteins is the causative mechanism. For this section, results of the functional studies are highlighted as mutations that cause RyRs to be either hypersensitive (more prone to open upon stimulation) or hyposensitive (requiring more stimulus to open). RyR mutations can be pathogenic either through hyper- or hypo-activity since alteration in Ca^{2+} homeostasis in either direction can cause aberrant muscle functions. Yet other mutations have exhibited no apparent alterations in the functional studies performed so far. The results are summarized in Table 1.

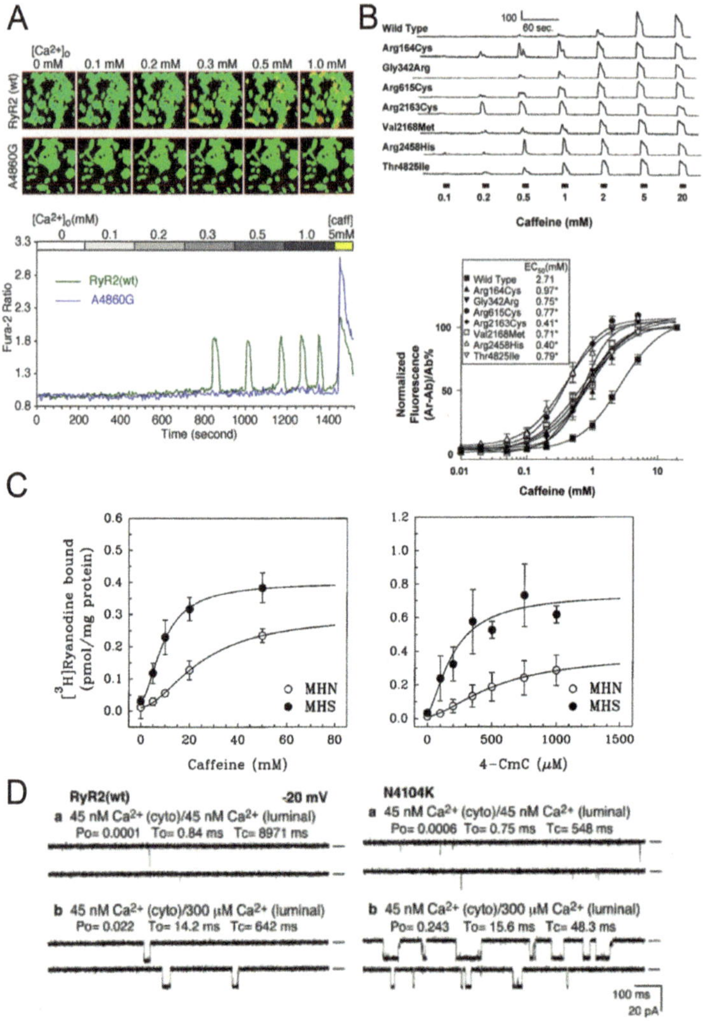

Figure 4. Representative figures from exemplary functional studies. (A) Single-cell fluorescent Ca^{2+} images of HEK-293 cells expressing RyR2 WT and A4860G at various extracellular $[Ca^{2+}]$ (*top*) and fura-2 ratios of representative RyR2 WT and A4860G cells (*bottom*)[110]. (B) Representative single-cell fluorescent traces of Ca2+ release stimulated by incremental doses of caffeine in dyspedic myotubes transfected with RyR1 WT and mutants cDNAs (*top*) and corresponding sigmoidal dose-response curves (*bottom*)[86]. (C) [^{3}H]ryanodine binding assay on SR vesicles from MHN (malignant-hyperthermia non-suceptible, or RyR1 WT) and MHS (malignant-hyperthermia suceptible, or RyR1 G2434R) individuals in presence of caffeine (*left*) and 4-CmC (*right*)[55]. (D) Single-channel activities of RyR2 WT and N4104K recorded in planar lipid bilayers with luminal $[Ca^{2+}]$ of 45nM (*a*) or 300nM (*b*). Downward strokes in the current traces denote channel-opening events[19].

Effect	Isoform	Mutations	Disease	References	Mutations	Disease	References
Hyperactive	RyR1	C35R	MH	[91, 94]	R2355W	MH	[58]
		R163C	MH/CCD/MmD	[61, 65-67, 85, 86, 91, 94, 103]	E2371G	MH	[82]
					G2375A	MH	[58]
		G248R	MH	[91, 94, 103]	G2434R	MH	[1,2,36]
		R328W	MH	[97]	R2435H	MH/CCD	[85, 91, 94]
		G341R	MH	[86, 91, 94]	R2435L	MH/CCD	[77, 88]
		H382N	MH	[83]	I2453T	MH/CCD	[57]
		I403M	MH/CCD	[91, 94]	R2454H	MH/CCD	[82]
		Y522S	MH/CCD	[60, 63, 64, 85, 87, 89, 91, 94, 120]	R2458C	MH	[91, 94]
					R2458H	MH	[86, 91, 94]
		R530H	MH	[82]	R2458H/R3348C	MH	[59]
		R552W	MH	[91, 94]	R2508C	MH/CCD	[102]
		A612P	MH	[59]	R2508G	MH	[83]
		R614C	MH	[47-52, 54, 86, 88, 89, 91, 94, 101, 116, 117, 129]	ΔR4214_F4216	CCD	[80]
					T4637A	CCD	[88]
		R614L	MH	[91, 94]	Y4796C	CCD	[87, 88]
		E1058K	MH	[83]	T4826I	MH	[76, 86, 103, 122]
		K1393R	MH	[83]	H4833Y	MH	[81, 103]
		R1679H	MH	[83]	R4861H	CCD	[78]
		R2163C	MH	[86, 88, 91, 94]	ΔF4863_D4869	CCD	[79]
		R2163H	MH/CCD	[85, 88, 91, 94]	R4893W	CCD	[78]
		R2163P	MH	[82]	A4894T	MH	[104]
		V2168M	MH	[86]	I4898T	CCD	[78, 89, 93]
		T2206M	MH	[56]	G4899R	CCD	[78]
		N2283H	CCD/MmD	[99]			
		N2342S	MH	[82]			
		ΔE2347	MH	[88]			
		A2350T	MH	[58, 96]			
	RyR2	ΔExon 3	CPVT	[115]	N2386I	ARVD2	[106, 109]
		A77V	CPVT/ARVD2	[115]	R2474S	CPVT	[48,125,54]
		R176Q	ARVD2	[106, 126-128]	T2504M	ARVD2	[106]
		R176Q/T2504M	ARVD2	[108, 109, 112, 115]	N4104K	CPVT	[19, 118, 119]
		E189D	CPVT	[113]	Q4201R	CPVT	[107, 108, 112]
		G230C	CPVT	[114]	R4497C	CPVT	[19, 68, 71, 72, 105, 118, 119, 123, 124]
		R420W	ARVD2	[115]			
		L433P	ARVD2	[108, 109, 115]	S4565R	CPVT	[111]
		S2246L	CPVT	[48,50,56-58]	V4653F	CPVT	[107, 112]
		R2267H	CPVT	[111]	I4867M	CPVT	[108]

Effect	Isoform	Mutations	Disease	References	Mutations	Disease	References
		P2328S	CPVT	[52, 54, 55]	N4895D	CPVT	[19]
Hypoactive	RyR1	S71Y/N2283H	CCD/MmD	[99]	I4898T	CCD	[7,12,13,46,70,73,74, 75]
		R109W/M485V	CCD/MmD	[99, 100]	G4899R	CCD	[87, 100, 103]
		C4664R	MH	[82]	G4899E	CCD	[98, 100]
		G4891R	CCD	[87]	A4906V	CCD	[87]
		R4893W	CCD	[87, 98]	R4914G	CCD	[87]
		A4894P	CNMDU1	[104]	ΔV4927_I4928	CCD	[80, 100]
	RyR2	L433P	ARVD2	[106]	A4860G	IVF	[110, 112]
		A1107M	CPVT	[115]			
		(T1107M)					
Uncertain effects	RyR1	I403M A1577T/	MH/CCD	[85]	G3938A (G3938D)	MH	[95]
		G2060C	CCD	[99]		MH	[92]
		R2939K	MmD	[90]	D3986A		
					(D3986E)		
	RyR2						

Table 1. Summary from functional studies on RyR disease-associated mutations. Mutations that alter RyR functions are listed as hyperactive or hypoactive. Mutations with no discernable change compared with wild type channel are listed as "uncertain." References to the functional studies are listed beside the corresponding mutations. (Δ) = deletion mutation. (/) = double mutation. Amino residue numbering is for human RyRs. (MH) = Malignant hyperthermia, (CCD) = central core disease, (MmD) = multi-minicore disease, (CNMDU1) = congenital neuromuscular disease with uniform type 1 fiber, (CPVT) = catecholaminergic polymorphic ventricular tachycardia, (ARVD2) = arrhythmogenic right ventricular dysplasia type 2, and (IVF) = idiopathic ventricular fibrillation.

The majority of the mutations in both RyR1 and RyR2 have been shown to make the channels hyperactive. This includes the first disease-associated mutation found in porcine stress syndrome, RyR1 R615C. Functional studies have revealed that RyR1 channels with this mutation have significantly lowered threshold for activation by [Ca^{2+}], caffeine, and halothane compared to wild-type channels, while having markedly increased threshold for inactivation by [Ca^{2+}], Ruthenium Red, or Mg^{2+} ions [47-52, 101, 116, 117, 129]. These results are characteristic of mutations that alter RyRs into hypersensitive channels [19, 55-59, 61, 63, 65, 67-69, 71, 73, 76-83, 85-89, 91, 93, 94, 96, 97, 102-109, 111-115, 118, 119]. RyRs that are hyperactive are often described as "leaky," and on top of their increased sensitivity towards activators or reduced sensitivity towards inhibitors, they often exhibit increased resting [Ca^{2+}] in the cytoplasm, reduced SR Ca^{2+} store content, or altered maximal Ca^{2+} release.

Although less common, some mutations in RyR have been demonstrated to reduce channel activity. [62, 74, 75, 80, 82, 84, 87, 89, 98, 100, 103, 104, 106, 110, 112, 115]. For example, the I4898T mutation in RyR1, associated with an unusually severe and highly penetrant form of CCD, has been shown to cause complete uncoupling of sarcolemmal excitation from SR Ca^{2+} release, in which activating signals from L-type Ca_V channels to RyR1 are uncoupled [84]. It has also been shown that the I4898T mutation leads to a complete loss of Ca^{2+} release induced by caffeine stimulation [89]. Many other CCD-associated mutations that are located at the predicted pore region of RyR1 (G4890R, R4892W, A4894P,

I4897T, G4898R, G4898E, A4905V, and R4913G) have also been shown to abolish E-C coupling and/or exhibit reduced sensitivity to activation by [Ca^{2+}], caffeine, or 4-CmC [62, 87, 98, 100, 103, 104]. Mutations that disrupt signaling between the L-type Ca_V and RyR are known as "E-C uncoupling" mutations. In RyR2, fewer mutations have thus far been associated with a reduction in activity, suggesting that a loss of function in RyR2 may be less tolerated than in RyR1. The A4860G mutation in RyR2 is associated with idiopathic ventricular fibrillation (IVF) and is located at the predicted inner pore helix. It has been shown to diminish response or increase the threshold for activation by SOICR [110, 112]. Furthermore, the mouse RyR2 A1107M mutation (corresponding to the T1107M mutation that is associated with hypertrophic cardiomyopathy in humans) has been shown to increase the threshold for Ca^{2+} release termination [115].

Effects of some other disease-associated mutations are less apparent. For instance, single channel measurements of RyR1 A1577T and G2060C mutant channel produced no discernible change in the activity of the channel compared to wild type [99]. Similarly, [^{3}H] ryanodine binding assays of RyR1 R2939K expressed in HEK-293 cells failed to show alteration in Ca^{2+} dependence and caffeine activation compared to wild-type channel [90]. In addition, RyR1 I404M expressed in dyspedic mice myotubes exhibited resting [Ca^{2+}] levels and SR Ca^{2+} content comparable to that of the wild type [85]. Furthermore, expressions of RyR1 D3987A and G3939A rabbit cDNA in HEK-293 cells, which correspond to the positions of MH-associated mutations D3986E and G3938D in humans, respectively, showed responses to activation by [Ca^{2+}], caffeine, and 4-CmC comparable to that of wild type [92, 95]. For these mutations where no clear functional effect has been observed, it is of course possible that they are not causative of the disease but, instead, simply represent polymorphisms. Alternatively, their effect may only become apparent in the native context, where particular regulatory mechanisms exist that are not captured by the model systems.

Overall, there is an apparent theme between RyR activity and disease phenotype. MH and CPVT are associated with RyRs that have an overall gain-of-function phenotype. On the other hand, CCD can be due to either a gain or a loss of RyR1 activity. Loss of function results in impaired Ca^{2+} release, and hence decreased contractility observed in CCD. The gain of RyR1 activity can lead to a general "leak" of Ca^{2+}, resulting in an overall lowered concentration of Ca^{2+} in the SR. The result is then an insufficient amount of Ca^{2+} being available for an E-C coupling event, again resulting in decreased contractility.

For those mutations with less clear effects, as well as those which have been shown to be causative for aberrant Ca^{2+} homeostasis, combining functional studies with structural investigations would provide further useful insight into the molecular basis of disease-associated mutations in RyRs.

4. Structural studies of RyRs

Structural biology has thrived in recent decades and provides researchers with powerful tools for exploring all aspects of life. Different structural techniques, covering the resolution range from 50 Å down to 1 Å, can reveal the structural details of various bio-molecules, from large protein/DNA/RNA complex to small peptides, which help to improve our understanding of the physiology and pathology of many biological systems.

However, the large size of the RyR and its membrane protein nature make it a very challenging target for structural studies. Most structural techniques require protein samples with high yield and purity, which is normally achieved by overexpression in recombinant systems combined with multi-step chromatography purification processes. The large size of the RyR makes the recombinant expression difficult because the folding of this giant requires the assistance of many chaperones which are often absent in non-native expression systems. The differences in the protein trafficking and post-translational modification systems may also affect the maturation of the recombinant RyR. The alternative way is to purify RyRs from native tissues, but the purification is not easy without artificial affinity tags. To further complicate the issue, the presence of a large exposed hydrophobic surface in the transmembrane region requires the addition of detergents to make the protein soluble during the purification. The denaturing property of the detergents usually makes the sample less homogenous and their presence also affects the crystal packing, both of which are undesirable for x-ray crystallography. The intrinsic dynamic feature of this multi-domain channel further increases heterogeneity of the sample and makes it harder to study.

Despite all the technical difficulties, during the last two decades, several structures of RyRs have been obtained using cryo-electron microscopy (cryo-EM) [130-141], NMR [142] and X-ray crystallography [143-148]. Some of these structures [142, 143] describe how regulatory proteins interact with small fragments (peptides) from RyRs and are not relevant to the theme of this book. Here we will focus on the structures of the full-length channel or large domains where disease mutations are localized, and show how the structural studies can reveal the molecular mechanism of a genetic disease. More details on the structural insights into RyR function have been described in a recent review paper [149].

4.1. Cryo-EM studies of RyRs

Electron microscopy has been able to obtain structural information on RyRs at near subnanometer resolution. The early studies using thin-section or negative stain electron microscopy discovered some "feet" structures (square-shaped densities) in the junction region between the SR and T-tubules in muscle tissues [150-157]. The identities of these "feet" were confirmed later when the purified RyRs were imaged by EM, showing similar densities [9]. The negative stain structures with improved resolution revealed that RyRs have a four-fold symmetry and can interact with four neighbouring molecules to form two-dimensional checkerboard-like lattices both in native tissue and in vitro [158-162], suggesting that RyRs may interact cooperatively during gating. The resolution was further improved by the cryo-EM technique [130-141], in which the protein samples are studied under cryogenic temperatures. So far the highest resolution reaches 9.6 Å for RyR1 in a reported closed state.

Many structural details can be appreciated from the cryo-EM structures. The overall shape of the RyR is like a mushroom with a large cap in the cytoplasmic domain (27 × 27 × 12 nm) and a small stem (12 × 12 × 6 nm) crossing the ER/SR membrane. Instead of a single rigid block, the large "cap" consists of fifteen individual globular regions per subunit with many solvent channels in between [163, 164] (Figure 5A,B). This arrangement maximizes the total exposed surface area, and RyRs thus form perfect scaffolds for many small molecules and protein regulators to dock. The number of transmembrane (TM) helices in the "stem" is still controversial at the current resolution. Five or six TM helices can be detected in the cryoEM maps [134, 141], but it has been suggested that the total number should be either 6 or 8 [165]. The last two TM helices create the pore-forming domain, which is homologous to the ones from tetrameric potassium channels and bacterial sodium channels [141].

Comparison of the RyR structures in the closed and open states reveals movement in both the "cap" region and "stem" region upon channel gating. An iris-like movement around the pore switches the channel between dilated and constricted conformations [166] (Figure 5C,D). Samso *et al.* systematically produced RyR structures in the closed and open states and found the inner helices in the TM region to kink in the open state, increasing the diameter of the pore by ~4 Å [132]. However, another group reported that the inner helics are already kinked in the closed state [141]. The discrepancy can be attributed to differences in sample preparation. Although the conditions may favor a closed or open channel when the RyR is in a membrane, this may not be the case after extraction with detergents. In addition, the amount of oxidation in the sample can also affect the open probability of the channel. It is therefore possible that the 9.6Å map represents an open, rather than a closed channel, and this would reconcile the discrepancies between both studies. So far, most cryo-EM studies are done on RyR1 due to its relatively high abundance. RyR2 and RyR3 have also been studied via cryo-EM [137, 138], albeit at lower resolution. The overall folding is similar for all three isoforms. The major difference between RyR1 and RyR2 is the clamp region on the corner of the "cap" [138], while a central domain (possibly corresponding to the residues 1303-1406 in RyR1), which is missing in RyR3, is the most divergent part between RyR1 and RyR3 [137]. These structural elements very likely contribute to the different properties of the three subtypes.

The cryo-EM studies of RyRs thus far do not provide the resolution to locate individual residues as X-ray crystallography does, but it can give clues about the approximate locations of individual domains through analysis of the difference densities from insertion of fusion proteins (such as GFP) or binding of antibodies for the particular domain. The locations of the three disease hot spots have drawn particular interest since these parts are certainly important for channel function, as the clustering of disease-associated mutations suggests. From the primary sequence analysis, it is clear that the third hot spot is in the transmembrane region ("stem") of the channel. Several insertion studies localize the N-terminal disease hot spot at the clamp region between the subdomain 5 and 9 [31, 167-169], and the central hot spot between the subdomain 5 and 6 [170], suggesting that these two hot spots interact with each other [171] (Figure 5A,B). Similar methods were also used to localize the divergent regions [172-176] and the phosphorylation sites [177, 178]. The accuracy of these studies varies depending on the resolution, linker length, insertion site selection and the size of the fusion protein or antibody. Difference densities analysis was also used to identify the binding sites of protein regulators, such as FKBP12/12.6 [133, 179-181], calmodulin [180, 182, 183], chloride intracellular channel 2 (CLIC-2) [184] and various toxins [185, 186].

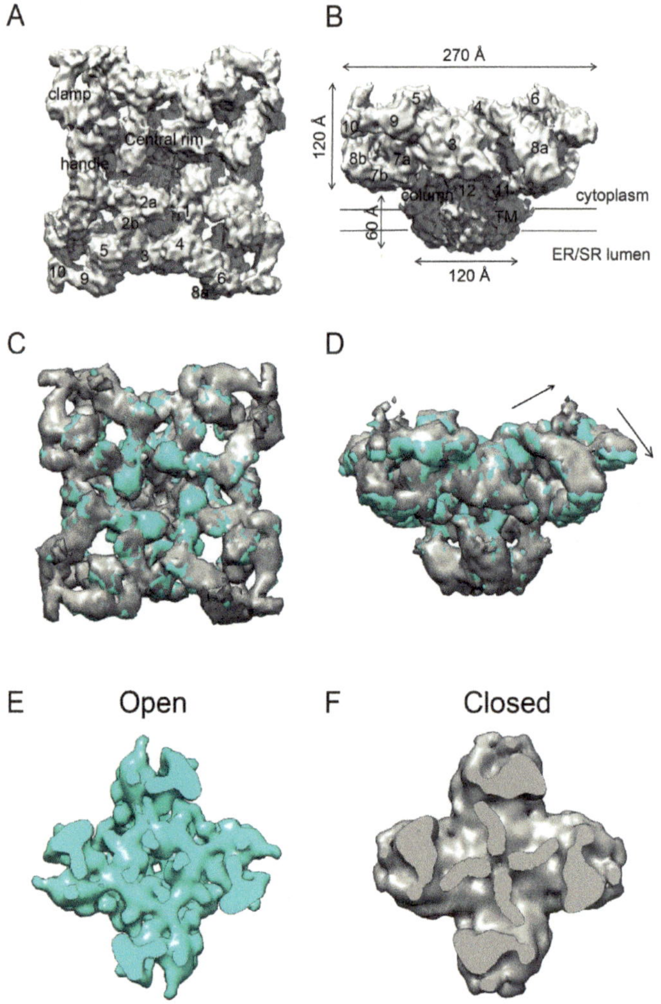

Figure 5. EM maps of RyRs. Top pannels show the top view (A) and side view (B) of the cryo-EM reconstruction of RyR1 in the closed state at 9.6Å (EMDB accession code 1275) [141]. The structural elements and the subregions are labeled. Middle pannels show the top view (C) and side view (D) of the superposition of the RyR1 cryo-EM maps in the closed (gray) and open (cyan) state. (EMDB accession codes 1606 and 1607) [132]. The structural change upon channel opening is indicated by the arrows. Bottom panels show a comparison of the transmembrane region of RyR1 in the open (E) (cyan EMDB accession codes 1606) and closed state (gray EMDB accession codes 1607).

4.2. X-ray crystallographic studies of RyRs

The crystallization of full-length RyRs is a very challenging task due to its large size, membrane protein nature and intrinsic flexibility. Improvement in techniques will likely reveal a high-resolution structure of intact RyRs in the future. The cryo-EM structures have revealed that the RyR is a large modular protein that consists of many small domains. Many efforts have therefore been made to crystallize individual domains or domain clusters that carry important functions.

The first few crystal structures of RyRs that have been solved are of the N-terminal domains (domain A) in RyR1 (residues 1-205) and RyR2 (residues 1-217) [144, 145]. Both display a β-trefoil folding motif (three groups of β-strands that form a triangle structure) that consists of twelve β strands and contains an extra α helix (Figure 6A,B). Domain A spans about one third of the N-terminal disease hot spot. A total of 23 and 9 mutations have been found so far in domain A of RyR1 and RyR2, respectively, many of which cluster in a loop between β strands 8 and 9. Several disease mutants of this domain have been analyzed either by NMR or x-ray crystallography, but none of them showed major structural changes [144, 145] (Figure 7A,B). The observation that most mutations are located on the surface of domain A indicates that they likely affect the interaction of domain A with other domains in RyR or auxiliary proteins.

A severe form of CPVT is caused by the deletion of the entire exon 3 (residues 57-91) from the *ryr2* gene [187, 188]. The structure of wild type domain A shows that exon 3 contributes to a loop region, the 3_{10} helix, β4 strand, and the α helix. One would expect that the complete absence of these structural elements will cause the misfolding of the domain and a loss-of-function phenotype. However, surprisingly, Δexon 3 is not strictly lethal. CPVT symptoms and functional studies suggest a gain-of-function phenotype instead [115]. Even more surprising, the mutant has a higher thermal stability compared to the wild type domain [145]. A crystal structure of RyR2 domain A with Δexon 3 revealed an unusual "structural rescue" scheme: a flexible loop following the exon 3 region replaces the deleted β4 strand and results in a similar overall fold of the domain [147] (Figure 7C). The α helix, however, is lost. The ability to "rescue" a β strand with a random loop segment is highly unusual and suggests that there has been evolutionary pressure to maintain the exact sequence of the flexible loop. Most likely, there is the possibility of alternative splicing, whereby exon 3 is naturally spliced in some cell types. This would represent a mechanism whereby the RyR activity can be fine-tuned in a tissue-specific manner [147]. So far, such a splice variant has not yet been reported.

Up to now, the largest reported crystal structure for all RyRs is for the N-terminal three domains (domain A, B and C, residues 1-559) of RyR1, which covers the majority of the N-terminal disease hot spot [146]. It shows a triangular arrangement of the three domains that interact with each other, mainly through hydrophilic interfaces. Domains A and B have similar β-trefoil folding motifs, while domain C has an armadillo-repeat structure consisting of a bundle of five α-helices (Figure 6C). A total of 76 mutations (RyR1+RyR2) have been identified in these domains. 17 of these are localized at the interfaces between domains A, B and

C (within one subunit). 9 mutations are buried inside the individual domains, and the remaining are on the surface of the ABC structure.

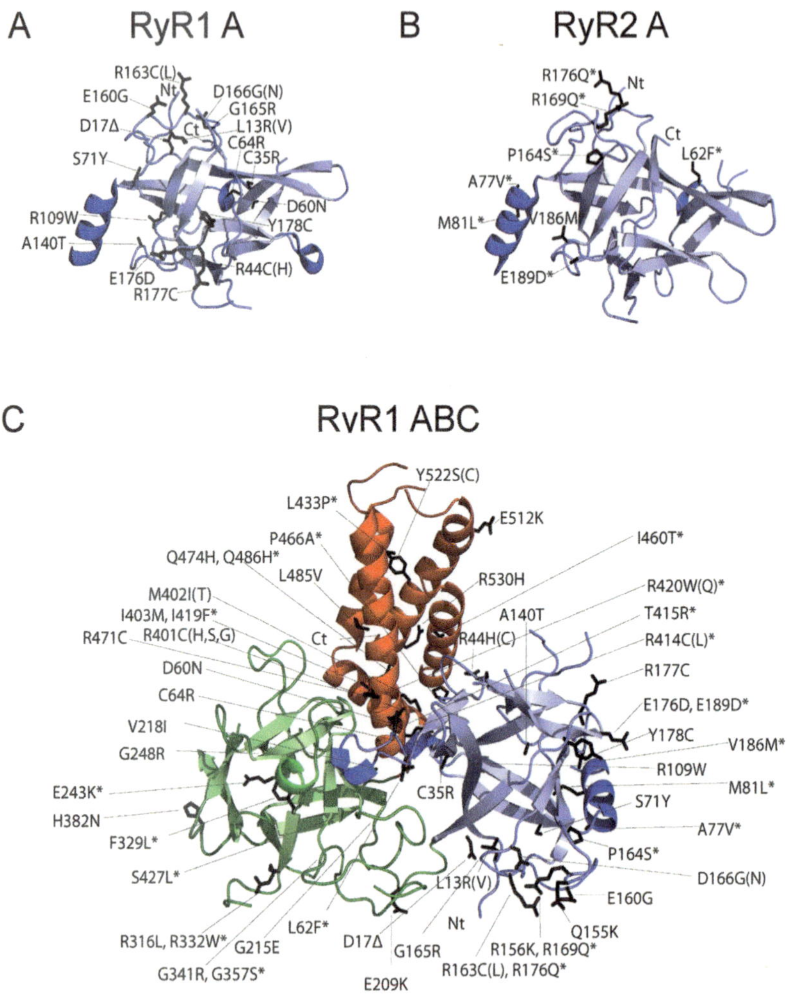

Figure 6. Crystal structures of RyR N-teminal hot spot domains. Shown are crystal structures of (A) RyR1 domain A (pdb: 3ILA), (B) RyR2 domain A (pdb: 3IM5), and (C) RyR1 domain ABC (pdb: 2XOA). α-helices and β-sheets are shown in dark and light colors, respectvely. RyR1 and RyR2 mutations are mapped on the strutural models, indicated by black sticks, and labeled. RyR2 mutations are distinguished from RyR1 mutations by *. Deletion mutations are labeled by Δ. The numbering is according to human RyR1 and RyR2 sequences. The N-terminal and C-terminal positions of the structures are labeled with Nt and Ct, respectively.

Although the EM structure itself usually does not provide the resolution to resolve the atomic positions, the combination of crystal structures and EM structures allows pseudo-atomic models to be built. Individual amino acid residues can thus be located within the overall 3D structure. The high-resolution crystal structures can be docked into the EM maps by matching their electron densities using complex 6 dimensional search algorithms [189-191]. The confidence of the solutions depends on the quality of the EM map, the size of the docked fragments and the agreement of conformations from the two structures. Sometimes a Laplacian filter, which uses an edge-detection algorithm to increase the sensitivity can increase the success rate when a small fragment is used as a search model [191]. Docking of the RyR1 ABC crystal structure into three different cryo-EM maps places it at the same location, the central rim region, forming a cytoplasmic vestibule around the four-fold symmetry axis (Figure 10) [146]. This solution contradicts previous results from insertion experiments which localize the N-terminal hot spot at the clamp region near the corner [167, 168]. The authors suggested that in the GFP-insertion study [168] the long linker and the native flexible loop make it possible for the inserted GFP to be present in a remote location [146]. In addition, the difference density observed in a GST-insertion study splits into two regions, one of which is indeed right beside the central rim region [167]. Interestingly, the location and orientation of domains ABC from the IP_3 receptor, a closely related Ca^{2+}-release channel, are remarkably similar to the docking solution of RyR1 ABC, which further validates the location of the N-terminal region [192].

Locating the N-terminal region within intact RyRs allows several new interfaces to be identified. As the ABC domains dock near the 4-fold symmetry axis, there is a direct interaction between domains A and B from neighboring subunits (Figure 10). In addition, there are five other interfaces between the ABC domains and other regions of RyR1. All the peripheric disease mutations identified in domains ABC are located in one of these six interfaces and none of them are exposed to the surface of the full-length channel, suggesting that they mainly affect the inter-domain interactions rather than interactions between the RyR and other proteins.

The activity of RyRs can be regulated by different types of kinases and phosphotases (Figure 1 and 2). It is believed that the chronic hyperphosphorylation of RyR2 by PKA can dissociate the binding of FKBP12.6 and cause heart failure [193-195], although this result has not been confirmed by other laboratories [118, 196, 197]. Two recent papers reported the structures of a domain containing the phosphorylation sites from all three RyR isoforms [148], and from RyR1 [198] (Figure 8A,B,C). The domain consists of two symmetric halves. Each half contains two α helices, one or more short 3_{10} helices, and a C-terminal β strand. Multiple phosphorylation sites were identified in this domain of RyR2 [148] and most cluster within the same loop. The RyR2 domain doesn't contain any reported disease mutations, but up to 11 disease mutations are found in the RyR1 domain. Interestingly, several disease mutations from this domain are also located close to the phosphorylation sites, suggesting that phosphorylation and disease mutations at this site may have the same effect (Figure 8A). One mutation, L2867G, reduces the melting temperature of the individual domain by 13°C and causes the aggregation of the domain at room temperature (Figure 7D). Several crystal structures for the other disease mutants were also reported in this study, showing that they affect surface properties and intradomain salt bridges (Figure 7E,F,G) [148]. Docking into the EM map places this domain in the clamp region, but none of the neighbouring domains have been identified thus far (Figure 10). Solving structures of other domains may place more pieces into this big jigsaw and increase our understanding of the isolated domains.

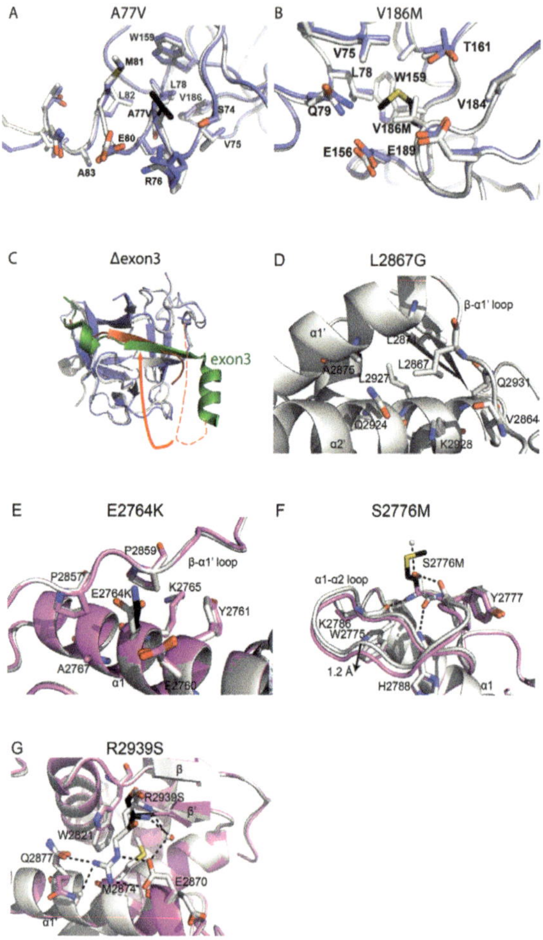

Figure 7. Disease mutant crystal structures. Superposition of the wild-type RyR domains (white) with the mutant structures (colors). Atoms are color coded, with nitrogens in blue, oxygens in red, and sulfurs in yellow. Hydrogen bonds are indicated by dashed lines. All mutants are from RyR1 except the Δexon3 mutant (C) which is from RyR2. (A) A77V, (B) V186M, (C) Δexon3, (D) L2867G mutant (only wild-type structure shown), (E) E2764K, (F) S2776M, (G) R2939S. The single residue mutations are indicated in black. In panel (C), exon 3 is shown in green, and the flexible loop that replaces exon 3 in Δexon3 structure (pdb: 3QR5), is shown in red.

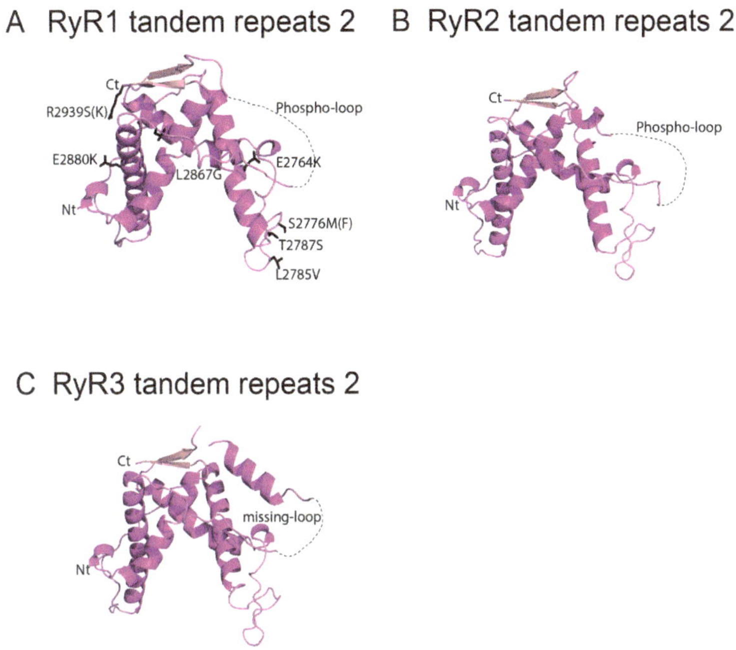

Figure 8. Crystal structures of RyR phosphorylation domains. (A-C) RyR1-3 phosphorylation (tandem repeats 2) domains (pdb: 4ERT, 4ETV, 4ERV, respectively). The phosphorylation loops in RyR1/2 and the corresponding loop in RyR3 are missing in the crystal structures, and indicated by dashed lines in the figures. α-helices and β-sheets are shown in dark and light colors, respectvely. RyR1 mutations are mapped on the strutural models, indicated by black sticks, and labeled. The numbering is according to human RyR1 sequence. The N-terminal and C-terminal positions of the structures are labeled with Nt and Ct, respectively.

4.3. Homology models for RyR domains

So far all the available crystal structures cover ~15% of the full-length RyR in total. There is still a big portion missing. One alternative way to obtain structural informaiton is to create homology models based on known structures using bioinformatics methods. Generally the reliability of a homology model depends on the sequence identities between two proteins, but protein 3D structures tend to be more conserved than their primary sequences during evolution [199]. As the largest ion channel, the evolution of modular RyRs involves the incorporation, loss and duplication of different domains. Protein sequence analysis identifies several domains that are present multiple times in RyR genes, including SPRY domains and tandem repeat domains.

The spore lysis A and RyR (SPRY) domains have been found in many different proteins from bacteria, archaea, viruses and eukaryotes. They are generally known as protein interaction domains [200]. There are three SPRY domains identified in metazoan RyR genes

(SPRY1,2,3) (Figure 3). In skeletal muscle, RyR1 (located in the SR membrane) and $Ca_V1.1$ (located in the plasma membrane) are thought to interact directly. Some biochemical evidence suggest that the RyR1 SPRY2 domain forms an interaction with one of the intracellular loops of $Ca_V1.1$, the so-called II-III loop [201]. Using the phyre2 engine [202], we built homology models for all three SPRY domains of RyR1, based on several known SPRY protein structures (Figure 9A,B,C). All these models show a signature β-sandwich (two stacked β-sheets) folding motif. Interestingly, all ten disease mutations identified in these three SPRYs are located peripherally when mapped into the models (Figure 9A,B,C). As before, it seems that mutations cluster at the surfaces of individual domains, likely affecting interactions with neighboring domains or RyR binding partners. This observation agrees with the known protein interacting properties of the SPRY domain. The mutations in these domains may weaken the interaction with other domains or proteins and change the channel activities.

Another domain fold present in RyRs is the so-called "RyR domain". The latter name is unfortunate, as it obviously is not the only domain present in RyRs. These domains are arranged in tandem repeats, and we will hereafter refer to them as "tandem repeat domains". Each repeat unit is about 100 residues in length, and there are two tandem repeats within each human *ryr* gene: one between SPRY1 and SPRY2, and the other at the central region (Figure 3). These repeat units are also present in bacteria, archaea and viruses, either in single form or in pair with itself or other proteins [203]. The phosphorylation domain mentioned above makes up the second tandem repeat [148]. Interestingly, in a crystal structure of a bacterial repeat domain (pdb code: 3NRT), a single domain dimerizes and presents a similar fold as the paired repeat domain shown in the phosphorylation domain structure. We created a homology model for the first tandem repeats from RyR1 based on these two protein structures [202]. (Figure 9D). Seven mutations are found on this tandem repeat. Five of these are located on the surface, likely affecting interactions with other domains or RyR binding partners. The remaining two are buried within the domain, and may thus affect the overall folding stability.

Although the total number of the TM helices in RyRs is not clear, from the secondary structure prediction, their last two TM helices clearly share homology with the pore-forming regions of potassium channels and bacterial voltage-gated sodium channels (Na_V). Because the pore-forming region is directly responsible for passage of Ca^{2+} ions through the SR membrane, any minor structural alteration in this region may directly interfere with the ion conduction. Indeed, up to 50 mutations (RyR1+RyR2) have been identified in this region, which consists of only 125 residues. The occurrence of one mutation per 2.5 residues makes the pore-forming region into a "super-hot" disease hot spot. We created a model for the RyR1 pore-forming domain based on several bacterial NaV structures (Figure 9E). Most mutations cluster in the top half (ER luminal side) of the domain. Interestingly, 31 out of 41 RyR1 mutations in this domain are associated with CCD, which can be caused by the loss-of-function of RyRs. Therefore, it seems that many mutations in the TM domain can directly block the ion conduction pathway and reduce channel activity, while mutations in the cytoplasmic domains tend to destabilize the closed state of the channel and make it "leaky".

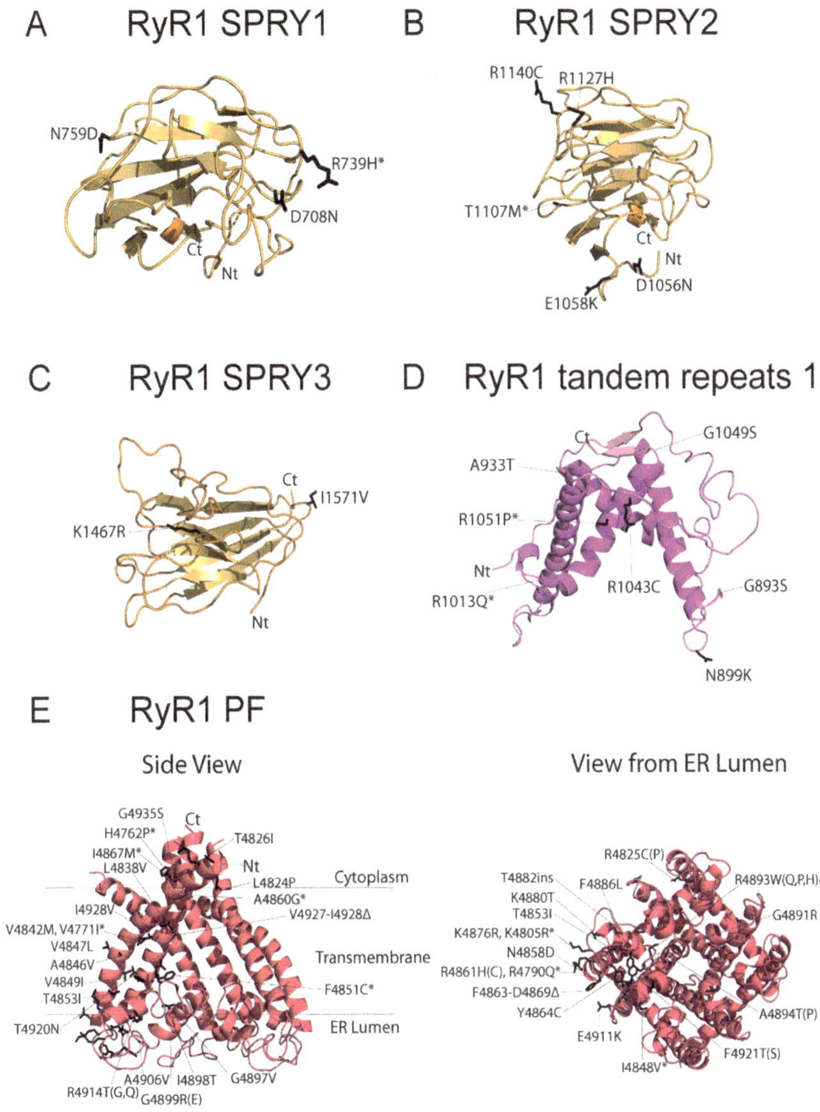

Figure 9. Homology structural models of RyR domains. Structural models were created by Phyre2 server [202]: (A-C) RyR1 SPRY 1-3, (D) RyR1 repeats 1, and (E) RyR1 pore-forming domain (PF). α-helices and β-sheets are shown in dark and light color, respectvely. RyR1 and RyR2 mutations are mapped on the strutural models, indicated by black sticks, and labeled. RyR2 mutations are distinguished from RyR1 mutations by *. Deletion mutations are labeled by Δ and insertion mutations are labeled by ins. The numbering is according to human RyR1 and RyR2 sequences. The N-terminal and C-terminal positions of the structures are labeled with Nt and Ct, respectively.

Like the previous studies with crystal structures, knowing the exact locations of these domains in the full length channel will deepen our understanding of the channel in the normal and disease states. But technically it is dangerous to dock homology models into the EM maps due to their limited accuracy. However, these models can still provide a good template to guide the design of the insertion sites for the EM studies, which will help to reveal the location of these domains and the corresponding disease mutations.

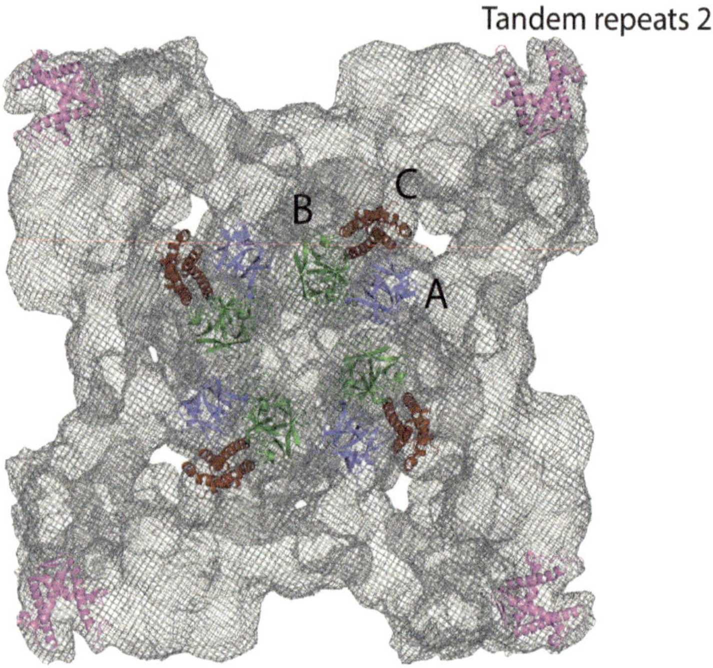

Figure 10. Pseudo-atomic models. Top view of the 9.6 Å RyR1 cryo-EM map (EMDB accession code 1275), showing the docked positions of the N-terminal disease hot spot (domain A (blue), B(green), C(red)) and the phosphorylation domain (purple) [141].

5. Conclusion

The available crystal structures and homology models represent ~32% of the full length RyRs. In the years to come, further crystallographic studies on predicted domains, and their localization into full-length RyRs will likely shed more light. Although obtaining well-diffracting crystals of intact RyRs may be an arduous task, this will ultimately be necessary to fully understand the function of RyRs in health and disease.

Author details

Zhiguang Yuchi, Lynn Kimlicka and Filip Van Petegem*

*Address all correspondence to: filip.vanpetegem@gmail.com

Department of Biochemistry and Molecular Biology, University of British Columbia, Vancouver, British Columbia, Canada

References

[1] Endo, M., M. Tanaka, and Y. Ogawa, Calcium induced release of calcium from the sarcoplasmic reticulum of skinned skeletal muscle fibres. Nature, 1970. 228(5266): p. 34-6.

[2] Fabiato, A., Calcium-induced release of calcium from the cardiac sarcoplasmic reticulum. The American journal of physiology, 1983. 245(1): p. C1-14.

[3] Block, B.A., et al., Structural evidence for direct interaction between the molecular components of the transverse tubule/sarcoplasmic reticulum junction in skeletal muscle. J Cell Biol, 1988. 107(6 Pt 2): p. 2587-600.

[4] Tanabe, T., et al., Regions of the skeletal muscle dihydropyridine receptor critical for excitation-contraction coupling. Nature, 1990. 346(6284): p. 567-9.

[5] Tanabe, T., et al., Restoration of excitation-contraction coupling and slow calcium current in dysgenic muscle by dihydropyridine receptor complementary DNA. Nature, 1988. 336(6195): p. 134-9.

[6] Rios, E. and G. Brum, Involvement of dihydropyridine receptors in excitation-contraction coupling in skeletal muscle. Nature, 1987. 325(6106): p. 717-20.

[7] Rogers, E.F., F.R. Koniuszy, and et al., Plant insecticides; ryanodine, a new alkaloid from Ryania speciosa Vahl. J Am Chem Soc, 1948. 70(9): p. 3086-8.

[8] Lai, F.A., et al., Purification and reconstitution of the calcium release channel from skeletal muscle. Nature, 1988. 331(6154): p. 315-9.

[9] Inui, M., A. Saito, and S. Fleischer, Purification of the ryanodine receptor and identity with feet structures of junctional terminal cisternae of sarcoplasmic reticulum from fast skeletal muscle. J Biol Chem, 1987. 262(4): p. 1740-7.

[10] Takeshima, H., et al., Primary structure and expression from complementary DNA of skeletal muscle ryanodine receptor. Nature, 1989. 339(6224): p. 439-45.

[11] Zorzato, F., et al., Molecular cloning of cDNA encoding human and rabbit forms of the Ca2+ release channel (ryanodine receptor) of skeletal muscle sarcoplasmic reticulum. J Biol Chem, 1990. 265(4): p. 2244-56.

[12] Otsu, K., et al., Molecular cloning of cDNA encoding the Ca2+ release channel (ryanodine receptor) of rabbit cardiac muscle sarcoplasmic reticulum. J Biol Chem, 1990. 265(23): p. 13472-83.

[13] Nakai, J., et al., Primary structure and functional expression from cDNA of the cardiac ryanodine receptor/calcium release channel. FEBS Lett, 1990. 271(1-2): p. 169-77.

[14] Hakamata, Y., et al., Primary structure and distribution of a novel ryanodine receptor/calcium release channel from rabbit brain. FEBS Lett, 1992. 312(2-3): p. 229-35.

[15] Lanner, J.T., et al., Ryanodine receptors: structure, expression, molecular details, and function in calcium release. Cold Spring Harb Perspect Biol, 2010. 2(11): p. a003996.

[16] Zalk, R., S.E. Lehnart, and A.R. Marks, Modulation of the ryanodine receptor and intracellular calcium. Annu Rev Biochem, 2007. 76: p. 367-85.

[17] Van Petegem, F., Ryanodine Receptors: Structure and Function. The Journal of biological chemistry, 2012.

[18] Palade, P., R.D. Mitchell, and S. Fleischer, Spontaneous calcium release from sarcoplasmic reticulum. General description and effects of calcium. J Biol Chem, 1983. 258(13): p. 8098-107.

[19] Jiang, D., et al., RyR2 mutations linked to ventricular tachycardia and sudden death reduce the threshold for store-overload-induced Ca2+ release (SOICR). Proc Natl Acad Sci U S A, 2004. 101(35): p. 13062-7.

[20] Ahern, G.P., P.R. Junankar, and A.F. Dulhunty, Subconductance states in single-channel activity of skeletal muscle ryanodine receptors after removal of FKBP12. Biophys J, 1997. 72(1): p. 146-62.

[21] Chelu, M.G., et al., Regulation of ryanodine receptors by FK506 binding proteins. Trends Cardiovasc Med, 2004. 14(6): p. 227-34.

[22] Ikemoto, T., M. Iino, and M. Endo, Enhancing effect of calmodulin on Ca(2+)-induced Ca2+ release in the sarcoplasmic reticulum of rabbit skeletal muscle fibres. J Physiol, 1995. 487 (Pt 3): p. 573-82.

[23] Tripathy, A., et al., Calmodulin activation and inhibition of skeletal muscle Ca2+ release channel (ryanodine receptor). Biophys J, 1995. 69(1): p. 106-19.

[24] Buratti, R., et al., Calcium dependent activation of skeletal muscle Ca2+ release channel (ryanodine receptor) by calmodulin. Biochem Biophys Res Commun, 1995. 213(3): p. 1082-90.

[25] Fuentes, O., et al., Calcium-dependent block of ryanodine receptor channel of swine skeletal muscle by direct binding of calmodulin. Cell calcium, 1994. 15(4): p. 305-16.

[26] Zalk, R., S.E. Lehnart, and A.R. Marks, Modulation of the Ryanodine Receptor and Intracellular Calcium. Annual Review of Biochemistry, 2007. 76(1): p. 367-385.

[27] Monnier, N., et al., Malignant-hyperthermia susceptibility is associated with a mutation of the alpha 1-subunit of the human dihydropyridine-sensitive L-type voltage-dependent calcium-channel receptor in skeletal muscle. Am J Hum Genet, 1997. 60(6): p. 1316-25.

[28] Rosenberg, H., et al., Malignant hyperthermia. Orphanet journal of rare diseases, 2007. 2: p. 21.

[29] Maclennan, D.H. and E. Zvaritch, Mechanistic models for muscle diseases and disorders originating in the sarcoplasmic reticulum. Biochim Biophys Acta, 2011. 1813(5): p. 948-64.

[30] Krause, T., et al., Dantrolene--a review of its pharmacology, therapeutic use and new developments. Anaesthesia, 2004. 59(4): p. 364-73.

[31] Paul-Pletzer, K., et al., Identification of a dantrolene-binding sequence on the skeletal muscle ryanodine receptor. J Biol Chem, 2002. 277(38): p. 34918-23.

[32] Zhao, F., et al., Dantrolene inhibition of ryanodine receptor Ca2+ release channels. Molecular mechanism and isoform selectivity. J Biol Chem, 2001. 276(17): p. 13810-6.

[33] Fujii, J., et al., Identification of a mutation in porcine ryanodine receptor associated with malignant hyperthermia. Science, 1991. 253(5018): p. 448-51.

[34] Gillard, E.F., et al., A substitution of cysteine for arginine 614 in the ryanodine receptor is potentially causative of human malignant hyperthermia. Genomics, 1991. 11(3): p. 751-5.

[35] Klingler, W., et al., Core myopathies and risk of malignant hyperthermia. Anesth Analg, 2009. 109(4): p. 1167-73.

[36] Robinson, R., et al., Mutations in RYR1 in malignant hyperthermia and central core disease. Hum Mutat, 2006. 27(10): p. 977-89.

[37] Denborough, M.A., X. Dennett, and R.M. Anderson, Central-core disease and malignant hyperpyrexia. British medical journal, 1973. 1(5848): p. 272-3.

[38] Jungbluth, H., et al., Minicore myopathy with ophthalmoplegia caused by mutations in the ryanodine receptor type 1 gene. Neurology, 2005. 65(12): p. 1930-5.

[39] Ferreiro, A., et al., Mutations of the selenoprotein N gene, which is implicated in rigid spine muscular dystrophy, cause the classical phenotype of multiminicore disease: reassessing the nosology of early-onset myopathies. Am J Hum Genet, 2002. 71(4): p. 739-49.

[40] Jurynec, M.J., et al., Selenoprotein N is required for ryanodine receptor calcium release channel activity in human and zebrafish muscle. Proc Natl Acad Sci U S A, 2008. 105(34): p. 12485-90.

[41] Kaindl, A.M., et al., Missense mutations of ACTA1 cause dominant congenital myopathy with cores. J Med Genet, 2004. 41(11): p. 842-8.

[42] Priori, S.G., et al., Mutations in the cardiac ryanodine receptor gene (hRyR2) underlie catecholaminergic polymorphic ventricular tachycardia. Circulation, 2001. 103(2): p. 196-200.

[43] Lahat, H., et al., A missense mutation in a highly conserved region of CASQ2 is associated with autosomal recessive catecholamine-induced polymorphic ventricular tachycardia in Bedouin families from Israel. American journal of human genetics, 2001. 69(6): p. 1378-84.

[44] Roux-Buisson, N., et al., Absence of triadin, a protein of the calcium release complex, is responsible for cardiac arrhythmia with sudden death in human. Human molecular genetics, 2012. 21(12): p. 2759-67.

[45] Pflaumer, A. and A.M. Davis, Guidelines for the diagnosis and management of Catecholaminergic Polymorphic Ventricular Tachycardia. Heart, lung & circulation, 2012. 21(2): p. 96-100.

[46] Watanabe, H., et al., Flecainide prevents catecholaminergic polymorphic ventricular tachycardia in mice and humans. Nat Med, 2009. 15(4): p. 380-3.

[47] Ohnishi, S.T., S. Taylor, and G.A. Gronert, Calcium-induced Ca2+ release from sarcoplasmic reticulum of pigs susceptible to malignant hyperthermia. The effects of halothane and dantrolene. FEBS Lett, 1983. 161(1): p. 103-7.

[48] Ohnishi, S.T., Effects of halothane, caffeine, dantrolene and tetracaine on the calcium permeability of skeletal sarcoplasmic reticulum of malignant hyperthermic pigs. Biochim Biophys Acta, 1987. 897(2): p. 261-8.

[49] Nelson, T.E., Abnormality in calcium release from skeletal sarcoplasmic reticulum of pigs susceptible to malignant hyperthermia. J Clin Invest, 1983. 72(3): p. 862-70.

[50] Mickelson, J.R., et al., Abnormal sarcoplasmic reticulum ryanodine receptor in malignant hyperthermia. J Biol Chem, 1988. 263(19): p. 9310-5.

[51] Mickelson, J.R., et al., Stimulation and inhibition of [3H]ryanodine binding to sarcoplasmic reticulum from malignant hyperthermia susceptible pigs. Arch Biochem Biophys, 1990. 278(1): p. 251-7.

[52] Fill, M., et al., Abnormal ryanodine receptor channels in malignant hyperthermia. Biophys J, 1990. 57(3): p. 471-5.

[53] Nelson, T.E., Halothane effects on human malignant hyperthermia skeletal muscle single calcium-release channels in planar lipid bilayers. Anesthesiology, 1992. 76(4): p. 588-95.

[54] Shomer, N.H., et al., Reconstitution of abnormalities in the malignant hyperthermia-susceptible pig ryanodine receptor. Am J Physiol, 1993. 264(1 Pt 1): p. C125-35.

[55] Richter, M., et al., Functional characterization of a distinct ryanodine receptor mutation in human malignant hyperthermia-susceptible muscle. J Biol Chem, 1997. 272(8): p. 5256-60.

[56] Wehner, M., et al., Increased sensitivity to 4-chloro-m-cresol and caffeine in primary myotubes from malignant hyperthermia susceptible individuals carrying the ryanodine receptor 1 Thr2206Met (C6617T) mutation. Clin Genet, 2002. 62(2): p. 135-46.

[57] Wehner, M., et al., The Ile2453Thr mutation in the ryanodine receptor gene 1 is associated with facilitated calcium release from sarcoplasmic reticulum by 4-chloro-m-cresol in human myotubes. Cell Calcium, 2003. 34(2): p. 163-8.

[58] Wehner, M., et al., Functional characterization of malignant hyperthermia-associated RyR1 mutations in exon 44, using the human myotube model. Neuromuscul Disord, 2004. 14(7): p. 429-37.

[59] Kaufmann, A., et al., Novel double and single ryanodine receptor 1 variants in two Austrian malignant hyperthermia families. Anesth Analg, 2012. 114(5): p. 1017-25.

[60] Chelu, M.G., et al., Heat- and anesthesia-induced malignant hyperthermia in an RyR1 knock-in mouse. FASEB J, 2006. 20(2): p. 329-30.

[61] Yang, T., et al., Pharmacologic and functional characterization of malignant hyperthermia in the R163C RyR1 knock-in mouse. Anesthesiology, 2006. 105(6): p. 1164-75.

[62] Zvaritch, E., et al., An Ryr1I4895T mutation abolishes Ca2+ release channel function and delays development in homozygous offspring of a mutant mouse line. Proc Natl Acad Sci U S A, 2007. 104(47): p. 18537-42.

[63] Durham, W.J., et al., RyR1 S-nitrosylation underlies environmental heat stroke and sudden death in Y522S RyR1 knockin mice. Cell, 2008. 133(1): p. 53-65.

[64] Andronache, Z., et al., A retrograde signal from RyR1 alters DHP receptor inactivation and limits window Ca2+ release in muscle fibers of Y522S RyR1 knock-in mice. Proc Natl Acad Sci U S A, 2009. 106(11): p. 4531-6.

[65] Bannister, R.A., et al., A malignant hyperthermia-inducing mutation in RYR1 (R163C): consequent alterations in the functional properties of DHPR channels. J Gen Physiol, 2010. 135(6): p. 629-40.

[66] Esteve, E., et al., A malignant hyperthermia-inducing mutation in RYR1 (R163C): alterations in Ca2+ entry, release, and retrograde signaling to the DHPR. J Gen Physiol, 2010. 135(6): p. 619-28.

[67] Feng, W., et al., Functional and biochemical properties of ryanodine receptor type 1 channels from heterozygous R163C malignant hyperthermia-susceptible mice. Mol Pharmacol, 2011. 79(3): p. 420-31.

[68] Liu, N., et al., Arrhythmogenesis in catecholaminergic polymorphic ventricular tachycardia: insights from a RyR2 R4496C knock-in mouse model. Circ Res, 2006. 99(3): p. 292-8.

[69] Lehnart, S.E., et al., Leaky Ca2+ release channel/ryanodine receptor 2 causes seizures and sudden cardiac death in mice. J Clin Invest, 2008. 118(6): p. 2230-45.

[70] Goddard, C.A., et al., Physiological consequences of the P2328S mutation in the ryanodine receptor (RyR2) gene in genetically modified murine hearts. Acta Physiol (Oxf), 2008. 194(2): p. 123-40.

[71] Fernandez-Velasco, M., et al., Increased Ca2+ sensitivity of the ryanodine receptor mutant RyR2R4496C underlies catecholaminergic polymorphic ventricular tachycardia. Circ Res, 2009. 104(2): p. 201-9, 12p following 209.

[72] Kashimura, T., et al., In the RyR2(R4496C) mouse model of CPVT, beta-adrenergic stimulation induces Ca waves by increasing SR Ca content and not by decreasing the threshold for Ca waves. Circ Res, 2010. 107(12): p. 1483-9.

[73] Suetomi, T., et al., Mutation-linked defective interdomain interactions within ryanodine receptor cause aberrant Ca(2)(+)release leading to catecholaminergic polymorphic ventricular tachycardia. Circulation, 2011. 124(6): p. 682-94.

[74] Boncompagni, S., et al., The I4895T mutation in the type 1 ryanodine receptor induces fiber-type specific alterations in skeletal muscle that mimic premature aging. Aging Cell, 2010. 9(6): p. 958-70.

[75] Loy, R.E., et al., Muscle weakness in Ryr1I4895T/WT knock-in mice as a result of reduced ryanodine receptor Ca2+ ion permeation and release from the sarcoplasmic reticulum. J Gen Physiol, 2011. 137(1): p. 43-57.

[76] Barrientos, G.C., et al., Gene dose influences cellular and calcium channel dysregulation in heterozygous and homozygous T4826I-RYR1 malignant hyperthermia-susceptible muscle. J Biol Chem, 2012. 287(4): p. 2863-76.

[77] Ghassemi, F., et al., A recessive ryanodine receptor 1 mutation in a CCD patient increases channel activity. Cell Calcium, 2009. 45(2): p. 192-7.

[78] Tilgen, N., et al., Identification of four novel mutations in the C-terminal membrane spanning domain of the ryanodine receptor 1: association with central core disease and alteration of calcium homeostasis. Hum Mol Genet, 2001. 10(25): p. 2879-87.

[79] Zorzato, F., et al., Clinical and functional effects of a deletion in a COOH-terminal lumenal loop of the skeletal muscle ryanodine receptor. Hum Mol Genet, 2003. 12(4): p. 379-88.

[80] Lyfenko, A.D., et al., Two central core disease (CCD) deletions in the C-terminal region of RYR1 alter muscle excitation-contraction (EC) coupling by distinct mechanisms. Hum Mutat, 2007. 28(1): p. 61-8.

[81] Anderson, A.A., et al., Identification and biochemical characterization of a novel ryanodine receptor gene mutation associated with malignant hyperthermia. Anesthesiology, 2008. 108(2): p. 208-15.

[82] Zullo, A., et al., Functional characterization of ryanodine receptor (RYR1) sequence variants using a metabolic assay in immortalized B-lymphocytes. Hum Mutat, 2009. 30(4): p. E575-90.

[83] Vukcevic, M., et al., Functional properties of RYR1 mutations identified in Swedish patients with malignant hyperthermia and central core disease. Anesth Analg, 2010. 111(1): p. 185-90.

[84] Avila, G., J.J. O'Brien, and R.T. Dirksen, Excitation--contraction uncoupling by a human central core disease mutation in the ryanodine receptor. Proc Natl Acad Sci U S A, 2001. 98(7): p. 4215-20.

[85] Avila, G. and R.T. Dirksen, Functional effects of central core disease mutations in the cytoplasmic region of the skeletal muscle ryanodine receptor. J Gen Physiol, 2001. 118(3): p. 277-90.

[86] Yang, T., et al., Functional defects in six ryanodine receptor isoform-1 (RyR1) mutations associated with malignant hyperthermia and their impact on skeletal excitation-contraction coupling. J Biol Chem, 2003. 278(28): p. 25722-30.

[87] Avila, G., K.M. O'Connell, and R.T. Dirksen, The pore region of the skeletal muscle ryanodine receptor is a primary locus for excitation-contraction uncoupling in central core disease. J Gen Physiol, 2003. 121(4): p. 277-86.

[88] Dirksen, R.T. and G. Avila, Distinct effects on Ca2+ handling caused by malignant hyperthermia and central core disease mutations in RyR1. Biophys J, 2004. 87(5): p. 3193-204.

[89] Brini, M., et al., Ca2+ signaling in HEK-293 and skeletal muscle cells expressing recombinant ryanodine receptors harboring malignant hyperthermia and central core disease mutations. J Biol Chem, 2005. 280(15): p. 15380-9.

[90] Zhou, H., et al., Multi-minicore disease and atypical periodic paralysis associated with novel mutations in the skeletal muscle ryanodine receptor (RYR1) gene. Neuromuscul Disord, 2010. 20(3): p. 166-73.

[91] Tong, J., et al., Caffeine and halothane sensitivity of intracellular Ca2+ release is altered by 15 calcium release channel (ryanodine receptor) mutations associated with malignant hyperthermia and/or central core disease. J Biol Chem, 1997. 272(42): p. 26332-9.

[92] Du, G.G. and D.H. MacLennan, Functional consequences of mutations of conserved, polar amino acids in transmembrane sequences of the Ca2+ release channel (ryanodine receptor) of rabbit skeletal muscle sarcoplasmic reticulum. J Biol Chem, 1998. 273(48): p. 31867-72.

[93] Lynch, P.J., et al., A mutation in the transmembrane/luminal domain of the ryanodine receptor is associated with abnormal Ca2+ release channel function and severe central core disease. Proc Natl Acad Sci U S A, 1999. 96(7): p. 4164-9.

[94] Tong, J., T.V. McCarthy, and D.H. MacLennan, Measurement of resting cytosolic Ca2+ concentrations and Ca2+ store size in HEK-293 cells transfected with malignant hyperthermia or central core disease mutant Ca2+ release channels. J Biol Chem, 1999. 274(2): p. 693-702.

[95] Du, G.G., et al., Mutations to Gly2370, Gly2373 or Gly2375 in malignant hyperthermia domain 2 decrease caffeine and cresol sensitivity of the rabbit skeletal-muscle Ca2+-release channel (ryanodine receptor isoform 1). Biochem J, 2001. 360(Pt 1): p. 97-105.

[96] Sambuughin, N., et al., Identification and functional characterization of a novel ryanodine receptor mutation causing malignant hyperthermia in North American and South American families. Neuromuscul Disord, 2001. 11(6-7): p. 530-7.

[97] Loke, J.C., et al., Detection of a novel ryanodine receptor subtype 1 mutation (R328W) in a malignant hyperthermia family by sequencing of a leukocyte transcript. Anesthesiology, 2003. 99(2): p. 297-302.

[98] Du, G.G., et al., Central core disease mutations R4892W, I4897T and G4898E in the ryanodine receptor isoform 1 reduce the Ca2+ sensitivity and amplitude of Ca2+-dependent Ca2+ release. Biochem J, 2004. 382(Pt 2): p. 557-64.

[99] Zhou, H., et al., Characterization of recessive RYR1 mutations in core myopathies. Hum Mol Genet, 2006. 15(18): p. 2791-803.

[100] Xu, L., et al., Single channel properties of heterotetrameric mutant RyR1 ion channels linked to core myopathies. J Biol Chem, 2008. 283(10): p. 6321-9.

[101] Jiang, D., et al., Reduced threshold for luminal Ca2+ activation of RyR1 underlies a causal mechanism of porcine malignant hyperthermia. J Biol Chem, 2008. 283(30): p. 20813-20.

[102] Migita, T., et al., Functional analysis of ryanodine receptor type 1 p.R2508C mutation in exon 47. J Anesth, 2009. 23(3): p. 341-6.

[103] Sato, K., N. Pollock, and K.M. Stowell, Functional studies of RYR1 mutations in the skeletal muscle ryanodine receptor using human RYR1 complementary DNA. Anesthesiology, 2010. 112(6): p. 1350-4.

[104] Haraki, T., et al., Mutated p.4894 RyR1 function related to malignant hyperthermia and congenital neuromuscular disease with uniform type 1 fiber (CNMDU1). Anesth Analg, 2011. 113(6): p. 1461-7.

[105] Jiang, D., et al., Enhanced basal activity of a cardiac Ca2+ release channel (ryanodine receptor) mutant associated with ventricular tachycardia and sudden death. Circ Res, 2002. 91(3): p. 218-25.

[106] Thomas, N.L., C.H. George, and F.A. Lai, Functional heterogeneity of ryanodine receptor mutations associated with sudden cardiac death. Cardiovasc Res, 2004. 64(1): p. 52-60.

[107] Lehnart, S.E., et al., Sudden death in familial polymorphic ventricular tachycardia associated with calcium release channel (ryanodine receptor) leak. Circulation, 2004. 109(25): p. 3208-14.

[108] Jiang, D., et al., Enhanced store overload-induced Ca2+ release and channel sensitivity to luminal Ca2+ activation are common defects of RyR2 mutations linked to ventricular tachycardia and sudden death. Circ Res, 2005. 97(11): p. 1173-81.

[109] Thomas, N.L., F.A. Lai, and C.H. George, Differential Ca2+ sensitivity of RyR2 mutations reveals distinct mechanisms of channel dysfunction in sudden cardiac death. Biochem Biophys Res Commun, 2005. 331(1): p. 231-8.

[110] Jiang, D., et al., Loss of luminal Ca2+ activation in the cardiac ryanodine receptor is associated with ventricular fibrillation and sudden death. Proc Natl Acad Sci U S A, 2007. 104(46): p. 18309-14.

[111] Tester, D.J., et al., A mechanism for sudden infant death syndrome (SIDS): stress-induced leak via ryanodine receptors. Heart Rhythm, 2007. 4(6): p. 733-9.

[112] Jones, P.P., et al., Endoplasmic reticulum Ca2+ measurements reveal that the cardiac ryanodine receptor mutations linked to cardiac arrhythmia and sudden death alter the threshold for store-overload-induced Ca2+ release. Biochem J, 2008. 412(1): p. 171-8.

[113] Jiang, D., et al., Characterization of a novel mutation in the cardiac ryanodine receptor that results in catecholaminergic polymorphic ventricular tachycardia. Channels (Austin), 2010. 4(4): p. 302-10.

[114] Meli, A.C., et al., A novel ryanodine receptor mutation linked to sudden death increases sensitivity to cytosolic calcium. Circ Res, 2011. 109(3): p. 281-90.

[115] Tang, Y., et al., Abnormal termination of Ca2+ release is a common defect of RyR2 mutations associated with cardiomyopathies. Circ Res, 2012. 110(7): p. 968-77.

[116] Treves, S., et al., Alteration of intracellular Ca2+ transients in COS-7 cells transfected with the cDNA encoding skeletal-muscle ryanodine receptor carrying a mutation associated with malignant hyperthermia. Biochem J, 1994. 301 (Pt 3): p. 661-5.

[117] Otsu, K., et al., The point mutation Arg615-->Cys in the Ca2+ release channel of skeletal sarcoplasmic reticulum is responsible for hypersensitivity to caffeine and halothane in malignant hyperthermia. J Biol Chem, 1994. 269(13): p. 9413-5.

[118] George, C.H., G.V. Higgs, and F.A. Lai, Ryanodine receptor mutations associated with stress-induced ventricular tachycardia mediate increased calcium release in stimulated cardiomyocytes. Circ Res, 2003. 93(6): p. 531-40.

[119] George, C.H., et al., Arrhythmogenic mutation-linked defects in ryanodine receptor autoregulation reveal a novel mechanism of Ca2+ release channel dysfunction. Circ Res, 2006. 98(1): p. 88-97.

[120] Boncompagni, S., et al., Characterization and temporal development of cores in a mouse model of malignant hyperthermia. Proc Natl Acad Sci U S A, 2009. 106(51): p. 21996-2001.

[121] Zvaritch, E., et al., Ca2+ dysregulation in Ryr1(I4895T/wt) mice causes congenital myopathy with progressive formation of minicores, cores, and nemaline rods. Proc Natl Acad Sci U S A, 2009. 106(51): p. 21813-8.

[122] Yuen, B., et al., Mice expressing T4826I-RYR1 are viable but exhibit sex- and genotype-dependent susceptibility to malignant hyperthermia and muscle damage. FASEB J, 2012. 26(3): p. 1311-22.

[123] Cerrone, M., et al., Bidirectional ventricular tachycardia and fibrillation elicited in a knock-in mouse model carrier of a mutation in the cardiac ryanodine receptor. Circ Res, 2005. 96(10): p. e77-82.

[124] Cerrone, M., et al., Arrhythmogenic mechanisms in a mouse model of catecholaminergic polymorphic ventricular tachycardia. Circ Res, 2007. 101(10): p. 1039-48.

[125] Kobayashi, S., et al., Dantrolene, a therapeutic agent for malignant hyperthermia, inhibits catecholaminergic polymorphic ventricular tachycardia in a RyR2(R2474S/+) knock-in mouse model. Circ J, 2010. 74(12): p. 2579-84.

[126] Kannankeril, P.J., et al., Mice with the R176Q cardiac ryanodine receptor mutation exhibit catecholamine-induced ventricular tachycardia and cardiomyopathy. Proc Natl Acad Sci U S A, 2006. 103(32): p. 12179-84.

[127] van Oort, R.J., et al., Accelerated development of pressure overload-induced cardiac hypertrophy and dysfunction in an RyR2-R176Q knockin mouse model. Hypertension, 2010. 55(4): p. 932-8.

[128] Mathur, N., et al., Sudden infant death syndrome in mice with an inherited mutation in RyR2. Circ Arrhythm Electrophysiol, 2009. 2(6): p. 677-85.

[129] Liang, X., et al., Impaired interaction between skeletal ryanodine receptors in malignant hyperthermia. Integr Biol (Camb), 2009. 1(8-9): p. 533-9.

[130] Hamilton, S.L. and Serysheva, II, Ryanodine receptor structure: progress and challenges. J Biol Chem, 2009. 284(7): p. 4047-51.

[131] Wagenknecht, T. and M. Samso, Three-dimensional reconstruction of ryanodine receptors. Front Biosci, 2002. 7: p. d1464-74.

[132] Samso, M., et al., Coordinated movement of cytoplasmic and transmembrane domains of RyR1 upon gating. PLoS Biol, 2009. 7(4): p. e85.

[133] Samso, M., X. Shen, and P.D. Allen, Structural characterization of the RyR1-FKBP12 interaction. J Mol Biol, 2006. 356(4): p. 917-27.

[134] Samso, M., T. Wagenknecht, and P.D. Allen, Internal structure and visualization of transmembrane domains of the RyR1 calcium release channel by cryo-EM. Nat Struct Mol Biol, 2005. 12(6): p. 539-44.

[135] Radermacher, M., et al., Cryo-electron microscopy and three-dimensional reconstruction of the calcium release channel/ryanodine receptor from skeletal muscle. J Cell Biol, 1994. 127(2): p. 411-23.

[136] Radermacher, M., et al., Cryo-EM of the native structure of the calcium release channel/ryanodine receptor from sarcoplasmic reticulum. Biophys J, 1992. 61(4): p. 936-40.

[137] Sharma, M.R., et al., Three-dimensional structure of ryanodine receptor isoform three in two conformational states as visualized by cryo-electron microscopy. J Biol Chem, 2000. 275(13): p. 9485-91.

[138] Sharma, M.R., et al., Cryoelectron microscopy and image analysis of the cardiac ryanodine receptor. J Biol Chem, 1998. 273(29): p. 18429-34.

[139] Serysheva, II, et al., Subnanometer-resolution electron cryomicroscopy-based domain models for the cytoplasmic region of skeletal muscle RyR channel. Proc Natl Acad Sci U S A, 2008. 105(28): p. 9610-5.

[140] Serysheva, II, et al., Electron cryomicroscopy and angular reconstitution used to visualize the skeletal muscle calcium release channel. Nat Struct Biol, 1995. 2(1): p. 18-24.

[141] Ludtke, S.J., et al., The pore structure of the closed RyR1 channel. Structure, 2005. 13(8): p. 1203-11.

[142] Wright, N.T., et al., S100A1 and calmodulin compete for the same binding site on ryanodine receptor. J Biol Chem, 2008. 283(39): p. 26676-83.

[143] Maximciuc, A.A., et al., Complex of calmodulin with a ryanodine receptor target reveals a novel, flexible binding mode. Structure, 2006. 14(10): p. 1547-56.

[144] Amador, F.J., et al., Crystal structure of type I ryanodine receptor amino-terminal -trefoil domain reveals a disease-associated mutation "hot spot" loop. Proceedings of the National Academy of Sciences, 2009. 106(27): p. 11040-11044.

[145] Lobo, P.A. and F. Van Petegem, Crystal structures of the N-terminal domains of cardiac and skeletal muscle ryanodine receptors: insights into disease mutations. Structure, 2009. 17(11): p. 1505-14.

[146] Tung, C.C., et al., The amino-terminal disease hotspot of ryanodine receptors forms a cytoplasmic vestibule. Nature, 2010. 468(7323): p. 585-8.

[147] Lobo, P.A., et al., The deletion of exon 3 in the cardiac ryanodine receptor is rescued by beta strand switching. Structure, 2011. 19(6): p. 790-8.

[148] Yuchi, Z., K. Lau, and F. Van Petegem, Disease mutations in the ryanodine receptor central region: crystal structures of a phosphorylation hot spot domain. Structure, 2012. 20(7): p. 1201-11.

[149] Kimlicka, L. and F. Petegem, The structural biology of ryanodine receptors. Science China Life Sciences, 2011. 54(8): p. 712-724.

[150] Shen, Y. and L. Tong, Structural evidence for direct interactions between the BRCT domains of human BRCA1 and a phospho-peptide from human ACC1. Biochemistry, 2008. 47(21): p. 5767-73.

[151] Revel, J.P., The sarcoplasmic reticulum of the bat cricothroid muscle. J Cell Biol, 1962. 12: p. 571-88.

[152] Franzini-Armstrong, C., STUDIES OF THE TRIAD : I. Structure of the Junction in Frog Twitch Fibers. J Cell Biol, 1970. 47(2): p. 488-99.

[153] Campbell, K.P., C. Franzini-Armstrong, and A.E. Shamoo, Further characterization of light and heavy sarcoplasmic reticulum vesicles. Identification of the 'sarcoplasmic reticulum feet' associated with heavy sarcoplasmic reticulum vesicles. Biochim Biophys Acta, 1980. 602(1): p. 97-116.

[154] Franzini-Armstrong, C., Membrane particles and transmission at the triad. Fed Proc, 1975. 34(5): p. 1382-9.

[155] Franzini-Armstrong, C., Structure of sarcoplasmic reticulum. Fed Proc, 1980. 39(7): p. 2403-9.

[156] Bonilla, E., Staining of transverse tubular system of skeletal muscle by tannic acid-glutaraldehyde fixation. J Ultrastruct Res, 1977(2): p. 162-5.

[157] Somlyo, A.V., Bridging structures spanning the junctioning gap at the triad of skeletal muscle. J Cell Biol, 1979. 80(3): p. 743-50.

[158] Ferguson, D.G., H.W. Schwartz, and C. Franzini-Armstrong, Subunit structure of junctional feet in triads of skeletal muscle: a freeze-drying, rotary-shadowing study. J Cell Biol, 1984. 99(5): p. 1735-42.

[159] Saito, A., et al., Preparation and morphology of sarcoplasmic reticulum terminal cisternae from rabbit skeletal muscle. J Cell Biol, 1984. 99(3): p. 875-85.

[160] Saito, A., et al., Ultrastructure of the calcium release channel of sarcoplasmic reticulum. J Cell Biol, 1988. 107(1): p. 211-9.

[161] Yin, C.C. and F.A. Lai, Intrinsic lattice formation by the ryanodine receptor calcium-release channel. Nat Cell Biol, 2000. 2(9): p. 669-71.

[162] Yin, C.C., et al., Two-dimensional crystallization of the ryanodine receptor Ca2+ release channel on lipid membranes. J Struct Biol, 2005. 149(2): p. 219-24.

[163] Orlova, E.V., et al., Two structural configurations of the skeletal muscle calcium release channel. Nat Struct Biol, 1996. 3(6): p. 547-52.

[164] Serysheva, I.I., et al., Subnanometer-resolution electron cryomicroscopy-based domain models for the cytoplasmic region of skeletal muscle RyR channel. Proceedings of the National Academy of Sciences, 2008. 105(28): p. 9610-9615.

[165] Du, G.G., et al., Topology of the Ca2+ release channel of skeletal muscle sarcoplasmic reticulum (RyR1). Proc Natl Acad Sci U S A, 2002. 99(26): p. 16725-30.

[166] Serysheva, II, et al., Structure of the skeletal muscle calcium release channel activated with Ca2+ and AMP-PCP. Biophys J, 1999. 77(4): p. 1936-44.

[167] Liu, Z., et al., Three-dimensional reconstruction of the recombinant type 3 ryanodine receptor and localization of its amino terminus. Proc Natl Acad Sci U S A, 2001. 98(11): p. 6104-9.

[168] Wang, R., et al., Localization of an NH(2)-terminal disease-causing mutation hot spot to the "clamp" region in the three-dimensional structure of the cardiac ryanodine receptor. J Biol Chem, 2007. 282(24): p. 17785-93.

[169] Paul-Pletzer, K., et al., Probing a putative dantrolene-binding site on the cardiac ryanodine receptor. Biochem J, 2005. 387(Pt 3): p. 905-9.

[170] Liu, Z., et al., Localization of a disease-associated mutation site in the three-dimensional structure of the cardiac muscle ryanodine receptor. J Biol Chem, 2005. 280(45): p. 37941-7.

[171] Ikemoto, N. and T. Yamamoto, Regulation of calcium release by interdomain interaction within ryanodine receptors. Front Biosci, 2002. 7: p. d671-83.

[172] Murayama, T., et al., Further characterization of the type 3 ryanodine receptor (RyR3) purified from rabbit diaphragm. J Biol Chem, 1999. 274(24): p. 17297-308.

[173] Benacquista, B.L., et al., Amino acid residues 4425-4621 localized on the three-dimensional structure of the skeletal muscle ryanodine receptor. Biophys J, 2000. 78(3): p. 1349-58.

[174] Liu, Z., et al., Three-dimensional reconstruction of the recombinant type 2 ryanodine receptor and localization of its divergent region 1. J Biol Chem, 2002. 277(48): p. 46712-9.

[175] Liu, Z., et al., Location of divergent region 2 on the three-dimensional structure of cardiac muscle ryanodine receptor/calcium release channel. J Mol Biol, 2004. 338(3): p. 533-45.

[176] Zhang, J., et al., Three-dimensional localization of divergent region 3 of the ryanodine receptor to the clamp-shaped structures adjacent to the FKBP binding sites. J Biol Chem, 2003. 278(16): p. 14211-8.

[177] Jones, P.P., et al., Localization of PKA phosphorylation site, Ser(2030), in the three-dimensional structure of cardiac ryanodine receptor. Biochem J, 2008. 410(2): p. 261-70.

[178] Meng, X., et al., Three-dimensional localization of serine 2808, a phosphorylation site in cardiac ryanodine receptor. J Biol Chem, 2007. 282(35): p. 25929-39.

[179] Wagenknecht, T., et al., Cryoelectron microscopy resolves FK506-binding protein sites on the skeletal muscle ryanodine receptor. Biophys J, 1996. 70(4): p. 1709-15.

[180] Wagenknecht, T., et al., Locations of calmodulin and FK506-binding protein on the three-dimensional architecture of the skeletal muscle ryanodine receptor. J Biol Chem, 1997. 272(51): p. 32463-71.

[181] Sharma, M.R., et al., Three-dimensional visualization of FKBP12.6 binding to an open conformation of cardiac ryanodine receptor. Biophys J, 2006. 90(1): p. 164-72.

[182] Wagenknecht, T., et al., Localization of calmodulin binding sites on the ryanodine receptor from skeletal muscle by electron microscopy. Biophys J, 1994. 67(6): p. 2286-95.

[183] Samso, M. and T. Wagenknecht, Apocalmodulin and Ca2+-calmodulin bind to neighboring locations on the ryanodine receptor. J Biol Chem, 2002. 277(2): p. 1349-53.

[184] Meng, X., et al., CLIC2-RyR1 interaction and structural characterization by cryo-electron microscopy. J Mol Biol, 2009. 387(2): p. 320-34.

[185] Samso, M., et al., Three-dimensional location of the imperatoxin A binding site on the ryanodine receptor. J Cell Biol, 1999. 146(2): p. 493-9.

[186] Zhou, Q., et al., Structural and functional characterization of ryanodine receptor-natrin toxin interaction. Biophys J, 2008. 95(9): p. 4289-99.

[187] Bhuiyan, Z.A., et al., Expanding spectrum of human RYR2-related disease: new electrocardiographic, structural, and genetic features. Circulation, 2007. 116(14): p. 1569-76.

[188] Marjamaa, A., et al., Search for cardiac calcium cycling gene mutations in familial ventricular arrhythmias resembling catecholaminergic polymorphic ventricular tachycardia. BMC Med Genet, 2009. 10: p. 12.

[189] Garzon, J.I., et al., ADP_EM: fast exhaustive multi-resolution docking for high-throughput coverage. Bioinformatics, 2007. 23(4): p. 427-33.

[190] Chacon, P. and W. Wriggers, Multi-resolution contour-based fitting of macromolecular structures. J Mol Biol, 2002. 317(3): p. 375-84.

[191] Wriggers, W. and P. Chacon, Modeling tricks and fitting techniques for multiresolution structures. Structure, 2001. 9(9): p. 779-88.

[192] Seo, M.D., et al., Structural and functional conservation of key domains in InsP3 and ryanodine receptors. Nature, 2012. 483(7387): p. 108-12.

[193] Marx, S.O., et al., PKA phosphorylation dissociates FKBP12.6 from the calcium release channel (ryanodine receptor): defective regulation in failing hearts. Cell, 2000. 101(4): p. 365-76.

[194] Wehrens, X.H., et al., Ryanodine receptor/calcium release channel PKA phosphorylation: a critical mediator of heart failure progression. Proc Natl Acad Sci U S A, 2006. 103(3): p. 511-8.

[195] Wehrens, X.H., et al., Ca2+/calmodulin-dependent protein kinase II phosphorylation regulates the cardiac ryanodine receptor. Circ Res, 2004. 94(6): p. e61-70.

[196] Jiang, M.T., et al., Abnormal Ca2+ release, but normal ryanodine receptors, in canine and human heart failure. Circ Res, 2002. 91(11): p. 1015-22.

[197] Zhang, H., et al., Hyperphosphorylation of the cardiac ryanodine receptor at serine 2808 is not involved in cardiac dysfunction after myocardial infarction. Circ Res, 2012. 110(6): p. 831-40.

[198] Sharma, P., et al., Structural Determination of the Phosphorylation Domain of the Ryanodine Receptor. FEBS J, 2012.

[199] Mackrill, J.J., Ryanodine Receptor Calcium Release Channels: An Evolutionary Perspective. 2012. 740: p. 159-182.

[200] van de Graaf, S.F., et al., Identification of BSPRY as a novel auxiliary protein inhibiting TRPV5 activity. J Am Soc Nephrol, 2006. 17(1): p. 26-30.

[201] Cui, Y., et al., A dihydropyridine receptor alpha1s loop region critical for skeletal muscle contraction is intrinsically unstructured and binds to a SPRY domain of the type 1 ryanodine receptor. Int J Biochem Cell Biol, 2009. 41(3): p. 677-86.

[202] Kelley, L.A. and M.J. Sternberg, Protein structure prediction on the Web: a case study using the Phyre server. Nat Protoc, 2009. 4(3): p. 363-71.

[203] Mackrill, J.J., Ryanodine receptor calcium release channels: an evolutionary perspective. Adv Exp Med Biol, 2012. 740: p. 159-82.

Chapter 6

The Genetics of Mental Retardation

Maria Puiu, Simona Dumitriu, Adela Chiriță-Emandi,
Raluca Grădinaru and Smaranda Arghirescu

Additional information is available at the end of the chapter

1. Introduction

Mental retardation(MR) was defined by the World Health Organisation as an intelligent quotient (IQ)<70 that is accompanied by adaptive limitations in two or more key skills areas, before the age of 18. General intellectual functioning is expressed by IQ. Typically, in children younger than 5 years old who present delays in the attainment of developmental milestones at the expected age, the term of "developmental delay" is used. Also, developmental delay is used before the age of 5,when IQ testing is reliable and valid and it takes into consideration learning and adaptive deficits which predict later intellectual disability.

Different classifications have been used to partition people with MR, the most frequent, accepted also by DSM IV (American Psychiatry Association) based on performances on standardised cognitive tests: mild (IQ 50-70), moderate (IQ 35-49), severe (IQ 20-34) and profound (IQ <20). [1]

According to this type of classification the level of difficulties and everyday life needs for the social and psychological support of a person affected by MR, can be established.

The definition and classification tend to accept the diagnosis of non-progressive form identifiable in small babies. In clinical practice, metabolic or neurodegenerative disorders may associate MR, frequently a progressive form, in children prior having normal development. Adrenoleukodystrophy manifests with progressive cognitive regression in boys, after a period of normal development. In addition, a pervasive developmental disorder manifested through cessation and regression of normal development, associating seizures and mycrocephaly in small girls is rather included in mental regression, only after a clear clinical picture in syndromal MR. The clinical association between MR and malformations, neurological dysfunctions such as epilepsy or cerebral palsy, sensorial deficits, other maladies or behaviour disturbances are usually earlier directed to evaluation and medical care.

Having such an impact on life, MR is one of the most frequent causes for genetic evaluation in babies in developped countries. Developmental screening addresses those who have developmental delays identifiable in primary care and need referral for furher evaluation.

2. The causes of mental retardation

MR has heterogeneous environmental and genetic causes acting invarious phases of pre, peri and postnatal development.

Prenatal	Environmental factors	-Deficiencies , such as iodine deficiency and folic acid deficiency -Severe malnutrition in pregnancy-Rh incompatibility -Using substances such as alcohol (maternal alcohol syndrome), nicotine, and cocaine during early pregnancy -Exposure to other harmful chemicals such as pollutants, heavy metals, and harmful medications such as thalidomide, phenytoin and warfarin sodium in early pregnancy -Maternal infections such as rubella, syphilis, toxoplasmosis, cytomegalovirus and HIV -Others such as excessive exposure to radiation
	Chromosomal abnormalities(cytogenetic techniques)	Trisomy 21 Partial trisomies (e.g., 4p, 9q) Aneusomies of the X chromosome Partial deletions (eg, 5p-/cri de chat) Translocations
	Cryptic chromosomal abnormalities(complex methods)	-Microdeletions or microduplications of chromosomal segments Wolf-Hirschhorn syndrome Pallister-Killian syndrome 18p deletion -Cryptic subtelomeric rearrangements (eg, deletions, duplications) -Cryptic interstitial rearrangements - microdeletion : ά-thalassemia with mental retardation ,Smith Magenis syndrome (deletie 17p11.2.) , Rubinstein-Taybi syndrome (16p13.3) -Cryptic interstitial rearrangements - duplications: 15q11-13 duplication: Kabuki Makeup syndrome -Contigous gene syndrome
	Mutation of a single gene	X-linked mental retardation Mowat-Wilson syndrome

		Cornelia de Lange syndrome Lissencephaly with cerebellar hypoplasia Walker–Warburg syndrome (also known as HARD syndrome) Muscle–eye–brain disease (MEB) Fukuyama congenital muscular dystrophy (FCMD) with type 2 lissencephaly Neurofibromatosis type 1 (NF1); Cerebral malformations
Perinatal	3rd trimester	Complications of pregnancy Diseases in mother such as heart and kidney disease and diabetes Placental dysfunction
	During delivery	Severe prematurity, very low birth weight, birth asphyxia Difficult and/or complicated delivery Birth trauma, vascular accidents
	Neonatal	Septicemia, severe jaundice, hypoglycemia
Postnatal (in infancy and childhood)	Traumatic, accidental, infectious	Brain infections such as tuberculosis, encephalitis, and bacterial meningitis Head injury Chronic lead exposure Severe and prolonged malnutrition Gross under stimulation
	MR that develops after a period of normal development	Lysosomal storage diseases Peroxizomal disorders Exposure to heavy metals, pesticide, malnutrition
	Multifactorial or complex inheritance MR	

Table 1. Causes of mental retardation in regards to development stage.

Current research has been directed to clarify the genetic base of what was accepted as 'idiopathic MR'. The initial reports about the implication of telomeric rearrangements in MR etiology created the necessity of a screening method. The prevalence of this type of modification was established at 5%, being higher in severe mental retardation group, nearly half of all being *de novo* mutations. The tendency to find a phenotype associated remained unfulfilled partly because of the reduced number of cases and partly because of the heterogeneity of the rearrangements. Deletion of the majority of end chromosomes were implicated in MR, some causing clinical recognizable syndromes such as Wolf-Hirchorn or Miller-Dieker syndromes.

By contrast, interstitial rearrangements are always clinically expressed by MR and cause recognizable phenotypic features. Submicroscopic deletions are responsible for the learning disabilities, velo-cardio-facial malformations from DiGorges syndrome (22q11 deletion), recognisable asymmetric cognition profile in Williams–Beuren syndrome (7q11.2 deletion) or cognitive and growth retardation from Smith–Magenis syndrome (17p11.2 deletion). The use of genomewide microarray-CGH has implicated interstitial chromosomal deletions or duplications in a significant part of unexplained MR so far.

MR can be part of a complex cognitive impairment in disorders caused by deregulations in imprinted genes. As examples, there are the Angelman syndrome and Prader Willi syndrome, both associated with microdeletions of the same region corresponding to 15q11.2–15q13, the paternally derived chromosome 15 causing PWS, and the maternally derived chromosome 15 causing AS.

A mutation in a single gene, should intervene in the biological mechanism of MR. A dysfunctional protein coded by this gene can deregulate functional cellular pathways or processes, influencing cellular connectivity, synaptic structure or function. As the result of this common genetic and physiopathological mechanism cerebral complex functions are impaired, the clinical expression being a limited ability to process information. Abnormalities of genes function may be implicated in almost any biological process that the cell conducts: DNA replication repair and recombination, translation, control of gene expression, membrane structure, membrane transport, energy conservation, cell communication, the cytoskeleton, cell life and division cycle. In an attempt of classify MR genes, two categories were taken into consideration: one including genes implicated in brain development, neurogenesis and neuronal migration, for which MR may be considered to be a secondary symptom due to brain malformation, and another one having those genes responsible for MR conditions without apparent brain abnormalities.

The list of indentified genes associated with MR is constantly growing. Using OMIM database entries and recent epidemiological studies the relative distribution of MR genes has been analysed. From the approximately 282 human MR genes, 16% reside on chromosome X, whereas its content represents only 3.37–4% of all known and predicted genes. The majority of known mutations in X-linked genes are loss-of-function mutations. Citation

X-linked forms of mental retardation are estimated to cause 10-20% of all inherited cases of mental retardation. The first gene to be identified was *FMR1* that causes fragile X syndrome and still remains the commonest single gene abnormality to be identified. The prevalence of many mutations isvery rare, many X-linked mental retardation disorders being present only in a limited number of patients. The future of microarray technology will enhance the diagnostic possibilities of cases suspected of X-linked mental retardation. Screening candidates are CGG repeat expansion in the fragile X-syndrome, the A140V and the mutation in the MECP2 gene.

2.1. Chromosomal abnormalities

Autosomal chromosom aneuploidies

Aberrations in autosomal chromosome number in live born babies are restricted to

aneuploidies: trisomy 13 (Patau's syndrome), 18 (Edward's syndrome) and trisomy 21 (Down syndrome), monosomy of any autosomal chromosome being lethal in the earliest stages of embryonic life. Malformations' severity can be lethal in the first week of life for newborns with Patau or Edward's syndrome; otherwise the level of functioning and cognitive development is severely affected.

Down syndrome(DS)

Down syndrome is the most frequent genetic cause of mental retardation. Results of standardized intelligence test IQ scores, in Down syndrome, may vary from low normal to severely retarded 85-20, dependent on the degree of cognitive deficits. Children with mosaicism may obtain scores with 10-30 point higher on IQ measurement that those with trisomy 21. [4,5] Longitudinal observation findings regarding cognitive development sustained that learning in children with Down syndrome may continue through late childhood and adolescence.

Early identified difficulties in achieving developmental milestones and learning disabilities, especially with language, create the opportunity of adequate education thus promoting a better social adaptation. Children with Down syndrome may present developmental stages similar to other children in the domain of sensoriomotor, adaptive and social interaction skills but with a slower rate.[2] Examination of developmental scores of young children with DS aresimilar with those of normal children, in Personal, Social and Adaptive Domains. Developmental scores are less similar in Communication and Cognitive Domains of the Battelle Developmental Inventory this being more evident as they approached 36thmonth. [3]

Neuropathological studies in Down syndrome showed that persistent hypocellularity to be one cause of intellectual disability. In DS individuals, cell density revealed reduced neuron number in late gestation (after weeks 19–23) by comparison with early gestation [6,7,8]. The same cellular reduction is maintained from the fetal age, through newborn period in the hippocampus, parahippocampalgyrus, cerebellum and neocortex. [6,7,9] Reduced volumes of the hippocampus, entorhinal, frontal, prefrontal, and temporal cortices, amygdala, cerebellum, brain stem nuclei, and mammillary bodies of the hypothalamus have been found in children and adults with DS. [10,11]

Autosomal structural anomalies

Wolf-Hirschhorn syndrome

Wolf-Hirschhorn syndrome(WHS) deletion of genetic material near the end of the short (p) arm of chromosome 4(4p-) the critical region- 4p16.3. The size of the deletion varies among affected individuals, larger deletions associate more severe intellectual disability and physical abnormalities than smaller deletions. A combination of Chromosomal microarray (CMA), FISH, and/or G-banded cytogenetic studies may be necessary for complete characterization of the chromosomerearrangement. [12]

The phenotype is dominated by prenatal and postnatal growth delay, a facial appearance of "Greek warrior helmet " with microcephaly, high forehead, broad bridge of the nose continuing to the forehead, hypertelorism, epicanthus, highly arched eyebrows, short philtrum, downturned mouth, micrognathia, and poorly formed ears, congenital heart and urinary defect and skeletal anomalies. [13] Central nervous system defects, sensorial defects (hearing and seeing), hypotonia and seizures complete the panel of intellectual disability. One third of the individuals with WHS have mild to moderate mental retardation. Battaglia et al [2008] found mild mental retardation in 10% of the patients, moderate in 25%, and severe/ profound in 65%. [14]

Phenotypic expression of WHS is related to the loss of multiple genes on the short arm of chromosome 4. From these, the lost of WHSC1, LETM1, and MSX1 is correlated with typical signs and symptoms of this disorder.

Cri du Chat syndrome

Cri du Chat syndrome (CdCS) is caused by a deletion of variable size occurring on the short arm of chromosome 5 (5p-). Localization of the deletion can be terminal, 5p terminal, in the majority of cases, but also we can find interstitial deletion, *de novo* translocation and familial translocation.

Imagistic findings in CdCS, especially MRI, were atrophy of the brainstem mainly involving the pons, cerebellum, median cerebellar peduncles and cerebellar white matter. [15]

Recent studies attempted to correlate genetic substrate with cognitive develop and behavioural pattern. The first assumption that any break point on chromosome 5 produces a typical phenotype of CdCS was modified by the newest studies results. In this way two distinct regions were implicated: one for the cat-like cry in 5p15.3 (between loci D5S13 and D5S760) and the other for dysmorphism, microcephaly, and mental retardation in 5p15.2 (between loci D5S23 and D5S791).

In 5p15.2 region, two separate subregions were also mapped: one for childhood facial dysmorphism and moderate mental retardation and the other for adult facial dysmorphism and severe mental retardation. The involvement in brain development and function, suggested by the presence of mental retardation may be sustained by the mapping of different genes (*SEMAF,CTNND2*) in this region.

CTNND2 gene codes a protein called delta-catenin involved in cell adhesion and movement. For example in a developing brain it is involved in neuronal migration, serving as a guide for nerve cell proper positions. In mature nerve cells delta-catenin has a role in synapses functioning. The disruption of these processes may be the fundament of the severe intellectual disability in individual who have CdCS and loss of CTNND2. [16]

SEMAF gene code a protein called Semaphorine F, in axonal guidance during neural development. The importance for axonal guidance and neuronal precursors migration during cortical development had been prooven in mice, suggesting that *SEMAF* may be responsible for some of the features of CdCS. [17]

Deletion of 5p15.3 was identified in individuals with speech delay but with no major intellectual impairment, also with subjects milder degree of cognitive impairment and fewer behavioural problems than those with deletion breakpoints in p15.2.[18] This region was implicated by abnormal gene expression in anomalous cerebral lateralisation which support the hypothesis of a separate region for the speech delay distal of p15.3 In general, individuals have delayed speech and language development, some never develop spoken language. Their receptive language is better than their expressive language, although both are delayed.

Subjects with deletion breakpoints in 5p15.3 had a milder degree of cognitive impairment and fewer behavioural problems than those with deletion breakpoints in p15.2. [19]

Pallister-Killian Syndrome

In people with Pallister-Killian mosaic syndrome (PKS) some cells have 2 extra copies of the short, p, arm of chromosome 12 fusionated as isochromosome 12p or i(12p). The genetic material from the isochromosome disrupts the normal course of development, causing the characteristic features of this disorder. The phenotypic expression is variable and also all affected children have mosaic tetrasomy 12p, onlythose who have a complete phenotype can be said to have PKS.

PKS is considered a neurodevelopmental disorder.PKS children experience learning disabilities some of them only mild but the majority severe to profound. Speech tends to be late, is often limited and sometimes absent. The learning processes may be influenced by the sensorial deficits (hearing and vision) and by the reduced interest for communication and the lack of eye contact reported by parents in the early years.

They have the ability to communicate their needs and preferences using gestures and vocal noises, since preschool and later they can attend special schools with dedicated support worker.

18p deletion

18p deletion or "18p-" means that part or the entire short arm of chromosome 18 is missing, or deleted, the individuals having only one of two copies of chromosome 18short arm. In some patients, this deletion is the only chromosomal change, in others can be the result of a more complex modification, for example an unbalanced translocation. People with an unbalanced translocation may have features of 18p- as well as features of the chromosome duplication. Atypical phenotype in a child with 18p- may is an argument to analyze the subtelomeric regions of all the chromosomes. [20]

Clinical phenotype at birth presents low weight, microcephaly, rectangular face, ptosis, epicanthal folds, low nasal bridge, hypertelorism, high-arched palate, prominent philtrum and large protruding ears. They may have low muscle tone – hypotonia and other neurological manifestation: a higher risk to associate holoprosencephaly, seizures and dystonia.

Holoprosencepahly may be severe in some newborn influencing survival, in others individuals milder forms causing brain minor changes, such as a missing corpus callosum, hydrocephalus or a change in the structure of the pituitary gland. Cerebral changes may be recognised in facial features such cleft lip and palate or hypotelorism or single incisor at the midline of the mouth.

Children may show delay in achieving milestones, mostly in the motor and verbal field. They may take longer to roll over, to sit, crawl and walk, and also language skills may develop later.

People with 18p- may manifest a variable degree of cognitive disabilities, tested IQ scores range from average to severe mental retardation.

Sex chromosomal aneuploidies

Turner syndrome(45X0)

Typically, genetic diagnosis of Turner syndrome had been done in adolescence, when puberty had fails to install. Although initially disregarded, many years after diagnosis the patients were considered to have mental retardation. Numerous researches showed lower Performance IQ than Verbal IQ and deficiency in nonverbal, visuo-spatial areas.

Psychosocial aspects of TS girls life seem to be impaired by low self-esteem, social isolation and peer relationships. Differences in appearance, short stature and the delay in the onset of puberty affect their self –esteem. They also may exhibit adjustment problems, anxiety and social immaturity.

A particular phenotype may be present to a significant number of patients with Turner syndrome called X ring Turner syndrome, having a X0 cell line, a ring X and almost every time a 46XX cell line. A study of Kuntsi et al., concluded that the presence of X ring chromsome leads to a reduction in cognitive performance, most of patients meeting criteria for mental retardation and special education. [21]

XXY Klinefelter syndrome(KS)

In boys with KS, the diagnosis may be established at birth or may be delayed to late childhood or adolescence since many of clinical features (delayed puberty, diminished or absent secondary sex characteristics, diminished testes) manifest in this period accompanied bycontinuousbehavioural problems and externalizing symptoms. Adults may be diagnosed during evaluation for infertilityor gynecomastia. [22] When present, mental retardation is usually mild. Verbal IQ scores measured in KS children are below average, while Performance IQ is normal.

Knowledgeabout increasing risk for specific developmental reading and having impaired verbal ability, in females with an extra X chromosome, the same hypothesis was raised about men. An exhaustive literature review of Rovert et al. concluded that KS children manifest deficit in verbal abilities and language processing. They presented a pattern of underachievement in school and a higher risk for dyslexia. [23]

IQ was found to be only 10-15 lower than the average peers in a control group of 13 years old boys. The level of intellectual deficit increases with the number of X chromosome, mental retardation being identified to individuals with more than four X

Other extra sex chromosome phenotypes

Clinical and developmental impact of a supernumerary sex chromosome led to the studies focused on establishing and recognising the physical and cognitive profiles of these disorders. Supernumerary X chromosome was proved to influence the cognitive development, with direct impact on language. Each extra X chromosome reduces the overall IQ by 15–16 points. [24] In this way, individuals affected by sex chromosome aneuploidy have a higher risk to develop mental retardation and significant psychopathology with every extra X chromosome. Since additional Y chromosomes are often accompanied by additional X chromosomes (48,XXYY, 49,XXXYY), it was difficult to pinpoint specific features in these phenotypes that are unique to either the X or Y chromosome. [23] Some differences have been observed althout:48, XXYY have higher scores in adaptive scales in daily living skills, socialization, and communication. The groups with 48,XXXY and 49,XXXXY have lower functioning cognitively compared to 48,XXYY, secondary to extra X. Every day living skills are impaired in this group, but also socialization, and communication.

	Clinical phenotype	IQs range	Behavioral phenotype
48,XXYY	tall, with long legs underdeveloped genitalia , hypergonadotropichypogonadism , gynecomastia	60 to 80	higher risk for internalizing and externalizing symptoms; anxiety and withdrawal aggressive and delinquent behaviors
48,XXXY	average to tall stature, facial dysmorphism: hypertelorism, flat nasal bridge, underdeveloped genitalia , hypergonadotropichypogonadism , gynecomastia	40 and 60	immaturity, passivity, with occasional irritability, temper tantrums, and outbursts
49,XXXXY	microcephaly coarse face, ocular hypertelorism, flat nasal bridge, and upslanting palpebral fissures underdeveloped genitalia , hypergonadotropichypogonadism ,	20 to 60	

Table 2. Clinical and behavioral phenotype in supernumerary sex chromosome disorders .

Volumetric studies demonstrated significantly reduced brain volumes in subjects with XXX and XXY, but not in XYY subjects, indicates that the presence of a extra X chromosome has a demonstrable effect on brain development. In the same direction the research on the presence of an extra Y chromosome couldn't be associated with significant volumetric brain differences relative to normal male controls. [25]

2.2. Contigous gene syndromes associated with cognitive deficits

In contiguous gene syndromes, the disorder is due to microdeletions or microduplications of chromosomal segments associated with clusters of single gene disorders. These disorders were recognized clinically prior to their cytogenetic localization. Usually the cytogenetic abnormalities are detected by high-resolution chromosome analysis like FISH, but there may be patients having submicroscopic molecular deletion. [26]

A particularity of contiguous gene syndromes is that loci that are physically contiguous with the deleted zone have an phenotypic impact. The clinical expression of the phenotype may vary from one individual to another depending on the extent of the deletion.

Since most of the patients of these contiguous syndromes many present a degree of mental retardation recommendation have been made for chromosome analyses to the patient with mental retardation and mendelian traits that are not usually associated with mental retardation.

PraderWilli syndrome(PWS)

PWS is caused by a chromosomal deletion on chromosome 15. Most cases of PWS (about 70 %) occur when the paternal region 15q11-q13is deleted in each cell. In another 25 % of cases, a person with PWS has two copies of chromosome 15 inherited from the mother – isodisomy (UDP). Rarely, PWS can also be caused by a chromosomal translocation, or by a mutation or other defect, that inactivates genes on the paternal chromosome 15. Approximately 1-5% of patients have neither deletion nor UDP, but a small deletion inthe centre controlling the imprinting process within 15q11-13.[27]Each of these genetic changes results in a loss of gene function in a critical region of chromosome 15. Due to imprinting, the maternally inherited copies of these genes are virtually silent, only the paternal copies of the genes are expressed. PWS results from the loss of paternal copies of this region.

On average people with PWS shows mild level of mental retardation, although individually their IQ scores may range from average to profoundly mentally retarded. Repeated studies since PWS had been discovered tried to establish a correlation between body mass index with IQ[28]. No significant relation has been found.

Specifically, the syndrome includes a particular eating behaviour (a compulsive search for food, non-selective non-discriminatory ingestion of large quantities of food and also, stealing food), irritability, reduced tolerance to frustration, stubbornness, anger, pinching skin, associated, in the vast majority of patients with mild mental retardation. Typically, the behavioural difficulties reach a peak in adolescence or in early adult life. Binge eating is the most severe and debilitating behaviour disorder, leading to obesity, diabetes and severe respiratory difficulties.

Usually, patients are happy and open to interpersonal networking, participating with interest in behavioural training. They can learn to structure their daily routine activities, rewards, breaks, boundaries and firm rules.

An extensive study focused on assessing self-aggressive, stereotyped and obsessive compulsive behaviour in individuals with PWS and showed that skin picking is found in 19.6% of individuals, with low frequencies of nose pinching, kicking and pulling nails and lips hair. From the compulsive behaviour category, the compulsive eating is the most common. Standardized assessments have identified high levels of depressive, anxiety and compulsive symptoms, with functioning impairment, which are not explained by developmental delays, difficulties in nutrition or by obesity in patients with PWS.

Angelman Syndrome (AS)

Is a neurological disorder with a heterogeneous genetic causality.

70% cases of AS occur when a segment of the maternal chromosome 15 containing this gene is deleted. In other cases, AS is caused by a mutation in the maternal copy of the UBE3A gene. AS results when a person inherits two copies of chromosome 15 from his or her father instead of one copy from each parent- uniparental disomy(UPD). AS may also be caused by a chromosomal rearrangement called a translocation, or by a mutation or other defect in the region of DNA that controls activation of the UBE3A gene. These genetic changes can abnormally turn off UBE3A or other genes on the maternal copy of chromosome 15.

UBE3A gene codes for a protein called ubiquitin protein ligase E3A. Ubiquitin protein ligases is implicated in the process of removing unnecessary protein from cells and maintaining the normal function of cells. In the brain UBE3A is expressed only from maternal allele [29], and it has a higher density in hippocampus and the Purkinje cells from the cerrebellum. Studies suggest that ubiquitin protein ligase E3A plays a critical role in the normal development and function of the nervous system.

The clinical picture comprises of psychomotor development delay, a joyful mood, hyper excitable personality, EEG recording anomalies and severe mental and language retardation. Apparent happiness is brand forthe syndrome, associated with a vague smile, rare specific laughs, exuberant background, hyperactive and stereotyped motor behaviour, and proactively social contact. Autistic symptoms lead to debates in diagnosis. The absence of expressive language, the reduced and inefficient use of nonverbal communication, motor and sensory stereotypes and sleep problems have all been correlated with low development profile and were considered by some authors as "co-morbid autistic disorder". Peters et al (2004) have found an association between AS and autistic spectrum disorders (according to DSM IV) in approximately one half of the evaluated cases. In addition, AS can be associated in various degree with ataxia, epilepsy and microcephaly.[30] Some children can develop severe myoclonic seizures, knowing that myoclonus with cortical origin is another manifestation of AS.

Williams syndrome (WS)

WS is characterized by particular facial appearance, with elfin appearance, cardiac abnormalities/malformations, connective tissue abnormalities, mental retardation or learning disorder, idiopathic infantile hypercalcemia, particular cognitive profile and an unusual personality profile.

The disorder is caused by a deletion of 1.5 megabase the long arm of chromosome 7, including the elastin gene (ELN). 16 genes were identified, so far, in the region 7q11.23. [31] The deleted region includes about 25 genes that probably contribute the manifestations of the syndrome. ELN gene deletion responsible for the synthesis of elastin, is associated with connective and cardiovascular anomalies, which are characteristic for the syndrome (supravalvular aortic stenosis, supravalvular pulmonary stenosis). Deletions of LIMK1, GTF2I, GTF2IRD1 genes are responsible for visual and spatial difficulties in these patients and the CYLN2 gene deletion is associated with particular behaviour, mental retardation and other cognitive deficiencies seen in patients with WS. The STX1A and LIMK1 gens are good candidates in investigating changes in cognitive or behavioural aspects of WS. LIMK1 gene was discussed in causal relationship with visual and spatial characteristics of WS [32], whereas the genes FZD9 and STX1A have been proposed to be involved in alterations of brain development. A more severe phenotype with lower cognitive ability is found in individuals with longer deletion (> 2.4 Mb) than typical deletion. Patients with a shorter deletion, that does not involve GTF2I (including those with de novo mutation) do not have intellectual disability, but have the specific WS cognitive phenotype.

Miller-Dieker syndrome

Miller-Dieker syndrome is characterized by lissencephaly and facial dysmorphy.The majority of the children have deletion of chromosome17p13.3.Children may present clinical features of Miller-Dieker syndrome by inheriting an unbalanced translocation.

The size of the deletion varies among affected individuals. The identified genes in this region, implicated in features of Miller-Dieker syndrome are: PAFAH1B1, responsible for the syndrome's characteristic sign of lissencephaly and YWHAE, which increases the severity of the lissencephaly.

Brain malformations cause abnormal muscle tone, spasticity or hypotonia, developmental delay, seizures severe intellectual disability, and feeding difficulties. PAFAH1B1 gene (also known as LIS1) provides instructions for making a protein is thought to be involved in directing the movement of nerve cells (neurokinesis) in the brain. Proper neuronal migration is essential for normal brain development and function. It also promotes neuronal migration by interacting with tubulin in microtubules. [33]

Decreased amount of PAFAH1B1 protein produced by the deletion of one copy of the PAFAH1B1 gene is responsible for many of the features of Miller-Dieker syndrome, including intellectual disability, developmental delay, and recurrent seizures (epilepsy). A decrease in neuronal migration caused by a lack of PAFAH1B1 protein is responsible for the lissencephaly.

YWHAE gene provides instructions for making the 14-3-3 epsilon (ε) protein, which is part of the large of a protein family involved in cell signalling. The 14-3-3ε protein helps to regulate a variety of processes including cell division and sensitivity to insulin in the body, in the brain being involved in neuronal migration by binding to other proteins involved in this process. It is thought that the 14-3-3ε protein is critical for proper neuronal migration and normal brain development. [34]

Di George syndrome

Is also referred as velocardiofacial syndrome and is caused by deletion of one copy of the 22q11.2 region resulting in abnormalities in the development of the third and fourth branchial arches, producing thymic hypoplasia, parathyroid hypoplasia, and conotruncal cardiac defects.

Children have frequently learning disabilities and behavioural problems. Developmental milestones are achieved later the peers of same age. In school age children IQ testing revealed scores that can range from average to mild retardation an a discrepancy between verbal and non-verbal IQ. The school performance may be lower than predicted by IQ testing secondary to weak executive functioning and low verbal abilities. They have also high scores in externalising symptoms secondary to attention deficit disorder, disinhibition and impulsivity, but also at internalising symptoms – shyness, anxiety and depression. In one longitudinal study, 20% of VCFS children in mid adolescence had significant prodromal psychotic symptoms. [35]

2.3. Monogenic mental retardation

Studies looking at single genes that may contribute to intellectual disability were started by reports of numerous families in which intellectual disabilities were common and transmitted in Mendelian pattern. In the some of them, the trait was inherited X-linked and was more frequent in males. The detailed analyses of _1000 Online Mendelian Inheritance in Man (OMIM) database entries and of the literature through September 2003 revealed 282 molecularly identified MR genes. [54]

Gene	Locus	Disorder	Protein function
CBP	16p13.3	Rubinstein–Taybi syndrome	CREB binding protein; chromatin-remodelling factor involved in Ras/ERK/MAPK signalling cascade
EP300	22q13.1	Rubinstein–Taybi syndrome	Transcriptional coactivator similar to CBP, with potent histone acetyl transferase: chromatin-remodelling factor
DNMT3B	20q11.2	ICF syndrome: immune deficiency associated with centromeric instability, facial dysmorphy and MR	DNA methyltransferase 3B, involved in chromatin remodelling
GTF2RD1	7q11.23	Williams syndrome	Transcription factors, potential regulator of c-Fos and immediate-early gene expression
CRBN	3p25	Nonsyndromic AR mental retardation	ATP-dependent protease; regulation of mitochondrial energy metabolism
CC2D1A	19p13	Nonsyndromic AR mental retardation	Unknown function, protein contains C2 and DM14 domains
UBE3A	15q11	Angelman syndrome	Ubiquitin–protein ligase E3A; protein degradation (proteasome): CNS development/function
RELN	7q22	Lissencephaly with cerebellar hypoplasia	Extracellular matrix (ECM) molecule, reelin pathway
VLDLR	9p24	Lissencephaly with cerebellar hypoplasia	Low-density lipoprotein receptor, reelin pathway
POMT1	9q34	Walker–Warburg syndrome (also known as HARD syndrome**)	Protein *o*-mannosyltransferase 1 (glycosylation of alpha-dystroglycan)

Gene	Locus	Disorder	Protein function
POMT2	14q24.3	Walker–Warburg syndrome	Protein o-mannosyltransferase 2 (glycosylation of alpha-dystroglycan)
POMGnT1	1p34	Muscle–eye–brain disease (MEB)	Protein o-mannose beta-1,2-n-acetylglucosaminyltransferase
Fukutin	9q31	Fukuyama congenital muscular dystrophy (FCMD) with type 2 lissencephaly	Homology with glycoprotein-modifying enzymes (no biochemical activity has been reported).
NF1	17q11	Neurofibromatosis type 1 (NF1); MR is present in 50% of NF1 cases	RasGAP function, involved in Ras/ERK/MAPK signalling transcription cascade; postsynaptic protein
Microcephalin	8p22-pter	Microcephaly vera	Cell cycle control and DNA repair
CDK5RAP2	9q33.1	Microchephalyvera	Mitotic spindle function in embryonic neuroblasts
ASPM	1q31.1	Microchephalyvera	Formation of mitotic spindle during mitosis and meiosis
CENPJ	13q12.2	Microchephalyvera	Localization to the spindle poles of mitotic cells

Table 3. Autosomal genes involved in MR disorders [31, 36]

X-linked mental retardation (XLMR)

Since the observations of L. Penrose, in 1983, of existence of a higher number of males than females with mental retardation in the population, several surveys were directed to elucidate the etiology of this report. The results indicated that many genes that determine mental retardation mapped for X chromosome. X-linked mental retardation (XLMR) was defined as a monogenic intellectual disability affecting mostly males, having a higher prevalence of MR relative to females.

The prevalence of XLMR had been estimated in different studied since 1980 the estimation made by Herbst and Miller, of 1.83 affected in 1000 males. [37] Since the X-linked disorders may be transmitted by an unaffected carrier mother, large families with numerous multigenerational individuals with mental retardation facilitated linkage studies and supported the idea of highly heterogeneous pathology.

Establishing the distribution of the level of cognitive deficit in the XLMR individuals group was considered a important socio-economic problem giving the extensive impact of MR not only for genetic and medical services but for social system. For mild mental retardation (IQ 70–50), the epidemiological studies found a ratio male- female of 1.9, indicating that 50% of all the cases of mild MR are due to XLMR. For this result it was considered that the excess of cases in males is due to XLMR. The same ratio is lower in moderate to severe MR (IQ<50), of

1.4, and making the same assumption than above we will conclude that 28.5% of all severely retarded males have XLMR. A percent of 10–16% from all severely retarded men is due to XLMR. Finally, in cohorts of mentally retarded males, the prevalence of the Fragile X syndrome was 2–2.5%,[38,39], 25% of all males with severe XLMR have having Fragile X syndrome.

Nonspecific ornonsyndromic XLMR include mental retardation caused by mutations of genes on the X chromosome without accompanying somatic, neurologic, biological, or behavioural manifestations which allows distinction from nonaffected male or from males with identified MR.

In other words, a nonprogressive intellectual disability, segregating in X linked manner that can be distinguished based on the knowledge of their causative gene. The studies of this type of XLMR were directed to establish the relation between X chromosome genes and the cognitive and adaptive functions and processes.

The difficulties in establishing a characteristic pedigree increased the difficulties in establishing the prevalence.

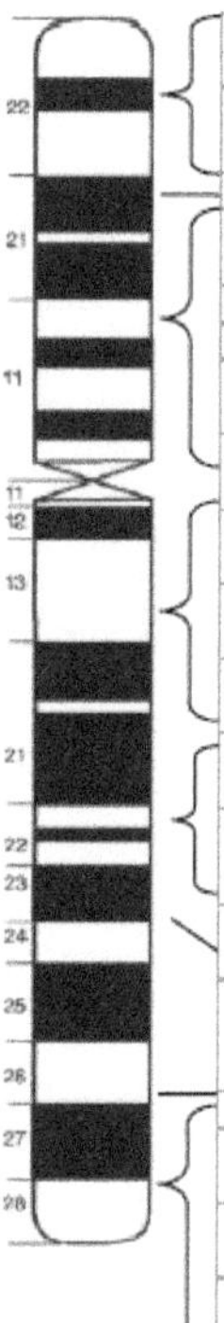

NLGN4	Cell adhesion
RSK2*	Signal transduction, protein serine/threonine kinase
IL1RAPL	Regulator of dense-core-granule exocytosis, signal transduction
TM4SF2	Membrane component, modulation of integrin-mediated signalling, possible role in synapse formation
ZNF41	Transcriptional regulator involved in chromatin remodelling
FTSJ1	Role in tRNA modification and RNA translation, methylation protein synthesis
PQBP1*	Transcription regulation
JARID1C*	Role in chromatin remodelling
FGD1*	Signal transduction, stimulation of neurite outgrowth
DLG3	Postsynaptic scaffolding protein linked to NMDA-type glutamatergic
ARX*	Transcription factor with possible role in the maintenance of specific neuronal subtypes in the cerebral cortex and axonal guidance in the floorplate, neuronal proliferation
ACSL4	Lipid metabolism, long-chain fatty-acid synthase, possible role in membrane synthesis and/or (FACL4) recycling
PAK3	Signal transduction, regulation of actin cytoskeleton, stimulation of neurite outgrowth
AGTR2	Brain-expressed angiotensin receptor 2
ARHGEF6	Integrin-mediated activation of Rac and cdc42, stimulation of neurite outgrowth
MECP2*	Transcriptional silencer of neuronal genes
FMR2	Transcriptional regulator, possibly involved in long-term memory and enhanced long-term potentiation
GDI1	Signal transduction, regulation of Rab4 and Rab5 pools, probably involved in the maturation of synaptic vesicles
SLC6A8*	Creatine transporter, required for maintenance of (phospho) creatine pools in the brain

* are implicated in syndromic XLMR

Figure 1. Gene function in nonsyndromic XLMR(Addapted after Hilger Ropers and Ben C. J, 2005)[40]

The description of an case as a nonsyndromic XLMR entity implies a complex evaluation including: growth, morphological features, neuromuscular development and function, behaviour, brain imaging, and laboratory testing. Affected males were not prove to have morphologic, neuromuscular, or behavioural manifestations that distinguish them from unaffected brothers or from other males with mental retardation. [40]. The degree of mental retardation could vary from mild to severe in the same family but is consistent. Carrier females may experience less severe learning problems. They also lack diagnostic findings on cranial imaging, biochemical studies, or cytogenetic analysis. Head circumferences and heights in affected males were most often in the normal range. Testicular volumes had been documented to be normal or enlarged.

Rett syndrome

Was described as a form of nonsyndromal XLMR. Mutation in gene MECP2 maps on chromosome Xq28.Rett syndrome it is frequently due to the deletion or insertion mutation in MECP2 gene. In 25% from the cases MECP2 large deletion were identified by PCR in girls with typical clinical picture. MECP2 gene is expressed in the brain in the neurons but not in the glia.

Rett syndrome was included in the chromatin modification disorders category because of the role of MECP2 in coding a protein that binds to chromatin and regulates transcription [41].

Clinical onset of the symptoms is early in the childhood, between 6-18 month, with loss of speech, behavioural changes, stereotypical behaviours, loss purposeful use of hands. The little girls affected tend to loss contact and interest for communication, and to occupy their time with repeated hand wringing, washing, or clapping motions. As they grew older microcephaly became evident, motor regression, seizures are added. They may also have an altered pattern of sleep and breathing difficulties.

Syndromic XLMR

Syndromic or specific XLMR implies that beside mental retardation the affected individuals present other manifestations that can include them in one of the categories:

1. syndromes, characterized by multiple congenital anomalies affecting organs and tissues but also including the brain,
2. neuromuscular conditions, with associated neurologic and/or muscular symptoms,
3. metabolic conditions and
4. dominant conditions [42] .

This attempt to classify XLMR has most a theoretical. Thus,because the same genes or even the same mutation can result in either a syndromic or a non-syndromic form of the disease. One example can be *ARX* gene found both in patients with non-syndromic X-linked mental retardation and in the syndromic X-linked West syndrome and Partington syndrome. [43]

The explanation may be that mutations in these genes in nonsyndromic XLMR families are presumed to cause only a partial loss of function of the encoded proteins, which could explain the absence of syndromic features

The classification from the 2007 XLMR gens update accept three classes to categorize XLMR conditions based on their clinical presentation:

a. syndromes, characterized by multiple congenital anomalies and defects in organs/tissues other than (but also including) the brain;

b. neuromuscular disorders, characterized by neurological or muscular symptoms (epilepsy, dystonia, spasticity, muscle weakness, and so on) but no malformations and

c. nonspecific conditions (MRX), where MR is the only consistent clinical manifestation among the affected individuals. [42]

The conditions associated with MR are recognizable on the basis of a distinctive clinical presentation and they can be considerate separate nosological entities, even if the causative gene or locus is unknown.

This distinction has mostly practical value.

Gene	Disorder	Clinical features	Protein function
FMR1	***Fragile X syndrome***	Facial anomalies, macroorchidism	mRNA processing, mRNA export from nucleus
ABCD1	***X-linked adrenoleukodistrophy***	Cognitive regression, spasticity, seeing loss, dementia, Addison disease	Membrane transporter, peroxisome
MAOA	***MAO-A-deficiency behaviour***	Aggressive and violent MAO	serotonin metabolism
OCRL1	***Lowe syndrome***	Short stature, cataracts, hypotonia, aminoaciduria, progressive renal disease	Signal transduction, lipid metabolism
GK	***Glycerol kinase deficiency***	Short stature, spasticity, osteoporosis	Nuclear translocation of the hyperglycerolaemia glucocorticoid-receptor complex
XNP	***ATR-X, Juberg–Marsidi syndrome, Carpenter syndrome, Holmes–Gang of gene syndrome, Smith–Fineman–Myers syndrome, Chudley–Lowry syndrome Spastic paraplegia***	Microcephaly, hypotonic facies, facial, urogenital and skeletal anomaliesthalassaemia, HbH inclusions, microcephaly, short stature, spastic diplegia	DNA helicase; chromatin remodelling, DNA methylation and regulation expression; regulator of cortical size

Gene	Disorder	Clinical features	Protein function
FGD1	***Aarskog–Scott syndrome***	Facial, digital and genital anomalies, short stature	RhoGEF; possible role in stimulation of actin polymerization
RSK2	***Coffin–Lowry syndrome***	Facial and skeletal anomalies	Serine-threonine protein kinase; CREB phosphorilation; long term memory
OPHN1	***Cerebellar hypoplasia or dysplasia***	Epilepsy, cerebellar anomalies	Negative control of rhoGTPases; and epilepsy stabilization of dendritic arbours
MECP2	***Rett syndrome*** ***Male fatal neonatal encephalopathy*** ***Progressive spasticity Spasticity*** ***NS-XLMR 57*** ***Angelman and Prader–Willi-like phenotypes***	Regression, epilepsy, acquired microcephaly, hand stereotypies, autism Hypotonia, apnea, epilepsy	Transcriptional silencer of neuronal genes
SLC6A8	***Creatine deficiency syndrome***	Epilepsy, facial anomalies	Creatine transporter, maintenance of (phospho) creatine pool in brain
FLNA	***Periventricular heterotopia*** ***Otopalatodigital syndrome I and II***	Epilepsy, brain anomalies, short stature, cleft palate, facial and skeletal anomalies	Actin-binding protein; neuriteoutgrowth;dendritic spine formation
ARX	***West syndrome*** ***Partington syndrome X-linkedlissencephaly, ambiguousgenitalia*** ***Proud syndrome***	Infantile spasms, regression, epilepsy, dystonia Lissencephaly, corpus callosum agenesis, epilepsy, ambiguous genitalia, Microcephaly, corpus callosum agenesis, urogenital anomalies	Transcription factor; neuronal proliferation/ differentiation of GABA-releasing neurons
CDKL5	***Infantile spasms***	Infantile spasms	Serine-threonine kinase; chromatin remodelling
SYN1	***Epilepsy, macrocephaly, aggression***	Epilepsy, macrocephaly, aggression	Synaptic-vesicle associated protein
SMS	***Snyder–Robinson syndrome***	Macrocephaly, palatal anomalies,scoliosis	Spermine synthase
PQBP1	***Renpenning syndrome, Sutherland–Haan syndrome, Hamel cerebro-palatocardiac syndrome, Golabi–Ito–Hall syndrome***	Microcephaly, short stature, slender habitus, long face, congenital heart defect, cleft palate	Polyglutamine-binding; mRNA splicing

Gene	Disorder	Clinical features	Protein function
PHF6	***Börjeson–Forssman–Lehmann syndrome***	Hypogonadism, obesity, facial anomalies, epilepsy	PHD zinc-finger protein; putative role in transcription
SLC16A2	***Thyroid and neurological abnormalities***	Hypotonia, spasticity, dystonia, abnormal thyroid tests	Monocarboxylate transporter; T3 transport into the cytoplasm
BCOR	***Lenz microphthalmia***	Microphthalmia, skeletal and urogenital anomalies	Transcriptional co-repressor; possible rolein modulation of histone acetylation and chromatin remodelling
PHF8	***Siderius–Hamel cleft lip or palate syndrome***	Cleft lip or palate	PHD zinc-finger protein; putative role in transcription
ATP6AP2	***Epilepsy***	Epilepsy	Renin receptor; activates ERK1 and ERK2
JARIDIC	***Microcephaly, spasticity, epilepsy, short stature, facial anomalies***	Microcephaly, spasticity, epilepsy, facial anomalies short stature,	Transcription factor;chromatin remodelling
IDS	***Hunter disease (MPZII)***	Short stature, skeletal and facial abnormalities, hearing loss	Metabolism, glycosaminoglycan metabolism
PLP1	***Pelizaeus-Merzbacher syndrome***	Nystagmus, truncalhypotonia and progressive spastic paraplegia, ataxia, and dystonia associated with CNS dysmyelination	Membrane component, myelin component
HPRT1	***SyndromeLesch-Nyhan***	Choreoathetosis, self-mutilation, hyperuricemia	Metabolism, purine ribonucleoside salvage
MID1	***Opitz syndrome***	Macrocephaly, facial anomalies, dysgenesis of corpus callosum, cardiac defects, hypotonia	Ubiquitin cycle, microtubule-associated complex
ATP7A	***Menkessyndrome***	Growth deficiency, sparse hair, limited movement, hypertonicity, seizures, arterial tortuosity, childhood death	Membrane transporter, copper-exporting ATPase activity

Table 4. Gene function in syndromic XLMR(Adapted after: Chellyet a.2006, [31]).

Fragile X syndrome

Fragile X syndrome is the most common form of XLMR, affecting approximately 25% of all families suffering from XLMR. It is caused by the loss of function of gene FMR1, which maps on chromosome Xq27.3, a55bp segment of DNA composed by repeats of the nucleotide CGG. CGG repeat is located in the 5®-untranslated region of FRM1.[44] Normal people have 6-55 copies, carriers have 55-230 copies and to not express the fragile site. In females carriers the FRAX repeats are expanded during meiosis. In affected males 230-1000 repeats are present and they express fragile X mental retardation. Repeat expansion associated with hypermethylation causing reduced or absent expression of FRM protein. The accumulation of untranslated FRM1 mRNA forms inclusion in neurons and glial cells of hippocampus and cerebral cortex causing the neurological manifestations of the syndrome. [45,32]

Clinical features include long narrow face, large and protruding ears, macroorchidism. Patients exhibit also moderate mental retardation, attention deficit, autistic symptoms, seizures and coordination problems.

Autism

First described as a behavioral disorder in children, in 1943 by Leo Kanner, was proven to affect mostly social interactions, the interest for relation, interaction and communication, the ability to decode facial expression and emotional message. It was suggested that autism has an organic basis sustained by the association with mental retardation (75%) and seizures (40%).

Evidence of concordance in twin studies, monozygotic- 60-92%, while in dizygotic twins range 0-10%, and the risk of recurrence higher than the general population in families with one autistic child brought into scientific interest the role of genetic factors in autism. [46]

Autism may occur in patients with monogenic diseases as tuberous sclerosis or Fragile X syndrome. Autistic like symptoms have also described in duplication of chromosome 15q11-13 [47] and deletion on chromosome 2q37.3 [48]

Between 1998 and 2004 an extended effort was carried out in the International Molecular Genetic Study of Autism Consortium. The goal of associating a chromosome with autism was not fulfilled but association studies have found positive association on chromosome 7q, especially with a missense mutation on the LAMB1 gene, and with 17q11.2 [49]

The presence of autistic symptoms in Rett syndrome directed the attention through MECP2 gene. As a result, MECP2 mutation was associated with a low percentage in autism. The same interest was raised by 15q11-13q, secondary to the presence of autistic features in individuals with Prader-Willi syndrome and Angelman syndrome. The result in this cases was a reduced expression of two genes in region 15q11-13q, UBE3A and GABRB3.

If the genomic regions play a role in autism, by genes defect or by common regulatory pathways are the preoccupation of further studies.

2.4. Mental retardation in metabolic disorders

The evolution of metabolic disorders may disrupt development of children with previous normal development. Genetic diseases presenting abnormal use or storage of different normal substances (protein, lipids, copper), these disordersmay manifest with a complex perturbation of cognition maturation and motor impairment.

DISORDER	CLINICAL FEATURES
Biotinidase Deficiency	Mental retardation, seizures, skin rash, loss of hair, death
Congenital Hypothyroidism	Mental retardation, other brain damage, growthdelay
Galactosemia	Severe brain damage, developmantal delay, kidney damage, eye abnormalities inneonates, death
ORGANIC ACIDEMIAS A condition in which the body cannot break down and get rid of certain organic acids and the metabolic acids accumulate in blood	
Glutaric Acidemia Type I	Neurological deterioration, muscle weakness or dystonic cerebral palsy, epilesy
Maple Syrup Urine Disease (MSUD)	Neonatal coma, convulsions, mental retardation, death
Malonic Aciduria	Developmental delay, vomiting, seizures, cardiomyopathy, hypoglycemia
Isovaleric Acidemia	Vomiting, lack of appetite, lethargy, neuromuscular irritability, hypothermia
Propionic Acidemia	Mental retardation, seizures, movement disorders, coma, sudden death
Methylmalonic Acidemias	Lethargy, vomiting and dehydration, respiratory distress, muscle weakness, coma, seizures, developmental delay
Multiple Carboxylase Deficiency	Seizures, immune system impairment, skin rashes, hair loss, hearing loss, mental retardation
2-Methyl-3- Hydroxybutyryl CoA Dehydrogenase Deficiency	Developmental delay
3-Methylglutaconyl CoA Hydratase Deficiency	Delayed motor development, short attention span, delayeddevelopment of speech
DISORDERS OF AMINO ACID METABOLISM A condition in which the body cannot break down several amino acids in protein foods and cannot get rid of ammonia, which has a toxic impact	
Arginase Deficiency	Developmental delay, seizures, hyperactivity, ataxia
Argininosuccinate Lyase Deficiency	Mental retardation, potential lethal coma, seizures, anorexia, vomiting, lethargy
Citrullinemia	Mental retardation, potential lethal, coma, seizures, anorexia, vomiting, lethargy
Homocystinuria	Heart disease, stroke, possible mental retardation, psychiatric problems

DISORDER	CLINICAL FEATURES
Phenylketonuria (PKU)	Severe mental retardation, seizures
FATTY ACID OXIDATION DISORDERS (FAOD) Problems with enzimes that breakdown of lipids from the food or from fat stored and production of Acetyl Co-A. The proces requires active transport across mitochondrial membrane	
Carnitine disorders Carnitine/Acylcarnitine Translocase deficiency (CAT) Carnitine Palmitoyl Tranferase deficiency Type I (CPT-I) Carnitine Palmitoyl Tranferase deficiency Type II (CPT-2) Carnitine Uptake Defect (CUD)	hypoglycemia, liver disease, sudden infant death(SIDS), encephalopathy, myopathy, cardiomyopathy.
Long chain fatty acid dehydrogenase disorders Long/Very Long Chain Acyl CoA Dehydrogenase deficiency (LCAD/VLCAD) Long Chain Hydroxy Acyl CoA Dehydrogenase deficiency (LCHAD)	hypoglycemia, hepatomegaly, myopathy, SIDS,Reye syndrome, and cardiomyopathy.
Medium chain fatty acid dehydrogenase disorders Medium Chain Acyl CoA Dehydrogenase deficiency (MCAD) Medium Chain 3-Ketoacyl CoA Thiolase deficiency (MCKAT) Multiple Acyl CoA Dehydrogenase deficiency (GA-II)	Children with MCAD are typically normal at birth and develop episodes of hypoketotic hypoglycemia, vomiting, lethargy, seizures associated with fasting.
Short chain fatty acid dehydrogenase disorders Short Chain Acyl CoA Dehydrogenase deficiency (SCAD) Short Chain Hydroxy Acyl CoA Dehydrogenase deficiency (SCHAD)	SCAD deficiency presents in the neonatal period with failure-to-thrive, hypotonia, and metabolis acidosis; hyperammonemia and lactic acidosis have been reported.
Glutaric acidemia (aciduria) types 1 and 2	Liver and muscle fat Macrocephaly, brain atrophy (type 1) Cortical dysplasias and heterotopias, polycystic kidneys (type 2)
MITHOCONDRIAL DISORDERS The illness result from deficiency of any mitochondria-located protein which is involved in energy metabolism. Variability in part due to variable numbers of affected mitochondria, and to the affected tissue, the most damaged cells of the brain, heart, liver, skeletal muscles, kidney and the endocrine and respiratory systems.	
Acute lactic acidosis Leigh syndrome	Depending on the type of tissues affected, symptoms may include:

DISORDER	CLINICAL FEATURES
MELAS MERF MIRAS Pyruvate Dehydrogenase Deficiency	loss of motor control muscle weakness and pain respiratory complications gastro-intestinal disorders and swallowing difficulties poor growth cardiac disease liver disease diabetes, seizures visual/hearing problems lactic acidosis developmental delays
GLYCOGEN STORAGE DISEASES Abnormal metabolism of glycogen	Hypoglycemia and ketosis (variable) Deposition of glycogen in tissues
MUCOPOLYSACCHARIDOSES Defective normal degradation leads to glycosaminoglycan accumulation	Because of maternal enzymes, patients normal at birth and then progress to disfigurement and disability, coarsened facial features short stature with disproportionately short trunk and skeletal dysplasia thickened skin ,organomegaly , hernias, excessive body hair, progressive joint stiffness Developmental delay Severe behavioral problems Hearing loss Communicating hydrocephalus
PEROXISOMAL DISORDERS This results in the over-accumulation of and branched chain fatty acids, such as	
Zellweger spectrum disorders Zellweger Syndrome Neonatal Adrenoleukodystrophy Infantile Refsum Disease	Destruction of the myelin (demyelination) leads to loss of white matter (leukodystrophy). Children may develop life-threatening problems in other organs and tissues, such as the liver, heart, and kidneys, adrenal glands
Chondrodysplasia Punctua spectrum	abnormal cartilage and bone development, chondrodysplasia punctata especially in the hands and feet, hearing loss and short stature, cardiac defects, and seizure disorders
LEUKODYSTROPHIES Genetically determined progressive disorders that affect the brain, spinal cord and peripheral nerves. The injury affect the white matter of the nervous system and is progressive, tends to get worse as the child gets older.	
Adrenoleukodystrophy Alexander's disease Canavan disease	

DISORDER	CLINICAL FEATURES
Cerebrotendinous Xanthomatosis Krabbe's disease	
Pelizaeus-Merzbacher disease	
LIPID STORAGE DISORDERS	
Various disorders have characteristic patterns of organ involvement, depending on particular substrate that is stored.	
Mutation causes abnormal enzyme function. Leads to glycosphingolipid accumulation in lysosomes	
Fabry disease	Progressive clinical manifestations neurodegenerative disease, organomegaly, skeletal abnormalities, pulmonary infiltrates
GM1 gangliosidosis	
Tay–Sachs disease	
Niemann-Pick disease	
GM2 gangliosidosis	
Gaucher disease	
Wolman disesse	
Fucosidosis	
Alpha-manosidosis	
Metacromatic leukodystropy	
Galactosialidosis	
MENKES SYNDROME	Alteration of copper metabolism. Children develop hypotonia, seisures, hypotermia, developmental and grow delay.
OCCIPITAL HORN SYNDROME	

Table 5. Metabolic diseases associated with MR or DD.

Researches led to the understanding of mental retardation in these diseases and to identification and implementation of the therapies, which prevent the consequences associated to the genetic defect. The positive results of therapies instituted in a timely manner put the basis of extensive screening programs for newborns designed to avoid irreversible changes in development processes.

2.5. Multifactorial inheritance and mental retardation

A clinical phenotype is frequently the result of a complexity of interaction between different pathways including many genes, proteins and environmental factors. Such diseases are of defective cellular migration (such as lissencephaly, heterotopias), neural tube defects, congenital hydrocephalus, myoclonic epilepsy, and narcolepsy. The experiences showed that these do not respect the Mendelian patterns of inheritance, althought genetic factors are implicated since a higher reccurence had been observed in some families.

The neural tube defect include spina bifida, anencephalyand any other defect that is a failure of closure of the neural tube and, in some cases, hydrocephalus associated to thedisturbance of the circulation of the cerebrospinal fluid.

Empirical data show that couples who have one child with a neural tube defect are at greater risk of having a second child with a neural tube defect thanother couples in the general population. Randomized controled data sustainned that maternal folic acid supplements lower the the number of children born with spina bifida. [50]. Later studies sustained mothernal folic acid supplement for many months, even years, before conception for women of having a child with a neural tube defect (a previous child with neural tube defect, mother taking antiepileptic medication).

Polymorphic DNA sequence variation could not sustain a single polymorphism in genes encoding enzymes involved in folate metabolism as a risk factor factor in all populations for neural tube defect. [51,52]

Genetic counselling for this families is important to take into consideration the neural tube defect isolated and those in which it forms part of asyndrome.

3. Establishing the diagnosis of mental retardation

Developmental disabilities may affect children in a single domain or in several arias of their life: global developmental delay, motor impairment, isolated speech and language delay, severe primary sensorial deficits and pervasive disabilities.

The earliest elucidation of the etiology of developmental delay may improve the quality of child life. In inborn errors of amino acids or organic acids, a correct diagnosis improves the evolution. Following an accurate clinical, biochemical, and sometimes molecular, a treatment could be initiated in this cases.

Even in the cases in which the diagnosis is not going to change the evolution for the child, a positive impact may have on the family. A team approach may empower parents to deal with disabilities and to search and choose proper medical, educational and social facilities.

The physician must be directed to evaluate child developmental level at every evaluation. A suspicion of mental retardation in any child may be raised in any child based on some clues: delayed speech, dysmorphic features (minor anomalies), difficult to manage temperament, hypotonia generally or of the extremities, clumsiness, general inability to do things for self and, not least, expressed concern by the parents.

1.Personal clinical history	length of pregnancy, premature onset of labour or rupture of the membranes, duration and course of labour, type of delivery and any complications, Apgar scores at one and (especially) five minutes should be reviewed, and birth weight length and head circumference measurements obtained and plotted on appropriate growth charts illnesses, feeding or sleeping difficulties in the newborn period and problems with sucking or swallowing, temperament

<table>
<tr><td></td><td>atypical course in child development
seizures</td></tr>
<tr><td colspan="2">Documented medical situations from prior evaluations may offer an objective perspective for the professionals.</td></tr>
<tr><td>2. Family history</td><td>existing cases of DD/MR
history of infertility or fetal loss
maternal health during gestation: use of drugs, tobacco, alcohol, sign of infections, hospitalisation, risk for sexually transmitted diseases</td></tr>
<tr><td>3. Dysmorphologic examination</td><td>unusualcranio-facial, skeletal, palmar crease patterns.
macrocephaly; microcephaly
genital anormalities</td></tr>
<tr><td colspan="2">Minor abnormalities, involving the face, ears, hands or feet may provide clues to developmental problems of possible prenatal origin. Most minor abnormalities are readily recognized even on cursory examination.(53)</td></tr>
<tr><td>4. Developmental evaluation</td><td>formal developmental screening
behaviour problems
ADHD
autism/autistic- like behaviours</td></tr>
<tr><td colspan="2">The formal test that address developmental delay have more domains: gross motor/fine, speech-language, cognition, social. For the physician it will be important to ask specific questions about the child's current developmental abilities at each visit.</td></tr>
<tr><td>5. Neurologic examination</td><td>-hypotonia, spasticity, ataxia
- seizures
- cerebral palsy</td></tr>
<tr><td colspan="2">An EEG can be obtained when a child with global developmental delay has a history or examination features suggesting the presence of epilepsy or a specific epileptic syndrome: Lennox-Gastaut syndrome, myoclonic epilepsy, Rett syndrome.
If available, MRI should be obtained in the presence of physical findings (e.g., microcephaly, focal motor findings).(53)</td></tr>
<tr><td>6. Endocrinologic examination</td><td>-growth delay
-obesity
-genital abnormalities
- clinical signs for hypotiroidy</td></tr>
<tr><td>7. Other clinical examination (cardiologist, orthopedicsurgeon, gynecologist, ophthalmologist, audiologist).</td><td>- heart malformations
-skeletal</td></tr>
<tr><td colspan="2">Children with global developmental delay may undergo appropriate vision and audiometric assessment at the time of their diagnosis. Vision assessment can include vision screening and a full ophthalmologic examination (visual acuity, extra-oculo-movements, funduscopic). Audiometric assessment can include behavioural audiometry or brainstem auditory evoked response testing when feasible. Transient evoked otoacoustic emissions are used as screening studies in newborns.</td></tr>
</table>

8. Karyotype	common cytogenetic abnormalities found included Down syndrome, sex chromosome aneuploidies (47, XXY), fragile X syndrome, and unbalanced translocations/deletion syndromes
9. FISH	microdeletion/microduplication abnormalities
10. Metabolic testing	testing amino and organic acids thyroid function IGF

Table 6. Clinical genetics evaluation of the child with suspicion of MR.

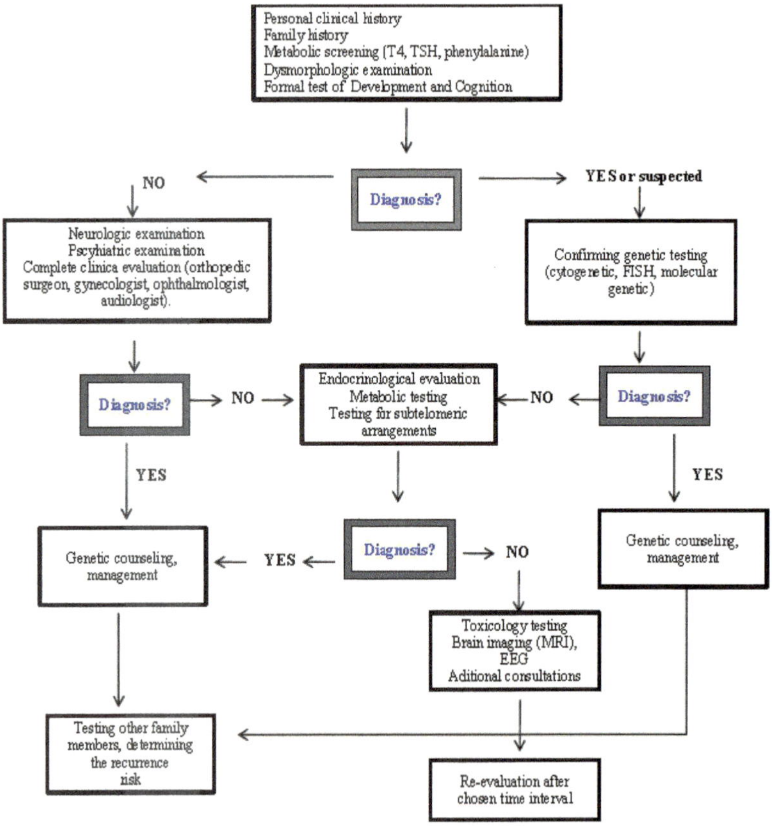

Figure 2. Algorithm of evaluation in DD/MR

Specific protocols for evaluation of children with DD/MR may be developed by every medical service based on the implication of a complex team and having as one of the objectives to keep the parents informed and facilitate the acquisition of the abilities and medical information that will make them able to manage their child at home.

4. Conclusion

Genetic factors have a major role in the etiology of mental retardation. In this chapter, we made a review of the genetic causes in mental retardation disorders, from chromosomal abnormalities, to contiguous gene syndromes, to monogenic mental retardation, to metabolic disorders that present with mental retardation and multifactorial inheritance.

Tremendous research strains were made to determine the genetic substrate along with the structural and functional impact of mental retardation. Firstly, efforts were targeted at understanding the cause and the natural history of the mental retardation disorders. Secondly, research aimed to precociously detect disorders (that can be treated), trough neonatal screening. Positive economic and social impact was shown by the extensive experience in screening, diagnosis and management of inborn errors of metabolism (PKU, hypothiroidism, organic acidemias). Unfortunately, most mental retardation syndromes do not have a treatment, and in these cases, the management is very difficult, expensive and lifelong. Thus, tailored professional support is needed for a family with a child with a mental retardation disease, in order to avoid social isolation and even isolation from the family. Access to interventions, based on developing skills and methods of coping, emotional management, support groups have reduced the negative impact on family functioning and established the base for development of resources in the community.

Author details

Maria Puiu[1,2*], Simona Dumitriu[1,2], Adela Chiriță-Emandi[1,2], Raluca Grădinaru[1] and Smaranda Arghirescu[1,2]

*Address all correspondence to: maria_puiu@umft.ro

1 University of Medicine and Pharmacy "Victor Babes" Timisoara, Romania

2 Emergency Hospital for Children "Louis Turcanu" Timisoara, Romania

References

[1] American Psychiatric Association. Diagnostic and statistical manual of mental disorders: DSM-IV [Internet]. *4th ed. Washington (DC): American Psychiatric Association; [cit-*

ed 2010 Mar 8]. 866 p. Weijerman ME, van Furth AM, van der Mooren MD, van Weissenbruch MM, Rammeloo L, Broers CJ, GemkeRJ.Eur J Pediatr., 169(10), 1195-9, Epub 2010 Apr 23. Prevalence of congenital heart defects and persistent pulmonary hypertension of the neonate with Down syndrome.

[2] Tingey, Carol. (1991). And Others Developmental Attainment of Infants and Young Children with Down Syndrome. *International Journal of Disability, Development and Education*, 38(1), 15-26.

[3] Dykens, E. M., Hodapp, R. M., & Evans, D. W. (2006). Profiles and development of adaptive behaviour in children with Down syndrome. *Down Syndrome Research and Practice*, 9(3), 45-50.

[4] Fishler, K., & Koch, R. (1991). Mental development in Down syndrome mosaicism. *American Journal on Mental Retardation*, 96, 345-351.

[5] Guidi, S., Bonasoni, P., Ceccarelli, C., et al. (2008). Neurogenesis impairment and increased cell death reduce total neuron number in the hippocampal region of fetuses with Down syndrome . *Brain Pathology*, 18(2), 180-197, View at Publisher View at Google Scholar View at Scopus.

[6] Golden, A., & Hyman, B. T. (1994). Development of the superior temporal neocortex is anomalous in trisomy 21. *Journal of Neuropathology and Experimental Neurology*, 53(5), 513-520.

[7] Weitzdoerfer, R., Dierssen, M., Fountoulakis, M., & Lubec, G. (2001). Fetal life in Down Syndrome starts with normal neuronal density but impaired dendritic spines and synaptosomal structure. *Journal of Neural Transmission* [61], 59-70.

[8] Jernigan, T. L., Bellugi, U., Sowell, E., Doherty, S., & Hesselink, J. R. (1993). Cerebral morphologic distinctions between Williams and Down syndromes. *Archives of Neurology*, 50(2), 186-191.

[9] Pinter, J. D., Eliez, S., Schmitt, J. E., Capone, G. T., & Reiss, A. L. (2001). Neuroanatomy of Down's syndrome: a high-resolution MRI study,. *American Journal of Psychiatry*, 158(10), 1659-1665.

[10] Noemí, Rueda., Jesús, Flórez., & Carmen-Cué, Martínez. (2012). Mouse Models of Down Syndrome as a Tool to Unravel the Causes of Mental Disabilities. *Neural Plasticity*, Article ID 584071, 26.

[11] Guidi, S., Ciani, E., Bonasoni, P., Santini, D., & Bartesaghi, R. (2011). Widespread proliferation impairment and hypocellularity in the cerebellum of fetuses with down syndrome. *Brain Pathology*, 21(4), 361-373.

[12] Battaglia, A., Carey, J. C., Viskochil, D. H., Cederholm, P., & Opitz, J. M. (2000). Wolf-Hirschhorn syndrome (WHS): a history in pictures. *ClinDysmorphol*, 9, 25-30.

[13] Battaglia, A., Filippi, T., & Carey, J. C. (2008). Update on the clinical features and natural history of Wolf-Hirschhorn (4p-) syndrome: experience with 87 patients and rec-

ommendations for routine health supervision. *Am J Med Genet Part C Semin Med Genet*, 148C, 246-51.

[14] Kagitani-Shimono, K., Imai, K., Otani, K., Kamio, N., Okinaga, T., Toribe, Y., Suzuki, Y., & Ozono, K. (2005). Epilepsy in Wolf-Hirschhorn syndrome (4p-). *Epilepsia*, 46, 150-5.

[15] Medina, M., Marinescu, R. C., Overhauser, J., & Kosik, S. K. (2000). Hemizigosity of delta-catenin (CTNND2) is associated with severe mental retardation in cri-du-chat syndrome. *Genomics*, 63, 157-164, 10.1006/geno.1999.6090.

[16] Simmons, A. D., Pueschel, A. W., Mc Pherson, J. D., Overhauser, J., & Lovett, M. (1998). Molecular cloning and mapping of human Semaphorin F from the Cri-du-Chat candidate interval. *BiochemBiophys Res Com*, 242, 685-691, 10.1006/bbrc. 1997.8027.

[17] Cornish, K., Green, A., & Cross, G. (1998). Defining the cognitive phenotype in cri-du-chat syndrome: the importance of careful characterisation of a 5p deletion before clinical predictions are made. *Genet Couns*, 9, 168-9.

[18] Marinescu, R. C., Johnson, E. I., Dykens, E. M., Hodapp, R. M., & Overhauser, J. (1999). No relationship between the size of the deletion and the level of developmental delay in cri-du-chat syndrome. Am J Med Genet.; 10.1002/(SICI)1096-8628(19990903)86:1<71::AID-AJMG14>3.0.CO;2-Y , 86, 66-70.

[19] Collins, M. S., & Cornish, K. (2002). A survey of the prevalence of stereotypy, self-injury and aggression in children and young adults with Cri du Chat syndrome. *J Intellect Disabil Res*, 46, 133-140, 10.1046/j.1365-2788.2002.00361.x.

[20] Thompson, R. W., Peters, J. E., & Smith, S. D. (1986). Intellectual, behavioral, and linguistic characteristics of three children with 18p-syndrome. *J DevBehav Pediatr*, 7(1), 1-7.

[21] Linden, M. G., Bender, B. G., & Robinson, A. (1995). Sex chromosome tetrasomy and pentasomy. *Pediatrics*, 96, 672-682.

[22] Rovet, J. (1996). The psychoeducational profile of boys with Klinefelter syndrome. *J Learn Disabil.*, Mar, 29(2), 180-96.

[23] Schwartz, I. D., & Root, A. W. (1991). The Klinefelter syndrome of testicular dysgenesis. *EndocrinolMetabClin North Am.*, Mar, 20(1), 153-63.

[24] Kuntsi, J. (2000). Ring-X chromosomes: their cognitive and behavioural phenotype. *Ann Hum Genet.*, Jul, 64(Pt 4), 295-305.

[25] South, S. T., Hannes, F., Fisch, G. S., Vermeesch, J. R., & Zollino, M. (2008a). Pathogenic significance of deletions distal to the currently described Wolf-Hirschhorn syndrome critical regions on 4p16.3. *Am J Med Genet C Semin Med Genet*, 148C, 270-4.

[26] Baldini, A. (2005). Dissecting contiguous gene defects: TBX1. *Curr Opin Genet Dev.*, Jun, 15(3), 279-84.

[27] Yagi, H., Furutani, Y., Hamada, H., et al. (2003). Role of TBX1 in human del22q11.2 syndrome. *Lancet*, 362, 1366-1373.

[28] Bearden, C. E., Jawad, A. F., Lynch, D. R., Soko, S., Kanes, S. J., Mc Donald-Mc Ginn, D. M., Saitta, S. C., Harris, S. E., Moss, E., Wang, P. P., Zackai, E., Emanuel, B. S., & Simon, T. J. (2004). Effects of a functional COMT polymorphism on prefrontal cognitive function in patients with 22q11.2 deletion syndrome. *Am J Psychiatry.*, Sep, 161(9), 1700-2.

[29] Inlow, J. K., & Restifo, L. L. (2004). Molecular and comparative genetics of mental retardation. *Genetics*, 166, 835-881.

[30] Peters, S. U., Beaudet, A. L., Madduri, N., et al. (2004a). Autism in Angelman's syndrome: implications for autism research. *Clin Genet*, 66, 530-6.

[31] Covic, , et al. (2011). Medical genetics. *Polirom.*

[32] Smith, M. (2005). Mental retardation and developmental delay: genetic and epigenetic factors,. *Oxford University Press.*

[33] Toyo-oka, K., et al. (2003). 14-3-3epsilon is important for neuronal migration by binding to NUDEL: a molecular explanation for Miller-Dieker syndrome. Nat Genet. Jul; , 34(3), 274-85.

[34] Spalice, A., et al. (2009). Neuronal migration disorders: clinical, neuroradiologic and genetics aspects. Acta Paediatr. Mar; Epub 2008 Dec 16., 98(3), 421-33.

[35] Baldini, A. (2004, May). DiGeorge syndrome: an update. *Curr Opin Cardiol.*, 19(3), 201-4, Review. PubMed citation.

[36] Mc Kinlay, Gardner. R. J., & Sutherland, G. R. (2004). Chromosome abnomalies and genetic counseling. *Oxford University Press.*

[37] Biancalana, V., et al. (2004). Five years of molecular diagnosis of Fragile X syndrome (1997a collaborative study reporting 95% of the activity in France. *Am. J. Med. Genet.*, 129A, 218-224.

[38] Grønskov, K., Hjalgrim, H., Nielsen, I. M., & Brondum-Nielsen, K. (2004). Screening of the ARX gene in 682 retarded males. *Eur. J. Hum. Genet.*, 12, 701-705.

[39] Pietro, Chiurazzi. (2008). XLMR genes: update2007. *European Journal of Human Genetics*, 16, 422-434, 10.1038/sj.ejhg.5201994, published online 16 January2008.

[40] Ropers., H. Hilger, & Hamel, Ben C. J. (2005). X-linked mental retardation. 10.1038/nrg1501, *Nature Reviews Genetics*, 6, 1-46.

[41] Yabut, O., Domagauer, J., & D'Arcangelo, G. (2010). Dyrk1A overexpression inhibits proliferation and induces premature neuronal differentiation of neural progenitor cells. *The Journal of Neuroscience*, 30, 4004-4014.

[42] Jamel, Chelly. (2006). Genetics and pathophysiology of mental retardation European Journal of Human Genetics. 14, 701-713, doi:10.1038/sj.ejhg.5201595.

[43] Herbst, D. S., & Mille,r, J. R. (1980). Nonspecific X-linked mental retardation II: the frequency in British Columbia. *Am J Med Genet*, 7, 461-469.

[44] Hilger, Ropers. ., & Hamel , Ben C. J. (2005). X-linked mental retardation Nature Reviews Genetics. (January) 10.1038/nrg1501 , 6, 46-57.

[45] Jacquemont, S. (2004). Aging in individuals with the FMR1 mutation. *Am J Ment Retard.*, Mar, 109(2), 154-64.

[46] Jacquemont, S. (2006). Fragile X-associated tremor/ataxia syndrome- FXTAS. *Schweiz Arch Neurol Psychiatr*, 157, 384.

[47] Dykens, E. M., Sutcliffe, J. S., & Levitt, P. (2004). Autism and 15q11-q13 disorders: behavioral, genetic, and pathophysiological issues. *Ment Retard Dev.Disabil.Res.Rev*, 10(4), 284-91.

[48] Smith, M., Escamilla, J. R., Filipek, P., Bocian, M. E., Modahl, C., Flodman, P., & Spence, M. A. (2001). Molecular genetic delineation of 2q37.3 deletion in autism and osteodystrophy: report of a case and of new markers for deletion screening by PCR. *Cytogenet Cell Genet*, 94, 15-22.

[49] Bonora, E., et al. (2005). Mutation screening and association analysis of six candidate genes for autism on chromosome 7q. *Eur J Hum Genet.*, Feb, 13(2), 198-207.

[50] Wald, N. (1991). Prevention of neural-tube defects-results of the Medical Research CouncilVitamin Study. *Lancet*, 338, 131-137.

[51] Relton, C. L., Wilding, C. S., Laffling, A. J., Jonas, P. A., Burgess, T., Binks, K., Tawn, E. J., & Burn, J. (2004). Low erythrocyte folate status and polymorphic variation in folate-related genes are associated with risk of neural tube defect pregnancy. *Mol Genet Metab.*, Apr, 81(4), 273-81.

[52] Relton, C. L., Wilding, C. S., Pearce, MS, Laffling, A. J., Jonas, P. A., Lynch, S. A., Tawn, E. J., & Burn, J. (2004). Gene-gene interaction in folate-related genes and risk of neural tube defects in a UK population. *J Med Genet.*, Apr, 41(4), 256-60.

[53] John, B. (2006). Moeschler and Michael Shevell, Clinical Genetic Evaluation of the Child With Mental Retardation orDevelopmental Delays. 10.1542/peds.2006-1006, *Pediatrics*, 117, 2304.

Chapter 7

Epilepsy and Genetics

Roya Vakili and Babak Kateby Kashy

Additional information is available at the end of the chapter

1. Introduction

Epilepsy is one of the most common neurological disorder, that affects approximately 50 million people in the world and 90% of epilepsy cases are seen in the less developed countries[1,2].Epilepsy and seizures affect nearly 3 million Americans of all ages.Inheritance as etiology for epilepsy has been suspected for centuries. Despite the frequency of seizure disorder and epilepsy little progress has been made in understanding the genetics and physiological basis of epilepsy until the past two decades.

There has been strong evidence of genetic influence in some epilepsy syndromes from twin studies. The monozygotic twins have identical genotype and dizygotic twins are genetically similar like any two siblings and environmental factors are held to minimum in these studies. There is consistentlyhigher concordance rates seen in monozygotic than dizygotic twins.The rates of concordance range from 10.8% in monozygotic twins with brain injuries to 70% in those without. In dizygotic twins the concordance rate is 3 to 10% [3,4].

Epilepsy is defined as recurrent unprovoked seizures[1].Seizures are unprovoked when there are no immediate precipitating factors (although an injury to the central nervous system may have occurred in the past) [5].Clinically epilepsy can be divided into two categories of seizure types: generalized and partial epilepsy. Generalized seizure refers to a condition when the entire brain is seizing from the onset of the event. Partial seizures describe condition when seizure activity starts from a localized brain region and has potential to spread to other areas of the brain.

The etiology of epilepsy can be divided into three categories, idiopathic, cryptogenic, and symptomatic. About 25% of epilepsies are associated with injuries to the central nervous system or gray matter like trauma, CNS infection, stroke, bleed, cerebral palsy, metabolic insults, etc. These types of epilepsy are classified as symptomatic according to the International Classification of Epileptic Syndromes. The remainder of cases are categorized as idiopathic or cryptogenic. The idiopathic epilepsies are of genetic origin. In the cryptogenic syndromes a specific etiology is unknown. However, in many instances in the cryptogenic group a genetic influence may remain a possibility [6,7].

An important consideration is that epilepsy is often multifactorial and can be result of both external and internal contributions. Even in symptomatic epilepsies genetics may be a responsible or contributing etiology. Seizures are seen in number of congenital neurodevelopmental disorders with cortical malformations. Tuberous sclerosis (TS) is a type of neurocutaneous disorder with associated malignant childhood epilepsy. These children may have West syndrome (hypsarrhythmia, mental retardation, and infantile spasm). About 50% of TS cases are familial and other half are sporadic mutation. It is a dominant mutation of two tumor suppressor genes TSC1 and TSC2 located on 9q34 and 16p13.3 that cause the disease [8].

Mutations in over 70 genes are found to be etiology for many types of epilepsy. Seizure is an episodic dysrhythmia of the cerebral cortex marked by abnormal network synchronization. Some of the inherited errors destabilize neuronal signaling by inflicting primary disorders of membrane excitability and synaptic transmission, whereas others do so indirectly by perturbing critical control points that balance the developmental assembly of inhibitory and excitatory circuits. Ion channels play a major role in generating and controlling neuronal excitability. The mutations of the ion channel can cause hyper- or hypo-excitability of neurons [9]. Usually channelopathies are associated with idiopathic epilepsy. Human inherited epilepsy disorders associated with ion channel mutations (Table 1) have been found in voltage- gated channels (Na+, K+, Ca2+, Cl-) and ligand-gated channels (nicotinic ACH receptors, GABA receptor) [10].

Epileptic disorder	Voltage-gated Ion channels	Gene, locus
Generalized epilepsy with febrile seizure plus type 1 (GEFS+)	Sodium channel, beta-1 subunit	SCN1B, 19q13.1
Generalized epilepsy with febrile seizure plus type 2 (GEFS+)	Sodium channel, alpha subunit	SCN1A, 2q24
Benign familial neonatal-infantile seizures (BFNIS)	Sodium channel, alpha subunit	SCN2A, 2q24
Benign familial neonatal convulsions	Potassium channel, alpha subunit	KCNQ2, 20q13.3 KCNQ3, 8q24
Juvenile myoclonic epilepsy Juvenile absence epilepsy Childhood absence epilepsy, type 3	Chloride channel	CLCN2, 3q27.1
Epileptic disorder	**Ligand-Gated Ion Channels**	**Gene, locus**
Autosomal dominant juvenile myoclonic epilepsy	GABA-A receptor, alpha 1 subunit	GABRA1, 5q34-q35
Autosomal dominant nocturnal frontal lobe epilepsy	Nicotinic acetylcholine receptor, Alpha-4 subunit	CHRNA4, 20q13.2-q13.3
Autosomal dominant nocturnal frontal lobe epilepsy	Nicotinic acetylcholine receptor, Beta-2 subunit	CHRNB2, 1q21

Table 1. Inherited epilepsy disorders and ion channel mutations.

Our knowledge in the field of epilepsy has evolved since the discovery of new specific inherited epilepsy syndromes. Causal mutations have been identified for some of these syndromes. They involve various ionic channels: Na+ channels in the generalized epilepsy with febrile seizures plus (GEFS+), benign familial neonatal infantile seizure is another channelopathy associated with Na channel mutation, nicotinic receptors in autosomal dominant nocturnal frontal lobe epilepsy (ADNFLE), K+ channels in benign familial neonatal convulsions, and GABA-A receptors in autosomal dominant juvenile myoclonic epilepsy. In addition, other paroxysmal neurological disorders like familial hemiplegic migraine and episodic ataxia a result of ion channel mutations and are sometimes associated with epilepsy [11].

More new genes associated with epilepsy has been reported the past several years and more mutations with electrophysiological information will emerge. The ion channelopathies linked to idiopathic epilepsies account for minority of cases. The ion channel mutation are common cause of rare monogenic idiopathic epilepsies [12]. The knowledge and understanding of genetics of epilepsy is growing rapidly perhaps with more detailed molecular dissection will have better definitions and explanation of the common epilepsy syndromes.

More and more genetic mutations are being found that contribute to development of epilepsy. Inheritance can be seen in the classical Mendelian fashion: autosomal dominant, autosomal recessive, X-linked or mitochondrial inheritance [13]. Familial epilepsies can be inherited in an autosomal dominant (AD), AD with an incomplete penetrance, or autosomal recessive (AR). Examples of mitochondrial inheritance include wider syndromes, such as "Mitochondrial encephalopathy, Lactic Acidosis and Stroke-like Episode Syndrome" (MELAS) and "Myoclonus Epilepsy with Ragged-Red Fiber Syndrome" (MERRF) [14].

However, in most cases the simple Mendelian model does not explain the familial distribution of most epilepsy. It is unclear how genetics and environment interact to influence the risk of developing different types or phenotypes of epilepsy syndromes. There is a large genetic influence in epilepsy perhaps the complexity stems from the fact that epilepsy is very heterogeneous, the important genetic and environmental factors may differ across clinically defined subsets or syndromes [5].

There have been familial genetic linkage studies conducted to understand genetics of familial epilepsy syndromes. Gene mutations have been found in multiple epilepsy syndromes including familial lateral temporal epilepsies, febrile seizures, generalized epilepsy with febrile seizures plus (GEFS+) and severe myoclonic epilepsy of infancy. Unfortunately, in many familial types of epilepsy genetic basis of the disease has not been identified including familial mesial temporal lobe epilepsy and photosensitive epilepsy [15, 16].

2. Generalized epilepsies

Generalized epilepsy with febrile seizures plus (GEFS+)

In 1997, Scheffer and Berkovic identified GEFS+ as a newly recognized autosomal dominant epilepsy syndrome [17]. They described a family that had 25 people with generalized epilepsy over 4 generations. Many individuals had febrile seizures past age 6 and/or had generalized afebrile seizures. The afebrile seizure types include atonic, myoclonic, absence and tonic-clonic seizures and in some partial seizures. Most phenotypes of GEFS+ have normal intelligence with normal neurological exam and normal brain imaging. In most individuals seizures stop by mid childhood and in some it persists. The genetic heterogeneity of GEFS+ has been well studied. The first locus was found on 19q13.1 (GEFS1) associated with gene (SCN1B) encoding sodium channel Beta 1 subunit. Missense mutations on SCN1A,found on locus 2q24, encoding for sodium-channel voltage gated alpha subunit account for most of the GEFS+ cases [18, 19]. Defects on SCN2A and GABA receptor subunit can cause the same or similar condition as well [4].

Febrile seizures are very common, about 5 to 10 % of children under age of 6 can be affected. The genetic cause of thisis oligo- or polygenic rather than monogenic. There are rare autosomal dominant pattern identified and gene loci described. The gene locations include FEB1 on chromosome 8q13-q21, FEB2 on19q, FEB3 on 2q 23-q24, FEB4 on 5q14a15, FEB5 on 6q22-q24 and FEB6 on 18p11.2 [20].

Autosomal Dominant form of Juvenile Myoclonic Epilepsy (JME)

This is a fairly common form of idiopathic generalized epilepsy. Patients with this disorder have early morning myoclonus and generalized tonic-clonic seizure. Age of onset is during adolescence. Patients have characteristic EEG showing generalized polyspike and wave discharges. Missense mutation of the gene GABRA1 encoding the alpha 1 subunit of the GABA-A receptor was recently found, locus 5q34-q35. This is not detected in the sporadic cases (21).

Childhood absence epilepsy (CAE)

Childhood absence epilepsy is a very common type of generalized epilepsy, making up about 8% of epilepsycases in school-aged children. The age of onset of seizures ranges from 4-13 years, with a peak at ages 6-7 years. There is family history of epilepsy in approximately 30% of patients. However, autosomal dominant pattern of inheritance with age-dependent penetrance is suspected. This is likely due to multifactorial pattern of inheritance involving interplay of the environment and genetics. The seizures are characterized by sudden impairment of consciousness lasting for several seconds. The EEG shows classic pattern of 3-Hz spike-wave discharge during the episodes [4].

One type of childhood absence epilepsy, ECA1, has been linked to 8q24, second type, ECA2, is caused by mutation in the GABRG2 gene on band 5q31.1. A third type, ECA3, is caused by a mutation of the chloride-channel gene CLCN2 on band 3q27. There have been reports of other epilepsy syndromes associated with voltage gated chloride channel mutation including, juvenile myoclonic epilepsy, juvenile absence epilepsy, and epilepsy with grand mal seizures on awakening [27]. The gene is CLCN2 which encodes chloride channel that is widely distributed in the nervous system and is involved in neuronal excitability.

3. Partial epilepsies

Familial nocturnal frontal lobe epilepsy

The genetics of this disorder was the first described for inherited idiopathic epilepsy. The age of onset for autosomal dominant nocturnal frontal lobe epilepsy (ADNFLE) is adolescence or young adulthood. Patients have brief motor seizures during non-REM sleep. The typical duration of seizures are less than 20 seconds with brief awakenings. Patients may have more prolong seizures. Patients usually complain of being tired during the day and underestimate the number of seizures. Auras are reported with these seizures including epigastric and sensory symptoms. A typical seizure may start with vocalization and grunting followed by hyper-kinetic movements or tonic contractions with clonic jerking. Treatment is with antiepileptic medication such as carbamazepine with reduction or cessation of seizures, but not all patients respond well to medication [4, 20].

First mutation in this disorder was identified in 1995, CHRNA4, and mapped to chromosome 20q13.3. More mutations and two other genes associated with this disorder (CHRNA2 and CHRNB2) have been found;these genes encode alpha 4 and beta 2 subunits of the neuronal nicotinic acetylcholine receptor (nAChR), respectively. The nAChR is member of large family of ligand-gated ion channels [22].

Benign familial neonatal convulsions (BFNC)

BFNC is an autosomal dominant inherited epileptic syndrome that occurs in the newborns, onset within first days of life and spontaneously disappears within few months, at most fourth month of life. Patient has frequent brief seizures in the form of tonic stiffening, apnea, clonic, and focal movements. In rare cases adulthood epilepsy occurs, less than 10%. Although it was thought to be a generalized seizure at first, video EEG monitoring found the disorder is partial type of epilepsy[23].

Mutations in the voltage gated potassium channel genes have been identified in BFNC on chromosome 20q13.3 (KCNQ2) and more rarely on chromosome 8q24 (KCNQ3). More than 40 mutations have been reported for KCNQ2 and three for KCNQ3 [24]. Potassium channels are most critical for maintaining resting membrane potentials and enable rapid repolarization after an action potential. Mutations in either KCNQ2 or KCNQ3 decrease function of the encodedpotassium channel.

Benign Familial Neonatal-Infantile Seizures (BFNIS)

This is an autosomal dominant epilepsy disorder characterized by focal afebrile seizures beginning age 2 days to 6 months and mean age of 11 weeks. The infants are normally developed. There have been 8 families reported to have this syndrome. Originally found in a large North American family. The mutation is in the sodium channel gene, SCN2A [25].

Benign familial Infantile Convulsions (BFIC)

This is another autosomal dominant inherited partial epilepsy syndrome. The seizures occur between 2 to 20 months and patient is in remission by age 3. Patient has clusters of afebrile partial seizures over few days. Patients respond well to antiepileptic medication. This is a genetically heterogeneous disorder and linked to chromosome 1q23, 2q24, 19q and 16q12q12 loci. It was first described in Japan and then in Italy [26].

Non-ion channel genes in epilepsy syndromes

Most epilepsy genes mentioned above were associated with channelopathies. In 2001 it was found that non-ion channel genes play a minorrole in etiology of idiopathic epilepsies. Autosomal Dominant Partial Epilepsy with Auditory Features (ADPEAF) or Familial Lateral Temporal Lobe Epilepsy (FLTLE)is a rare type of genetic epilepsy caused by mutation in the LGI1 gene (leucine-rich glioma inactivated gene 1) on chromosome 10q24. This mutation modulates excitatory neurotransmission. The clinical features of this disorder include complex partial seizures from the temporal lobe with auditory auras (identifiable voices, music, buzzing,roaring, and ringing), ictal aphasia, visual disturbance and secondary generalized tonic-clonicseizures. The age of onset is variable usually occurs in young adulthood. Usually the seizures can be well controlled on antiepileptic medications, some patients have spontaneous remission in their 30s and later [28,29].

Progressive myoclonus epilepsy (PME)

PMEs are collection of rare neurogenetic syndromes, and seizures are a predominant feature of these disorders. Patients usually have triad of myoclonic seizures, tonic-clonic seizures, and progressive neurological decline often associated with dementia and ataxia. The pathophysiology of these disorders is more diverse and mutations detected may affect many functions such as metabolic, mitochondrial function, and cell migration. Most PMEs are autosomal recessive in inheritance [30]. Examples of these disorders include Unverricht-Lundborg disease, Lafora body disease, myoclonic epilepsy with ragged red fibers, dentatorubral-pallidoluysian atrophy, and neuronal ceroid lipofuscinoses.

Unverricht-Lundborg disease

Unverricht-Lundborg disease also known as the Baltic myoclonic epilepsy, because of its high prevalence in that region is a typical example of progressive myoclonus epilepsy. It is characterized by generalized seizures, myoclonus, and progressive neurological deterioration including dementia and ataxia. The disease was first described by Unverricht in Estonia in 1891 and by Lundborg in Sweden in 1903. The onset of disease is between ages of 6 and 18. It is autosomal recessive disease mapped on to chromosome 21q22.3. At this time few point mutations have been identified in the CSTB gene (Cystatin B). Cystatin B is found to be involved in normal maintenance of neuronal structure and loss of it in mouse models caused increased proteolysis, apoptosis, and gliosis [31]

Lafora body disease

Lafora body disease is a polyglucosan storage disease, first described in 1911 by Lafora and Glueck. It is an autosomal recessive disease; linkage to chromosome 21 and chromosome 6p23-25 have been found. The gene encoding novel protein tyrosine phosphatase called Laforin has been identified. Laforin is involved in development and maturation of neuronal networks [32]. This is a rare neurodegenerative disease most patients with this disease do not live past their 20s. Onset of symptoms late childhood or adolescence and become progressively worse over time

Myoclonic epilepsy and ragged-red fiber disease (MERRF)

This is a mitochondrial disease that affects individuals before age of 20. Patients have ataxia, hearing loss, poor night vision, and myoclonic seizures.This is maternally-inherited mutation at position 8344 in the mitochondrial genome in over 80% of cases. Lactic acidosis and ragged-red fibers on muscle biopsy are diagnostic. Clinical presentation of mitochondrial disorders is very heterogeneous ranging from impairment in single tissue to encephalopathies, myopathies, cardiomyopathies and other complex multisystem disorders [14, 33].

Dentatorubural-pallidoluysian atrophy (DRPLA)

DRPLA is a rare autosomal dominant disorder. The symptoms of this disease start in infancy to early childhood.The disease is from the trinucleotide (CAG) expansion on chromosome 12p. Patients presents with ataxia, myoclonus, dementia and seizures. The severity of the clinical manifestation depends on the length of the unstable trinucleotide repeat [34].

Neuronal ceroidlipofuscinoses (NCL)

NCL are autosomal recessive neurodegenerative disorders result in storage of lipopigments in brain and other issues. It is a type of lysosomal storage disease. Clinical manifestation includes behavioral changes, seizures, visual problems, decline in mental function, and loss of motor function. There are different subtypes according to age of onset, pathology and genetic linkage.

Infantile NCL (CLN1) presents at about 12 months with developmental regression, myoclonus, ataxia, and visual problems. The genetic defect in CLN1 is identified in the palmitoyl-protein thioesterase gene (35). Late infantile NCL (CLN2) have similar clinical findings as CNL1 by age 2-4 years, patient may have intractable epilepsy. The gene found in most cases is in chromosome 11p15. Juvenile NCL (CLN3) also known as Batten disease is the most common neurodegenerative disorder of childhood. Clinical finding includes visual loss at age 5 to 10years and gradual mental decline and seizures. CLN3 maps on chromosome 16p12.1. The CLN3 protein alters metabolism of proteins important for cell function. Adult NCL (CLN4) is a rare subtype and distinguished from others by absence of ocular manifestation. CLN5 and CLN6 are variants of the late-infantile NCL. [4, 36]

4. Pharmacogenetics and epilepsy

There is an inherited variance in drug sensitivity among patients; people react to the same medication differently. Pharmaco-dynamics and kinetic mechanism may be able to determine person's response to medication or adverse reaction. Genetic differences of receptor subunit may influence response to antiepileptic medications. Studies have shown that response to benzodiazepine can be genetically altered [37]. Current advances made in genetics can allow modulations of channel function. Targeting channels may be a successful way to produce antiepileptic medications. Certain antiepileptic drugs affect different ion channels. Dilantin is an example of antiepileptic drug that inhibits voltage gated NA channel. There is hypothesis that alteration of the channel after mutation of a subunit may alter responsiveness to this medication [38]. However, some GEFS+ patients respond well to Dilantin so the mutation does not alter effectiveness of the medication. More systemic studies need to be completed to better understand this and this may be an important area of investigation [11].

Pharmacokinetics can affect drug resistance in epilepsy. Multidrug resistance (MDR) means resistance to structurally and functionally different agents. The MDR-1 gene encodes a membrane protein, p-glycoprotein, which functions to transport molecules across membranes. Increased expression of this is seen in brains of patients with intractable epilepsy [39].

5. Conclusion

As field of genetics of epilepsies continues to advance the genetic heterogeneity of epilepsy syndrome has become more apparent.There is heterogeneity in etiology and clinical manifestation of epilepsy[40]. In addition, different genes and mutations may cause the same seizure phenotype. The discovery of dysfunction of ion channels, channelopathies, account for many forms of inherited or idiopathic epilepsies as ion channels are critical for normal neuronal excitation. The progress made in understanding genetic of epilepsies will contribute to our ability to recognize and diagnose diseases, provide genetic counseling, potentially find new treatments and anticonvulsant medications.

Author details

Roya Vakili* and Babak Kateby Kashy*

*Address all correspondence to:

*Address all correspondence to:

Michigan State University, Department of Neurology; Metro Health Neuroscience, Wyoming, MI, USA

References

[1] World Health Organization. (2009). Epilepsy. Retrieved January 5, 2012.

[2] Chang, B. S., & Lowenstein, D. H. (2003). Epilepsy. *N. Engl. J. Med.*, 349(13), 1257-66.

[3] Treiman, L. J., & Treiman, D. M. (2001). Genetic aspects of Epilepsy. In:Wyllie, E (Ed). The treatment of Epilepsy: Principles and Practice. Lippincott Williams and Wilkins, Philadelphia;, 115-129.

[4] Kaneko, S., Okada, M., Iwasa, H., Yamakawa, K., & Hirose, S. (2002). Genetic of epilepsy: current status and perspectives. *Neuroscience Research.*, 44, 11-30.

[5] Ottman, R. (1997). Genetic Epidemiology of Epilepsy. *Epidemiol Rev.*, 19(1), 120-128.

[6] Tomoum, H. Y. (2003). Genetics of Epilepsy. *Egyptian Journal of Medical Human Genetics.*, 4(2), 89-94.

[7] Johnson, M. R., & Sanders, J. W. (2001). The Clinical Impact of Epilepsy Genetics. *Journal of Neurology, Neurosurgery, and Psychiatry.*, 70, 428-430.

[8] Kullman, D. M. (2002). Genetics of Epilepsy. *Journal of Neurology Neurosurgery Psychiatry.*, 73(2), 32-35.

[9] Lerch, H., Jurkat-Rott, K., & Lehmann-Horn, F. (2001). Ion channels and epilepsy. *American Journal of Medicinal Genetics*, 106, 146-159.

[10] George, A. L., & Jr , . (2004). Inherited Channelopathies Associated with Epilepsy. *Epilepsy Curr.*, 4(2), 65-70.

[11] Kurian, M., & Picard, F. (2006). Inherited Epilepsy Syndromes and Channelopathies. *Epileptologie*, 75-85.

[12] Mulley, J. C., Scheffer, I. E., Petrou, S., & Berkovic, S. F. (2003). Channelopathies as a genetic cause of epilepsy.". *Curr Opin Neurol.*, 16(2), 171-6.

[13] Sisodiya, S., Cross, J. H., Blümcke, I., Chadwick, D., Craig, J., Crino, P. B., Debenham, P., Delanty, N., Elmslie, F., Gardiner, M., Golden, J., Goldstein, D., Greenberg, D. A., Guerrini, R., Hanna, M., Harris, J., Harrison, P., Johnson, M. R., Kirov, G., Kullman, D. M., Makoff, A., Marini, C., Nabbout, R., Nashef, L., Noebels, J. L., Ottman, R., Pirmohamed, M., Pitkänen, A., Scheffer, I., Shorvon, S., Sills, G., Wood, N., & Zuberi, S. (2007). Genetics of epilepsy: epilepsy research foundation workshop report,. *Epileptic Disord.*, 9(2), 194-236.

[14] Hirano, M., Kunz, W., & Dimauros, S. (2001). Mitochondrial Disease. In Epilepsy: A Comprehensive Textbook, (ed.J.J. Engel and T.A. Pedley). Lippincott Williams and Wilkins, Philadelphia;, 2621-2630.

[15] Striano, P., de Falco, A., Diani, E., Bovo, G., Furlan, S., Vitiello, L., Pinardi, F., Striano, S., Michelucci, R., de Falco, F. A., & Nobile, C. (2008). A Novel Loss-of-Function LGI1 Mutation Linked to Autosomal Dominant Lateral Temporal Epilepsy. *Archives of Neurology.*, 65, 939-942.

[16] Kasteleijn-Nolst, Trenité. D. G. A. (2006). Photosensitivity, visually sensitive seizures and epilepsies. *Epilepsy Research.*, 70, 269-279.

[17] Scheffer, I. E., & Berovic, S. F. (1997). Generalized epilepsy with febrile seizures plus. A genetic disorder with heterogenousphenotypes. *Brain*, 120, 479-490.

[18] Sugawara, T., Tsurubuchi, Y., Agarwala, K. L., Ito, M., Fukuma, G., Mazaki-Miyazaki, E., Nagafuji, H., Noda, M., Imoto, K., Wada, K., Mitsudome, A., Kaneko, S., Montal, M., Nagata, K., Hirose, S., & Yamakawa, K. (2001). A missense mutation of the Na+ channel alpha II subunit gene Na1 in a patient with febrile and afebrile seizures causes channel dysfunction. *ProcNatlAcadSci U S A.*, 98(11), 6384-9.

[19] Catterall, W. A., Dib-Hajj, S., Meisler, M. H., & Pietrobon, D. (2008). Inherited Neuronal Ion Channelopathies: New Windows on Complex Neurological Diseases. *J Neurosci.*, 28(46), 11768-11777.

[20] Steinlein, O. (2008). Genetics and epilepsy. *Dialogues in Clinical Neuroscience.*, 10(1), 29-38.

[21] Bianchi, M. T., Song, L., Zhang, H., & Macdonald, R. L. (2003). Two different mechanisms of disinhibition produced by GABA-A receptor mutations linked to epilepsy in humans. *J Neurosci*, 22, 5321-5327.

[22] Aridon, P., Marini, C., Di Resta, C., Brilli, E., De Fusco, M., Politi, F., Parrini, E., Manfredi, I., Pisano, T., Pruna, D., Curia, G., Cianchetti, C., Pasqualetti, M., Becchetti, A., Guerrini, R. ., & Casari, G. (2006). Increased Sensitivity of the Neuronal Nicotinic Receptor [alpha]2 Subunit Causes Familial Epilepsy with Nocturnal Wandering and Ictal Fear. *The American Journal of Human Genetics*, 79, 342-350.

[23] Singh, N. A., Charlier, C., Stauffer, D., et al. (1998). A novel potassium channel gene, KCNQ2, is mutated in an inherited epilepsy of newborns. *Nature Genetics.*, 18, 25-29.

[24] Rogawski, M. A. (2000). KCNQ2/KCNQ3 K+ channels and the molecular pathogenesis of epilepsy: implications for therapy. *Trends Neurosci.*, 23(9), 393-8.

[25] Kaplan, R. E., & Lacey, D. J. (1983). Benign familial neonatal-infantile seizures. *American Journal of Medical Genetics.*, 16(4), 595-599.

[26] Vigevano, F., Fusco, L., Di Capua, M., Ricci, S., Sebastianelli, R., & Lucchini, P. (1992). Benign infantile familial convulsions. *Europ J Pediat.*, 151, 608-612.

[27] Haug, K., Warnstedt, M., Alekov, A. K., Sander, T., Ramirez, A., Poser, B., Malijevic, S., Hebeisen, S., Kubisch, C., Rebstock, J., Horvath, S., Hallmann, K., & Heils, A. (2003). Mutations in CLCN2 encoding a voltage-gated chloride channel are associated with idiopathic generalized epilepsies. *Nat Genet*, 33, 527-532.

[28] Andermann, F., Kobayashi, E., & Andermann, E. (2005). Genetic focal epilepsies: state of the art and paths to the future. *Epilepsia.*, 46(10), 61-7.

[29] Pisano, T., Marini, C., Brovedani, P., Brizzolara, D., Pruna, D., Mei, D., Moro, F., Cianchetti, C., & Guerrini, R. (2005). Abnormal phonologic processing in familial lateral temporal lobe epilepsy due to a new LGI1 mutation. *Epilepsia.*, 46(1), 118-23.

[30] Kaneko, S., & Wada, K. (1988). Molecular genetics studies of epilepsies. *Brain Nerve.*, 50, 1071-1077.

[31] Lieuallen, K., Pennacchio, L. A., Park, M., Myers, R. M., & Lennon, G. (2001). Cystatin B-deficient mice have increased expression of apoptosis and glial activation genes. *Human Molecular Genetics.*, 10, 1867-1871.

[32] Ganesh, S., Agarwala, K. L., Amano, K., Suzuki, T., Delgado-Escueta, A. V., & Yamakawa, K. (2001). Regional and developmental expression of Epm2a gene and its evolutionary conservation. *Biochem Biophys Res Commun.*, 283(5), 1046-53.

[33] Shoffner, J. M., Lott, M. T., Lezza, A. N., Seibel, P., Ballinger, S. W., & Wallace, D. C. (1990). Myoclonic epilepsy and ragged-red fiber disease (MERRF) is associated with a mitochondrial DNA tRNA(Lys) mutation. *Cell.*, 61(6), 931-937.

[34] Koide, R., Ikeuchi, T., Onodera, O., Tanaka, H., Igarashi, S., Endo, K., Takahashi, H., Kondo, R., Ishikawa, A., Hayashi, T., et al. (1994). Unstable expansion of CAG repeat in hereditary dentatorubral-pallidoluysian atrophy (DRPLA). *Nat Genet.*, 6(1), 9-13.

[35] Vesa, J., Hellsten, E., Verkruyse, L. A., Camp, L. A., Rapola, J., Santavuori, P., Hofmann, S. L., & Peltonen, L. (1995). Mutations in the palmitoyl protein thioesterase gene causing infantile neuronal ceroidlipofuscinosis. *Nature.*, 376(6541), 584-7.

[36] Tripathi, M., & Jain, S. (2002). Genetics of Epilepsy. *Current Science.*, 82(6), 671-677.

[37] Mc Kernan, R. M., et al. (2000). Sedative but not anxiolytic properties of benzodiazepines are mediated by the GABAA receptor a1 subtype. *Nature Neuroscience,* 3, 587-592.

[38] Lucas, P. T., Meadows, L. S., Nicholls, J., & Ragsdale, . (2005). An epilepsy mutation in the β1 subunit of the voltage-gated sodium channel results in reduced channel sensitivity to phenytoin. *Epilepsy Research.*, 64, 77-84.

[39] Tishler, D. M., Weinberg, K. I., Hinton, D. R., Barbaro, N., Annett, G. M., & Raffel, C. (1995). MDR1 gene expression in brain of patients with medically intractable epilepsy. *Epilepsia.*, 36(1), 1-6.

[40] Berg, A. (2001). Introduction to the Epilepsies. In Epilepsy: A Comprehensive Textbook, (ed.J.J. Engel and T.A. Pedley). Lippincott Williams and Wilkins, Philadelphia;, 761-766.

Chapter 8

Molecular Bases of Ataxia Telangiectasia: One Kinase Multiple Functions

Venturina Stagni, Simonetta Santini and
Daniela Barilà

Additional information is available at the end of the chapter

1. Introduction

Ataxia Telangiectasia (A-T) is an autosomal recessive hereditary progressive neurodegenerative and multisystem disease characterized by cerebellar ataxia, telangiectasia, recurrent sinopulmonary infections, variable immunologic defects among which a significantly higher incidence of leukaemia and lymphoma and type 2 diabete. This disorder has been clearly linked to the loss of expression of the serine/threonine kinase ATM (Ataxia Telangiectasia Mutated), a central player of the DNA Damage Response (DDR). Several clinical features of A-T patients, as well as the pleiotropic phenotypes observed in Atm deficient mice, can be associated to a defective DDR. Moreover, ATM deficient cellular models display radiosensitivity and failure to activate cell cycle checkpoints in response to DNA damaging agents. Emerging evidences indicate that ATM kinase may be involved in several additional signalling pathways, among which the signalling cascades triggered by oxidative stress, hypoxia, autophagy, metabolic changes, growth factors and death receptors, suggesting that the endangerment of these functions in the absence of ATM activity may importantly contribute to the development of A-T pathology.

The aim of this chapter is to provide a schematic, although exhaustive, description of the signalling cascades that may modulate and may be modulated by ATM kinase activity. Data obtained from different model systems, including *in vitro* and *in vivo* studies, human and mouse models will be integrated. The chapter will be subdivided in paragraphs to improve the readability and to emphasize different aspects of the genetic, molecular and functional features of this pathology. The structure of the protein as well as its primary function in the DDR will be discussed. However, particular emphasis will be given to the enrolment of ATM to other signalling pathways and to the molecular mechanisms that ensure ATM kinase activity regulation. Finally, we will deeply discuss the functional links between ATM kinase and cancer, immune system defects and neurodegeneration.

2. Ataxia telangiectasia pathology

Ataxia-telangiectasia (A-T) [1], is a multisystem neurodegenerative syndrome that occurs early in childhood. A-T is an autosomal recessive disease with an estimated frequency in the range of one per 40000 to one per 300 000 births. At birth, infants generally appear normal and begin walking at a normal age (approximately age 1 year); however, by age 2–3 ataxia (loss of muscle co-ordination) becomes visible and generally by age 10 patients are confined to a wheelchair (for a recent review [2]). Clinically, A-T presents with uncoordinated or ataxic movements that are often associated with ocular telangiectasia (dilated blood vessels of the eye). Ataxia generally precedes telangiectasia, which is described as the chronic dilation of a group of capillaries causing elevated, dark red blotches on the skin or eyes. The prominent neurological sign of A-T is an inexorable loss of cerebellar function, and progressive dysarthria (speech defects) and choreoathetosis (abnormal body movements). Studies have shown a gradual decrease in granular and Purkinje cells, which are large branching cells of the nervous system and are located in the cerebellum. Characteristic eye movement abnormalities also feature strongly in A-T, and these might be related to cerebellar dysfunction. Although, the hallmark of clinical presentation is a debilitating progressive neurodegeneration, other characteristics are associated with A-T, such as extreme radiosensitivity, immunodeficiency (frequently manifested as decreased or absent IgA, IgE and IgG2), cancer predisposition (particularly lymphoma and leukaemia), insulin-resistant diabetes and premature aging.

Clinical diagnosis of A-T is relatively easy once the characteristic neurodegeneration and ocular telangiectasia have developed. In these cases the diagnosis can usually be confirmed by finding an elevated serum α-fetoprotein level, although so far it is not clear why α-fetoprotein remains high in A-T patients since there is no obvious liver damage. In young children where ataxia and/or telengiectasia did not occur yet, the diagnosis is still challenging. A-T pathology has been clearly linked to the loss of function of the product of the ATM gene. Most patients are compound heterozygotes with different mutations in the two ATM alleles. The identification of the ATM gene has facilitated diagnosis, although the large dimensions of the gene and the lack of mutational hot spots, prevent mutational analysis for clinical screening. Additional confirmatory laboratory test results include absence of the ATM protein on immunoblots, lack of ATM protein kinase activity, increased frequency of chromosomal breaks after exposure to γ-radiation, radioresistant DNA synthesis and decreased colony survival after γ-radiation. None of these methods is 100% specific or 100% sensitive, and clinical correlation is essential. The two most common causes of death are chronic lung disease (about one-third of cases) and cancer (about one-third of cases) (reviewed in [2]).

3. Genetic and molecular bases of A-T: From ATM gene to ATM protein

Ataxia–telangiectasia (A-T) is a rare autosomal recessive disorder caused by deficiency of the Ataxia–Telangiectasia Mutated (ATM) protein kinase. A-T patients generally lack functional ATM protein due to missense or nonsense mutations in the ATM gene, which has been identified by positional cloning strategy in 1995 [3].

These mutations occur throughout the entire coding sequence of the gene and overall lead to the production of truncated or unstable ATM variants [4]. The human ATM gene is located at 11q22-23 and covers 160 kb of genomic DNA; the gene product, ATM protein, is produced from a 13 kb transcript that codes for a 350 kDa protein.

ATM protein belongs to the phosphatidylinositol 3 kinase-like kinase (PIKK) family of Ser/Thr-protein kinases, which includes ATR (ataxia–telangiectasia and RAD3-related), DNA-PKcs (DNA-dependent protein kinase catalytic sub-unit) and mTOR (mammalian target of rapamycin), and many others. The proteins that are members of this family show a conserved domain organization in their C-terminal portion, which includes the presence of a kinase domain, flanked by a FAT domain (conserved sequence in FRAP, ATM and TRAPP proteins), that precedes the catalytic domain, and a FATC domain (FAT-C-terminal) that is located at the very C-terminal of the protein. Interestingly the FAT and the FATC domain have been proposed to play a role in the conformational maintenance of the catalytic domain and therefore in the control of the functionality of these kinases [5]. This model is also supported by the identification in these domains of several post-translational modifications that play a role in the modulation of ATM activity. Among these, S1981 in the FAT domain, a major autophosphorylation site that modulates the assembly of the inactive dimeric conformation [6], and C2991 in the FATC, whose acetylation contributes to the modulation of S1981 phosphorylation and to ATM kinase activation [7].

The N terminus of ATM is composed of HEAT (Huntingtin, Elongation factor 1A, protein phosphatase 2A A-subunit, TOR) repeats [8]. Moreover, several motifs that allow ATM interaction with other proteins have been mapped in the N-terminal region of ATM. Among these, sequences for the interaction with NBS1, c-Abl, p53, which play an essential role in the regulation and in the execution of ATM function, as well as with chromatin. The protein is heavily subjected to several post-translational modifications, among which phosphorylations and acetylation, that overall play a role in the modulation of ATM kinase activity as described in the next paragraph (for recent reviews on ATM [9] [10]).

4. ATM function: The DNA damage response

ATM function in the DNA damage response has been deeply investigated by several groups. Several excellent reviews in this topic are currently available [9, 11-13]. For this reason this paragraph will only briefly summarize the state of the art on this issue.

ATM has been first identified as an essential component of the DNA damage response, a complex of signalling cascades that ensures the maintenance of genomic stability. The occurrence of a DNA damage triggers cell cycle arrest and the initiation of the repair process. Alternatively, the cell that contains the damaged DNA may undergo apoptosis or senescence. The molecular mechanisms that allow the choice among these responses have not been clearly elucidated yet, although the common idea is that apoptosis or senescence are initiated in case the damage in not repairable. Genetic defects that perturb these mechanisms almost invariably cause severe syndromes that are characterized by the degeneration of specific tissues (especially the nervous and immune system), sensitivity to specific DNA-damaging agents and predisposition to cancer (reviewed in [11], see next paragraph on "DNA damage response and other genomic instability syndromes"). Different types of DNA damage may trigger different types of DNA repair responses (for a recent review see [13]).

In particular, ATM is major player of the cellular response to Double Strand Breaks which represent the most toxic type of DNA lesion, elicited mainly by ionizing radiation (IR or γ-radiation) and other genotoxic stresses. DSBs occur also during physiological processes such as meiotic recombination and the assembly of the T-cell receptor and immunoglobulin genes via V(D)J recombination, in T cells and B cells, respectively. The central role of ATM in the DDR to DSBs has been strongly suggested by some observations derived from A-T patients or Atm KO mice as well as from Atm deficient cells. Indeed A-T cells are highly sensitive to IR, and are characterized by failure of checkpoint induction in response to IR. As already pointed out, ATM deficiency leads both in human and mice to immune system defects (see also next paragraph on "Functional links between ATM kinase and the immune system defects") as well as to genomic instability and to higher incidence of cancer development (see also next paragraph on "Functional links between ATM kinase and cancer").

Within minutes after the induction of DSBs, most ATM molecules become vigorously active and participate to checkpoints activation, as well as to DNA repair and to the induction of senescence or apoptosis [14]. Overall, the signalling cascades that allow ATM to participate and modulate all these responses have been only partially elucidated and rely on the ability of ATM to trigger the phosphorylation of a large number of substrates, among which several kinases, that amplify the signal, and transcription factors, DNA repair components and other that execute the different responses (see also next paragraph on "Identification of ATM substrates: proteomic studies"). The activation process includes ATM recruitment to the DSBs, which is mediated by the MRN complex and by the damaged DNA (see next paragraph on "Molecular mechanisms that ensure the modulation of ATM kinase activity"). Activation of this pathway includes a plethora of phosphorylation and ubiquitination events triggered by ATM kinase, among which the activation of c-Abl kinase which in turn modulates the activity of Rad51 and Rad52 proteins and the phosphorylation of histone H2AX which marks the DSBs. Therefore activated ATM participates directly to the repair of the DNA lesion. In particular, ATM modulates Homologous Recombination (HR) and contributes to repair also through its interplay with other PI3K-like kinases such as ATR and DNA-PK.

Activated ATM is also released from the damaged DNA and may therefore trigger the cell cycle checkpoints activation. ATM may modulate cell cycle arrest as well as the apoptotic or senescence induction. For these responses, among the others, a crucial effector of ATM signalling is p53 transcription factor. ATM may modulate p53 functionality by directly phosphorylating p53 on S15 (promoting p53 transcriptional activity) as well as via the activation of Chk2 kinase, which in turn triggers p53 phosphorylation on S20 (impairing p53 interaction with Hdm2 ubiquitin ligase, therefore promoting its stabilization). Moreover ATM may direcly phosphorylate and modulate Hdm2 and may also modulate HIPK2 and therefore p53 phosphorylation on S46, which enhances p53 apoptotic activity. To summarize, the interplay between ATM and p53 is a good example of the complexity of the signalling cascades that modulate the balance and the integration of the different checkpoints with the apoptotic response.

An exhaustive picture of the signalling cascades through which ATM modulates cell cycle, cell death and DNA repair is beyond the scope of this chapter and it is available in these suggested reviews [9, 11-13].

4.1. DNA damage response and other genomic instability syndromes

A-T belongs to a group of human diseases that are collectively known as "genomic instability syndromes", each of which results from a defective response to a specific DNA lesion [11]. Genetic defects that affect specific DNA damage response pathways lead to syndromes that combine various degrees of tissue degeneration, growth and developmental retardation, premature signs of ageing, chromosomal instability, sensitivity to the corresponding DNA-damaging agents and cancer predisposition. The prominent genomic instability syndromes – Xeroderma pigmentosum (XP), Cockayne's syndrome, Trichothiodystrophy (TTD), Bloom's syndrome (BS), Werner's syndrome (WS), Rothmund–Thompson syndrome (RTS), Fanconi's anemia (FA), Nijmegen breakage sindrome (NBS), ataxia-telangiectasia-like disease (ATLD) - are all autosomal recessive and display defects in the main damage-response pathways, each of which is activated by a different class of damaging agent (see for an exhaustive review [11])

4.2. Identification of ATM substrates: Proteomic studies

It has been shown that ATM and ATR kinases mainly phosphorylate a subset of Serine and Threonine resisdues located inside the S/T-Q motif [15]. Antibodies that allow the identification of proteins phosphorylated on S/T-Q residues have been generated and are commercially available. These tools allowed therefore the development of several proteomic studies aimed to an exhaustive identification of ATM/ATR substrates in cells treated with IR. Matsuoka and colleagues performed a large-scale proteomic analysis of proteins phosphorylated in response to DNA damage on consensus sites recognized by ATM and ATR and identified more than 900 regulated phosphorylation sites encompassing over 700 proteins. Functional analysis of a subset of this data set indicated that this list is highly enriched for proteins involved in the DDR [16]. Mu and colleagues performed a similar study and identified proteins that belong to the ubiquitin-proteasome system (UPS) to be required in mammalian DNA damage checkpoint control, particularly the G1 cell cycle checkpoint, thus revealing protein ubiquitylation as an important regulatory mechanism downstream of

ATM/ATR activation for checkpoint control [17]. Other proteomic studies where aimed to the analysis of the phosphoproteome dinamic changes, dependent or independent on ATM, involved in the DNA damage response [18, 19]. Recently, a comparative analysis of ATM deficient and proficient lymphoblastoid cells by label-free shotgun proteomic experiments has been conducted. This study provided an insight on the functional role of ATM deficiency in cellular carbohydrate metabolism's regulation [20].

Overall proteomic approaches, identified several changes dependent on ATM expression and activity increasing the comprehension of the DNA damage response. More intriguingly, these studies identified as possibile substrates or effectors of ATM several proteins whose known functions are not linked to the DDR, supporting the idea that ATM may perform several other functions in addition of its well known role in the DDR.

5. ATM kinase: Other functions

First evidences that induce scientists to postulate a more general signaling role for ATM, independent from DNA damage, rise from several observations made on A-T patients as well as from a series of abnormalities of ATM-deficient cells.

First of all, cerebellar degeneration, ataxia and telangienctasia in A-T patients fit less well with the assumption that exclusive function of ATM is in DDR. It is evident, for example, that post-mitotic neurons of the cerebellum are less dependent on the DNA damage response-associated cell-cycle regulation mediated by ATM [21]. Furthermore, some A-T patients develop insulin-resistant diabetes [22, 23]. This feature is also part of the clinical profile of the metabolic syndrome and cannot be explained by the aberrant DNA damage signaling activation.

Importantly, ATM-deficient cells exhibit some abnormalities, which are difficult to ascribe only to the role of ATM in DNA damage response [12]. These alterations include:

-reduced internalization of phytohaemagglutinin (PHA), defective Ca^{2+} mobilization, depolarization in response to extracellular K^{+};

- decreased duration of Ca^{2+} and Na^{+} firing;
- increased growth factor demand and defective signalling through the epidermal growth factor (EGF) receptor;
- occurrence of markers for oxidative stress such as protein nitrosylation, increased thiol conjugates, and lipid peroxidation.

Finally, although ATM is primarily localized to the nucleus, it has been shown that a minor fraction of the protein is present in the cytoplasm of various cell types [24]. First evidence for a cytoplasmic form is the discovery of ATM association with both peroxisomes and endosomes [25, 26]. In neurons of the cerebellum, ATM is equally distributed between the nucleus and the cytoplasm [27, 28], which further suggests additional roles for ATM also outside the nucleus. ATM activation in the cytosol has been described upon insulin treatment [29] or, more recently, upon oxidative stress induction [30].

All of these observations provide evidence for additional and unexplored ATM functions mainly linked to its extranuclear localization. However, only in the last years different groups start to investigate more deeply and systematically the molecular mechanism and the biological significance of these new functions. In this section a summary of these studies will be provided.

5.1. ATM and oxidative stress

Cells living in an oxygen-rich environment are constantly challenged by oxidative stress. Oxidative stress is defined as an imbalance between cellular oxidants and antioxidants in which the production of Reactive Oxygen Species (ROS) exceeds the anti-oxidative capacity. ROS include the superoxide anion radical ($\bullet O^{-2}$), hydrogen peroxide (H_2O_2), and the hydroxyl radical ($_\bullet OH$). Together with other reactive nitrogen species (RNS), these ROS are the major mediators of oxidative stress. Numerous exogenous and endogenous stress stimulators can disrupt cellular homeostasis and evoke oxidative stress. Physical factors (ultraviolet light and ionizing radiation), oxygen level changers (hypoxia and subsequent reoxygenation) and chemical factors (hydrogen peroxide and chemotherapeutic reagents) are some of the possible exogenous sources of ROS. Several potential endogenous sources of ROS exist within the cell. ROS generated as byproducts and normal metabolites during aerobic metabolism in mitochondria are the primary sources of ROS. In conclusion ROS produced by both endogenous and exogenous sources either directly or indirectly activate antioxidant machinery and physiological stress signaling pathways.

Over the past two decades, evidence has accumulated that links ATM deficiency to increased oxidative stress in cells, which is thought to play a key role in neurodegeneration, metabolic dysregulation and oncogenesis [31].

Cells from individuals affected by A-T syndrome have constitutive oxidative stress and this altered oxidative stress has long been linked to A-T as both a cause and a consequence of the disease [10].

Because treatment of ATM-null mice with antioxidants can ameliorate intrinsic defects in stem cell renewal [32, 33] and delay their tumor onset [34, 35], it has been suggested that increased accumulation of intracellular ROS associated with ATM dysfunction contributes to the clinical features of this pathology [31, 36, 37].

Although, the increased oxidative damage associated with ATM deficiency has largely been attributed in the past to the defects in the DDR pathway, the basis for this phenomenon remains unclear, and recent data have provided some possible new clues that are independent of DDR. For example, a potential role for ATM in the control of an antioxidant response via the pentose phosphate pathway (PPP) has been reported and may be relevant in ATM null tissues showing increased oxidative stress [38]. The authors demonstrated that ATM regulates the PPP by inducing glucose-6-phosphate dehydrogenase (G6PD) activity, which in turn promotes NADPH (Nicotinamide Adenine Dinucleotide Phosphate) production and nucleotide synthesis. Consistently, ATM might contribute to maintain the reducing power of the cellular environment by promoting NADPH production. Moreover ATM can modulate ROS also through modulation of mithocondria activity (see next paragraph "ATM and Mitochondria").

Although, it has been recognized since several years that ATM is activated also by oxidative stress (as H_2O_2), the biochemical mechanisms underlying the response of ATM to oxidative stress were described only recently. Guo and colleagues proposed that ATM functions as a redox sensor in the cytoplasm and, as such, may regulate global cellular responses to oxidative stress [39]. ATM activation by oxidative stress involves the formation of a disulfide bridge between cysteine (C2991) residues to form a ATM dimer [39] (described in the following paragraph "Molecular mechanisms that ensure the modulation of ATM kinase activity"). Importantly, this mode of ATM activation can occur independently of the MRN complex, suggesting a role for ATM in signaling other than direct DNA damage.

Notably, ionizing radiations that generate DNA DSBs can also produce ROS that inactivate key DNA repair. Hence, ATM oxidative activation may allow cells to respond to DNA DSBs and maintain genetic integrity under these toxic conditions. ATM appears to function as a key nodal point, bringing together DNA damage response and also the response to oxidative stress [40]. Clearly, further analysis of the importance of oxidative stress–induced activation of ATM will illuminate the possible contribution of this feature toward specific aspects of the A-T phenotype.

A possible role of ATM in vascular stability has long been suspected because of the manifestation of telangiectasia (dilated blood vessels) and vascular leakiness in both patients with ataxia telangiectasia and aged ATM-deficient mice. Recently, Okuno and colleagues demonstrated a very interestingly correlation between oxidative stress–induced activation of ATM and the occurrence of telangiectasia [41]. In this papers the authors demonstrated that ROS substantially accumulates in newly formed immature vessels and activates ATM. Loss of ATM in endothelial cells minimizes pathological ocular and tumor neoangiogenesis as a consequence of defective oxidative defense rather than an impaired DDR [41]. This paper provides the first evidence for a link between a clinical feature of A-T and DNA damage independent function of ATM kinase.

5.2. ATM and mitochondria

Mitochondria play an important role in ATP synthesis and apoptosis and are also the major source of intracellular ROS. A number of human diseases are linked to mutations of the mitochondrial genome. Among these are premature ageing, cancer, diabetes mellitus, and a variety of syndromes involving the muscles and the central nervous system [42]. A-T is similar to other progressive neurological disorders that are characterized by oxidative stress and intrinsic mitochondrial dysfunction [43].

Different studies, using immortalized cell lines established from patients with A-T, have reported that cells lacking ATM function exhibit alterations in mitochondrial homeostasis, including defects in mitochondrial structure, decreased membrane potential, and respiratory activity [44, 45].

An important step in the control of mitochondrial function is the biogenesis of these organelles, which involves mitochondrial DNA (mtDNA) replication and mitochondrial mass increase. Due to limited coding capacity of mtDNA, mitochondria rely largely on nuclear genes (over 1000 genes) for their proliferation. Mitochondrial biogenesis therefore requires complex coordination between the nuclear and mitochondrial genomes [46]. Upon energy depletion, activated AMPK turns off ATP-consuming processes such as synthesis of lipids, carbohydrates, and proteins, and turns on ATP-generating pathways including mitochondrial biogenesis [47].

Interestingly ATM has been implicated in the mitochondrial biogenesis pathway mediated through AMPK activation [48, 49] supporting a role of ATM in mitochondrial functions.

It is of interest also that several ATM substrates show mitochondrial translocation (CREB, p53) and affect mitochondrial functions (HMGA1) [10]. Moreover A-T cells have lower cytochrome c oxidase activity than normal cells, which could explain their reduced respiratory activity; interestingly, treatment of normal cells with an ATM inhibitor also results in reduced cytochrome c oxidase activity [50]. While there are numerous external sources of ROS, the great majority of ROS within eukaryotic cells derives from the mitochondrion as by-products during the generation of adenosine triphosphate (ATP), through the process of oxidative phosphorylation. These evidence lead to postulate that mitochondrial dysfunction may be responsible for elevated ROS production and oxidative stress of A-T cells [10, 45].

However, there are some inconsistencies between these studies, such as discrepancies in the nature of mitochondrial DNA content abnormalities. Recently Valentin-Vega and colleagues clarify this point and report that *in vivo* loss of *ATM* results in striking mitochondrial dysfunction in thymocytes, leading to elevated mitochondrial number and increased mitochondrial ROS production. The increase in mitochondrial content is associated with defects in the intracellular destruction of abnormal mitochondria (mitophagy). Therefore, they conclude that ATM has major role in modulating mitochondrial function and ROS generation *in vivo* and *in vitro* and suggest that decreased mitophagy, rather than increased mitochondrial biogenesis, is associated with the increased mitochondrial content [51].

5.3. ATM, hypoxia and autophagy

Although maintenance of oxygen homeostasis is an essential cellular and systemic function, it is only within the past few years that the molecular mechanisms underlying this fundamental aspect of cell biology started to be elucidated and their connections to development, physiology and pathophysiology have been established. HIF-1 (hypoxia-inducible factor 1) is the transcriptional activator that functions as a master regulator of oxygen homeostasis [52]. Recently, advances in delineating upstream signal transduction pathways leading to the induction of HIF-1 activity, and expression of downstream target genes, have been made and these lead to significant contribution to the understanding of oxygen homeostasis regulation [52]. Interestingly low oxygen tension or hypoxia is a common feature of all solid tumors [53]. It is strongly associated with tumor development, malignant progression, metastatic outgrowth, and resistance resistance to therapy and is considered an independent prognostic indicator for poor patient prognosis in various tumor types [53].

In this context it is well established that ATM is activated under hypoxic conditions not only in a DNA damage dependent way [54] but also through an MRN-independent mechanism in the absence of DNA damage. Phosphorylated ATM is found in a diffuse pattern in the nucleus [55]. The mechanism of ATM activation is not clear: although acute hypoxia induces release of ROS from mitochondria [56], this is not essential for ATM activation under these conditions [55]. Recently Mongiardi and colleagues have demonstrated that ATM may function as an oxygen sensing protein. In particular they demonstrated that A-T cells exhibit a blunted response to mild hypoxia, being defective in upregulating HIF-1α. The disability of ATM-negative cells to upregulate HIF-1α is a consequence of an impaired sensing of oxygen variations [57]. In addition, ATM is a direct regulator of the transcription factor complex HIF-1, a heterodimer of HIF-1α and HIF-1β subunits that regulates metabolism, mitochondrial function and angiogenesis under hypoxic conditions [58]. ATM phosphorylation of HIF1α on Ser696 stabilizes the protein under hypoxic conditions, which promotes mTORC1 inhibition and growth suppression. Moreover authors suggest that suppression of ATM may significantly contribute to the signalling through which TORC1 activity can remain elevated in hypoxic tumor [58].

Interestingly mTORC1 negatively regulates autophagy a catabolic process in which cells deliver cytoplasmic components for degradation to the lysosome [59]. Concomitant with mTORC1 repression by ROS, autophagy increased in cells treated with H_2O_2. Consistently Alexander and colleagues demonstrated that ATM signaling in response to ROS also leads to mTORC1 inhibition and is involved in the consequential induction of autophagy[60]. Whether autophagy is activated as a survival mechanism in response to ROS or functions in an ATM-driven programmed cell death pathway remains to be explored.

5.4. ATM and metabolic syndrome

Metabolic syndrome is a cluster of metabolic abnormalities and related clinical syndromes among which the most relevant ones are insulin resistance and atherosclerosis [61]. Insulin resistance along with visceral adiposity, dyslipidemia and chronic subclinical proinflammatory state are the main characteristic features of metabolic syndrome. The role of ATM in the regulation of metabolism is emerging as a very interesting topic. A-T patients have an increased risk of developing type 2 diabetes and display growth impairments associated with insulin resistance and glucose intolerance [22, 23]. Diabetic complications are not considered a primary characteristic associated with A-T owing to their late onset and the fact that most A-T patients succumb to the disease early in life. However, several studies have demonstrated a relationship between ATM and metabolic signaling pathways. For example, there is a close interplay between ATM and insulin pathway (reviewed in [10]). The identification of cytoplasmic ATM as an insulin-responsive protein provides the first indication that a defective response to insulin could be related to the development of insulin resistance and type 2 diabetes in A–T patients [29]. Moreover ATM is required for AKT phosphorylation at Ser473 and for translocation of the cell's surface glucose transporter 4 (GLUT4) in response to insulin stimulation [62]. These results suggest that reduced expression of ATM may trigger the development of insulin resistance because of the consequent downregulation of AKT activity. Recent evidence indicates that the effects of ATM on insulin function and glucose metabolism may be mediated through p53 phosphorylation [63]. Deletion of the p53- encoding gene, or its mutation to generate p53 variants that lack the primary ATM phosphorylation site, results in elevated ROS levels, glucose intolerance, insulin resistance, reduced AKT phosphorylation and reduced expression of sestrin proteins, which are involved in the regulation of intracellular antioxidants [63]. These effects can be rescued by the addition of dietary antioxidants, suggesting that ATM affects insulin function and glucose metabolism by regulating intracellular ROS levels through p53 phosphorylation. Moreover Schneider and colleagues discovered a new relationship between ATM deficiency and metabolism in mice, looking specifically at aspects of the metabolic syndrome such as insulin resistance, adiposity, blood pressure, circulating cholesterol and lipid levels, and atherosclerosis. They have shown that transplantation of bone marrow with $ATM^{-/-}ApoE^{-/-}$ mice increases atherosclerosis, whereas activation of ATM in $ATM^{+/+}ApoE^{-/-}$ mice alleviates the vascular disease. The results indicate that ATM deficiency causes insulin resistance, resembles the metabolic syndrome, and increases vascular disease [64]. Interestingly, ATM has recently been identified as a functional target of metformin, a drug widely used in the treatment of type 2 diabetes [65]. Metformin is a very interesting drug because reduces insulin resistance and increases glucose uptake in skeletal muscle, but the mechanism of its action is not fully understood. ATM seems to function upstream of metformin- induced AMPK activation, because treatment of rat hepatoma cells with an ATM inhibitor reduced AMPK activation and phosphorylation following metformin treatment [65]. However the role of ATM downstream metformin treatment is very controversial and several research groups are currently trying to clarify this point [66].

5.5. ATM and growth factors

Growth factors regulate essential processes in cells as cell proliferation, motility, survival and morphogenesis. Several growth factors activate receptor tyrosine kinases (RTK), leading to activation of cellular signaling pathways as PI3K/AKT signalling, which promotes cell survival, and the mitogen-activated protein (MAP) kinase cascade [67].

First evidences of functional interactions between ATM and growth factor–mediated signaling are:

- the observation that cultured A-T cells display an increased demand for growth factors in the media compared to wt cells;
- the identification of ability ATM as a mediator of the insulin-mediated signaling, which in turn regulates AKT signaling [29, 62].

Moreover, it has been recently shown that also MEK/ERK signaling is modulated by ATM [68] and that inhibition of ATM activity inhibits cell proliferation and induces apoptosis in cancer cell lines with overactive AKT [69]. Collectively, these studies suggest that ATM may modulate prosurvival signaling downstream growth factor stimulation. Recently, ATM activation has been identified also downstream the growth factor receptor HER2 in a breast cancer mouse model [70]. Thus, it is clear that the ATM is activated upon growth factor stimulation, but the mechanism of this activation is still unknown. It is tempting to speculate that ROS production induced by growth factor stimulation could be responsible for activation of cytoplasmic ATM. Another hypothesis is that ATM could be indirectly activated by hyperproliferation induced by growth factor signaling.

ATM can also regulate the expression of some growth factor receptors an in particular of some Receptor Tyrosine Kinases (RTKs). For example, the expression of the insulin-like growth factor 1 receptor (IGF1R) is reduced in ATM-deficient cells, and the radiosensitivity of A-T cells, following IR treatment is affected by IGF1R expression levels; both effects can be rescued by ATM cDNA expression [71]. More recently, De Bacco and colleagues demonstrated that DNA damage induces ATM dependent transcription of the growth factor receptor MET and this regulation contributes to radioresistance of MET-dependent tumors [72].

Interestingly RTKs signaling is often aberrantly regulated in different type of tumors, so overall these data suggest also a functional role for ATM in RTKs-dependent tumor progression. In this regard, a possible role of ATM inhibition in cancer therapy will be discussed in the paragraph "Functional links between ATM kinase and cancer".

5.6. ATM and death receptors

The observation that A-T patients display an increased rate of lymphoma and leukaemia onset, has been largely explained by the identification of ATM as a major modulator of the DNA damage response and by the central role that physiological DNA damage plays in the development of the immune system [73-75] (see next paragraph "Functional links between ATM kinase and the immune system defects").

Other important modulators of the immune system development and function are death receptors such as Fas (CD95/APO-1) and Tumour necrosis factor (TNF)-Related Apoptosis-Inducing Ligand (TRAIL). The death receptor system is essential for the regulation of the lymphoid system homeostasis [76]. It is assumed that the negative selection process of B as well as T cells in the germinal center (GC) and thymus, respectively, depends on Fas system [77, 78]. Mice lacking functional Fas expression suffer from autoimmunity and increased incidence of B cell lymphomas [79, 80]. Patients with mutations that impair the function of proteins involved in Fas-dependent apoptosis develop the autoimmune lymphoproliferative syndrome (ALPS), which predisposes them to autoimmune disorders and to lymphoma development [81, 82]. Finally, Fas mutations where identified in lymphomas, in particular those deriving from GC B cells(reviewed in [83]).

Fas (CD95/APO-1) is a transmembrane protein belonging to the tumor necrosis factor superfamily. Upon binding of Fas ligand or agonistic antibodies, the Fas receptor recruits several cytosolic proteins to form the death-inducing signalling complex (DISC). This is necessary to catalyze Caspase-8 activation, which triggers the caspase cascade [84]. Caspase-8 activation is absolutely required to trigger receptor-activated apoptotic response and its catalytic activity has to be tightly regulated to avoid inappropriate activation and undesired cell death. This regulation is ensured by FLIP proteins, which are structurally similar to Procaspase-8 and can therefore compete with Procaspase-8 for binding to DISC, thus preventing Caspase-8 activation and the following apoptotic cascade [85].

Taking into account the linkage between Fas impairment and the development of immune system tumors that are more also frequent in A-T patients, we asked whether any relationship exists between Fas and ATM signaling pathways. We could show that ATM deficiency results in a significant resistance of lymphoid cells derived from A-T patients to Fas-induced apoptosis. Interestingly, loss of endogenous ATM kinase activity results in the aberrant upregulation of FLIP protein levels. Consistently, ATM kinase activation downregulates FLIP protein levels providing a novel mechanism to modulate Fas sensitivity. Interestingly, Hodgkin Lymphoma cells that are characterized by Fas-resistance and by FLIP overexpression, may be sensitized to Fas upon ATM kinase expression, which triggers FLIP downregulation. These data point to ATM as a novel player in Fas-induced apoptosis and suggest a novel molecular mechanism for the increased lymphoma susceptibility of A-T patients and for the development of B cell lymphoma [86]. These observations have been further extended also to TRAIL receptor. ATM modulates TRAIL sensitivity similarly to what described for Fas [87]. This observation provides a rational for the employment of several DNA damaging agents largely used in chemotherapy, to enhance TRAIL sensitivity, by triggering ATM activation which in turn drives FLIP protein downregulation [87]. This is consistent with the identification of ATM and Chk2 activation downstream death receptor stimulation [88]. ATM would therefore represent a crucial interplay between the modulation of DNA damage response and death receptor induced apoptosis (reviewed in [89]).

6. Molecular mechanisms that ensure the modulation of ATM kinase activity

ATM activation has been at first identified as a response to DSBs DNA damage. ATM is recruited to DSBs and activated by DNA damage through interactions with the MRE11–RAD50–NBS1 (MRN) complex, which is bound to DNA ends at the site of the break. The activated ATM is important for the initiation of DNA end resection that is an essential step to initiate DNA repair via the homologous recombination pathway (reviewed in [11]). *In vitro* experiments have shown that ATM activation in response to DSBs requires the interaction with free ends DNA and with the MRN complex [90]. In this context, it has been proposed that ATM protein exists as an inactive dimer in which the catalytic domain of one molecule is engaged in an intermolecular interaction with the FAT domain of the other molecule. DSBs triggers autophosphorylation on S1981, a serine residue located within the FAT domain, and this phosphorylation causes the release of the intermolecular interaction leading to release of an active monomer [6]. The mutation of the autophosphorylation site disrupts ATM signaling in human cells [91, 92]. Nevertheless, the functional significance of ATM autophosphorylation is still debated as mouse models and in vitro studies have shown that ATM autophosphorylation is not required for ATM activation by DNA damage or oxidation [30, 90, 93, 94]. However, ATM autophosphorylation at Ser1981 is at present considered a hallmark of ATM activation and several antibodies that specifically recognize ATM when phosphorylated on S1981 are commercially available and commonly employed to detect the occurrence of ATM activation. Moreover, additional DSBs-induced ATM autophosphorylation sites, Ser367, Ser1893 and Ser2996, have been identified and have been shown to be required for ATM signaling in human cells [91, 92]. Global phosphoproteomic screens of the DNA damage signalling network independently confirmed the identification of these autophosphorylation sites. Furthermore these studies also revealed additional ATM phosphorylation sites [16-19]. An updated list of ATM phosphorylation sites is avaivable at PhosphoSite database http://www.phosphosite.org/proteinAction.do?id=1393&showAllSites =true.

Several phosphatases have been identified as important modulators of ATM activity, consistently with the central role that the regulation of phosphorylation plays in the modulation of ATM kinase activation in response to DNA damage. PP2A, PP5 and WIP1 phosphatases regulate ATM activity [95-97]. PP2A directly modulates the state of phosphorylation of S1981 [95]. Conversely PP5 interacts with ATM in a DNA-damage-inducible manner and its activity sustains ATM activation [96]. Wip1 phosphatase has been identified as a novel player of the ATM-dependent signaling pathway, as it directly dephosphorylates Ser1981. Deficiency of Wip1 resulted in activation of ATM kinase, while its overexpression triggers the downregulation of the ATM-dependent signaling cascade after DNA damage [97].

The activity of other kinases may also contribute to the modulation of ATM kinase activity. It has been shown that Cdk5 (cyclin-dependent kinase 5), activated by DNA damage, directly phosphorylates ATM at S794 in postmitotic neurons. This phosphorylation precedes and is required for ATM autophosphorylation at S1981, and sustains ATM kinase activition and signaling. The downregulation of Cdk5-ATM interplay attenuates DNA damage-induced neuronal cell cycle reentry and expression of p53 targets PUMA and Bax, protecting neurons from DNA damage-induced cell death [98]. Similarly, c-Abl, a non receptor tyrosine kinase previously identified as a target and effector of ATM kinase activity in the DNA damage response [99, 100], has been recently identified as important modulator of ATM kinase activation. DNA damage triggers ATM kinase dependent inducion of c-Abl activity, which in turn triggers ATM tyrosine phosphorylation. This phosphorylation is required to enhance ATM autophosphorylation on S1981 and ultimately to sustain ATM activity, allowing the apoptotic response [101].

It has also been shown that DNA damage induces the rapid acetylation of ATM. This acetylation depends on the Tip60 histone acetyltransferase (HAT). Suppression of Tip60 blocks ATM kinase activation and prevents the ATM-dependent phosphorylation of p53 and Chk2. [7]. The systematic mutagenesis of lysine residues identified a single acetylation site at K3016, which is located in the highly conserved C-terminal FATC domain [102]. K3016 acetylation is required for the DNA damage induced autophosphorylation on S1981. The acetylation of ATM on lysine 3016 by Tip60 is therefore a key step linking the detection of DNA damage and the activation of ATM kinase activity.

Recent studies have identified a completely different mechanism for ATM activation in response to oxidative stress. According to the proposed models ATM would be present as inactive monomers (reviewed in [10]). Oxidation triggers the assembly of an active dimer in which the two monomers are covalently linked by intermolecular disulfide bonds [30, 39]. C2991, located in the C-terminal FATC domain, has been identified as a crucial residue for ATM activation by oxidation, as a C2991L mutant cannot be activated by H_2O_2. The interplay between the molecular mechanisms that trigger ATM activation in response either to DSBs or to oxidative stress has not been clearly investigated yet. It has been shown that the S1981A mutant is still competent for activation in response to oxidation. Similarly, the C2991L mutant is competent for DNA damage induction. ATM activation in response to these two different stresses triggers the ATM-dependent phosphorylation of an overlapping subset of substrates although significative differences have also been identified. As an example, although low levels of H_2O_2, which specifically trigger oxidative stress, drive the phosphorylation of p53 and Chk2 proteins, similarly to what observed in response to DNA damage, they fail to mediate histone H2AX and KAP1 phosphorylation which seem to be peculiar for the DSBs response [30]. Importantly, the distinction between ATM activation mediated through oxidation and that mediated by DNA damage is difficult, because oxidative stress and ROS production may usually induce DNA damage, and indeed ATM is often exposed to both these stresses simultaneously. IR treatment is able to trigger both DNA damage and oxidative stress suggesting that the large number of substrates identified by proteomic approaches aimed to characterize the global pattern of ATM substrates in this context probably represent targets from both the DNA repair and oxidation pathways. This observation may provide an explanation for the identification, among more that 700 substrates of ATM, of proteins clearly involved not only in the control and execution of cell cycle checkpoints and DNA rapair, but also in many other pathways such as the insulin signaling [16].

A-T has a pleiotropic phenotype that affects multiple systems, and most likely the complex clinical features arise from the synergistic effects of a defective DNA damage response and oxidative stress in the absence of ATM. It is intriguing to speculate that a subset of clinical features associated with A-T might be mainly due to defects in ROS response by ATM, whereas other features might primarily result from the impairment of a functional DNA damage response. Interestingly, some A-T patients present a form of ATM with a truncated C-terminal region (R3047X), that therefore lacks C2991 ([10] and references therein). Although these patients develop ataxia similarly to the others, their cells are less sensitive to IR compared to other A-T cells. Moreover, one patient that expresses the R3047X variant does not display immunodeficiency ([10] and references therein). Future studies will clarify whether the variability of the clinical features displayed by A-T patients may arise from different mutations which impact differently on the different functions performed by ATM.

At present the occurrence of other post-translational modification that may modulate ATM activation by oxidative stress has not been investigated. Future systematic proteomic experiments will also define the complete profile of the oxidative stress dependent ATM substrates. These studies will clarify the differences and the similarities among the different mechanisms of activation of ATM kinase and their potential cross-regulation.

7. Functional links between ATM kinase and cancer

7.1. ATM expression and cancer

ATM is considered one of the principle guardians of the genome as a consequence of its principle role in the coordination and execution of the DNA damage response. According to this function, ATM is generally defined as a tumor suppressor gene. Several *in vitro* and *in vivo* evidences support this idea. First of all ATM deficiency is clearly associated with an increased onset of tumorigenesis both in human and in mouse models. Indeed, about 20% of A-T patients display a significantly higher incidence in the development of leukaemia and lymphoma, according to the decreased ability of A-T cells to correctly handle the physiological double strand brakes occurring during the maturation of the immune system (reviewed in [73, 75]). Consistently, Atm -/- mice develop lymphoma and leukaemia within the first three months of life and die of malignant thymic lymphoma by 4–5 months of age [103-105]. Several reports also describe an increased rate in the development of solid tumors for the heterozygous relatives of A-T patients compared to the whole population. In particular a link between ATM heterozygosity and a higher predisposition to breast cancer onset has been well established (reviewed in [106]). In 1987 it has been proposed that relatives of A-T patients might be at increased risk of cancer and in particular breast cancer [107]. Later on, several other epidemiologic studies support the same conclusion [108]. A large study conducted on 1160 relatives of 169 A-T patients, estimated the overall relative risk of breast cancer in carriers to be 2.23 (95% CI = 1.16-4.28) compared to the general population [109]. Although this observation was of importance to A-T families, it was immediately clear that it might have a much wider significance, as it has been estimated that about 1% of the whole population might be carriers of an *ATM* gene mutation.

The frequency of ATM variants in human breast cancer has been largely investigated by several laboratories. Unfortunately, the results of these studies were often inconclusive mainly because of the low number of cases included in each study as well as for the technical difficulties linked to the sequencing *of ATM* gene(reviewed in [75]). More recently, 76 rare sequence variants in the ATM gene have been analyzed in a case-control family study of 2,570 cases of breast cancer and 1,448 controls. The risk estimates from this study suggest that women carrying the pathogenic variant, ATM c.7271T > G, or truncating mutations have a significantly increased risk of breast cancer with a penetrance similar to that conferred by germline mutations in BRCA2 [110].

Consistently with the observation that loss of ATM expression or heterozygosity may enhance cancer predisposition, some reports also describe loss of ATM expression in some tumor samples in the whole population. In particular ATM expression is strongly reduced or lost in some leukaemia and lymphoma [73, 111-113]. The modulation of ATM expression levels in breast cancer has been largely investigated. Several reports, demonstrate the occurrence of low levels of ATM expression in breast cancer. In particular, it has been proposed that ATM may be aberrantly reduced or lost in BRCA1/BRCA2-deficient and ER/PR/ERBB2-triple-negative breast cancer [114, 115].

Several molecular mechanisms, alternative to the occurrence of genetic mutations that lead to loss or reduction of ATM expression, have been identified. ATM is down-regulated by N-Myc-regulated microRNA-421 and this may play a role in neuroblastoma [116]. Over-expression of miR-100 is responsible for the low-expression of ATM in the human glioma cell line M059J [117]. Furthermore, it has been shown that miR-18a is upregulated in cell lines as well as in patients' tissue samples of breast cancer. miR-18a triggers the downregulation of ATM expression by directly targeting the ATM-3'-UTR and abrogated the IR-induced cell cycle arrest [118].

Alternatively, ATM promoter methylation has been shown to epigenetically trigger ATM expression downregulation in cancer. The ATM gene is aberrantly methylated and silenced in locally advanced breast cancer [119] and aberrant methylation has been correlated with low levels of ATM expression and increased radiosensitivity in colorectal cancer and glioblastoma cell lines [120, 121].

7.2. ATM and the DDR as barrier to tumor development

Recent evidence from both cell culture, animal models and analysis of clinical specimens show a correlation between oncogene activation or loss of tumor suppressor expression and the occurrence of DNA replication stress and induction of the DNA Damage Response(DDR) (reviewed in [122]). The key initial observations that inspired the hypothesis that tumorigenic insults may drive DDR activation as a sort of barrier that delays or prevent cancer progression in vivo, were:

1. The occurrence of activated DNA damage signalling in a subset of human cancer cell lines, especially those defective for p53 function.
2. The occurrence of activated DNA damage response, exemplified by Thr68 phosphorylation on Chk2 protein, in clinical specimens of large subsets of human and lung carcinomas [123].

These results suggested that some disease-associated event (not occurring in the adjacent normal tissue) led to activation of the DDR. Therefore, it has been postulated that oncogenic events may trigger DNA damage and the consequently activation of ATM-Chk2 signaling cascade. To test whether this activation may represent a barrier to the transformation process two sets of experimental approaches have been conducted. The first one, was to develop cell culture models of conditional oncogene activation, while the second was to extend the analysis of the occurrence of the DDR to a large panel of human tumor biopsies derived from various type of cancers at various stages, especially from premalignant and pre-invasive lesions which represent very early stages of cancer progression. Two studies jointly provided evidence for a role of the DDR machinery as an inducible barrier against cancer in clinical specimens from various tissues [124, 125]. The authors found that according to their hypothesis, tumor cells in clinical specimens from various tissue (and not cells located in the adjacent normal tissue) show a costitutive activation of checkpoints kinases such as ATM and Chk2, phosphorylated H2AX and p53 and foci formation by the DDR proteins such as 53BP1. Importantly, in the early pre invasive lesions, the DDR activation preceded occurrence of mutations or loss of expression of DDR component, consistently with the idea that the DDR barrier generates a sort of selective pression for these mutations that would allow the escape from the barrier and consequently drive cancer progression. The DDR activation was also well recapitulated in human cell culture models following oncogene expression, as well as in xenograft models [124, 125]. One key question related to the induction of the DDR as a barrier to tumor development is the mechanistic basis on the induction of DNA damage in cancer. It has been postulated that oncogene expression triggers DNA replication stress, including replication forks collapse and subsequent formation of DSBs [124-127]. Additional events that may contribute to the induction of DDR in this context are telomere erosion and ROS generation (reviewed in [122]). It has been shown that, the activation of DDR is required for the oncogene-mediated induction of senescence [126, 127], a state of permanent growth arrest refractory to physiological proliferation stimuli, that would counteract tumor progression (reviewed in [128].

7.3. ATM kinase inhibition and cancer therapy

The central function of ATM in the DNA damage response and in the modulation of IR- sensitivity, suggested that the modulation of its activity may be exploited for cancer therapy. For this reason a great effort is still ongoing to develop and improve ATM kinase inhibitors and to define the conditions in which their employment could be beneficial for the cancer therapy. A major obstacle in the development of a specific inhibitor of ATM catalytic activity is linked to the high similarity among the kinase domains of the PI3K-like family proteins. For a long time caffeine has been largely employed to modulate ATM/ATR kinase activity. It has been shown that depending on its concentration caffeine may be able to equally block ATM and ATR activities (10 μM) or, alternatively, to selectively interfere with ATM activity (5 μM) [129, 130]. Later on, screening a small molecule compound library developed for the phosphatidylinositol 3'-kinase-like kinase family, an ATP-competitive inhibitor, 2-morpholin-4-yl-6-thianthren-1-yl-pyran-4-one (KU-55933), that inhibits ATM with an IC_{50} of 13 nmol/L and a Ki of 2.2 nmol/L. KU-55933 has been identified. KU-55933 shows specificity with respect to inhibition of other phosphatidylinositol 3'-kinase-like kinases. Inhibition of ATM by KU-55933 resulted in the ablation of IR-dependent phosphorylation of several ATM targets, including p53, H2AX, NBS1, and SMC1 and sensitize cells to the cytotoxic effects of ionizing radiation and to the DNA double-strand break-inducing chemotherapeutic agents, etoposide, doxorubicin, and camptothecin. Inhibition of ATM by KU-55933 also caused a loss of ionizing radiation-induced cell cycle arrest. By contrast, KU-55933 did not potentiate the cytotoxic effects of ionizing radiation on ataxia-telangiectasia cells, nor did it affect their cell cycle profile after DNA damage [131]. More recently, it has been developed an improved analogue of KU-55933, named KU-60019, with Ki and IC_{50} values half of those of KU-55933 [68]. KU-60019 is 10-fold more effective than KU-55933 at blocking radiation-induced phosphorylation of several ATM targets in human glioma cells. KU-60019 inhibits the DNA damage response, reduces AKT phosphorylation and prosurvival signaling, inhibits migration and invasion, and effectively radiosensitizes human glioma cells [68]. A library of 1500 compounds was selected based on known kinase inhibitor templates and calculated kinase pharmacophores from the Pfizer proprietary chemical file. These compounds were screened with potential inhibitors being identified by a decreased ability of purified ATM kinase to phosphorylate GST-p53[1–101] substrate. This screening approach identified the compound CP466722 as a potential novel ATM inhibitor. The ATM-related kinase, ATR, was not inhibited by CP466722 *in vitro*, although inhibitory activities against Abl and Src kinases were reported [132]. CP466722 was not toxic and importantly, inhibition of cellular ATM kinase activity was rapid and completely reversed by removing CP466722. Interestingly, clonogenic survival assays demonstrated that transient inhibition of ATM is sufficient to sensitize cells to ionizing radiation and suggests that therapeutic radiosensitization may require ATM inhibition for short periods of time [132]. Despite the large effort made so far to improve the specificity and the efficacy of these type of inhibitors, these compounds still deserve further investigation as none of them can be used in *in vivo* studies in animal models because of their elevated toxicity. The identification of ATM as a novel player of other signalling cascades, not related to the DNA damage response, raised also the question that its ability to prevent tumorigenicity may be strictly dependent on the specific tumor context. In particular several studies identified ATM activity as a promoter of AKT phosphorylation and activity, which in turn sustains proliferation and cellular transformation [133] [62] [69]. These reports are consistent with the observation that ATM may be activated downstream Receptor Tyrosine Kinases [29, 134], as well with the observation that AKT may be activated in response to DNA damage [68, 135, 136]. Furthermore, ATM activition in response to IR has been shown to promote the expression of MET receptor tyrosine kinase [72]. MET, in turn, promotes cell invasion and protects cells from apoptosis, thus supporting radioresistance. Drugs targeting MET increase tumor cell radiosensitivity and prevent radiation-induced invasiveness. Overall, these observations suggest that in some conditions, ATM activity may sustain tumorigenicity by modulating the levels of the receptor as well as by sustaining AKT activation. Therefore its inhibition may be enhance cancer therapy efficacy. However, the inhibition of ATM may be beneficial or conversely detrimental to cancer therapy, depending on the specific context [137], suggesting that extreme caution should be taken in this regard. Further investigation will clarify this issue.

8. Functional links between ATM kinase and the immune system defects

A-T patients display several immunological dysfunctions (reviewed in [75]). The central role of ATM kinase in the control and execution of the DNA Damage Response (DDR), along with the observation that DNA damage occurs physiologically to ensure the development and the functionality of the immune system, strongly suggest that most of the immune defects linked to A-T may arise from defects in the DDR. The activation of the DDR is an important component of the V(D)J recombination, a genetically programmed DNA rearrangement process occurring during the early development of lymphocytes that results in assembly of highly diversified antigen receptors essential to functional lymphocytes. Defects in repair proteins involved in rejoining V(D)J recombination-induced DSBs preclude the generation of antigen receptors, profoundly compromising T- and B-cell development and causing severe immune deficiencies. The role of ATM in V(D)J recombination has been largely investigated. Immunoglobulin class switch recombination has been shown to be impaired in Atm-deficient mice [138]. Moreover, during the V(D)J recombination ATM participates to the stabilization of DNA double-strande-break complexes [139]. ATM may also function directly in end joining, end processing or end protection [140]. A recent study reported also the persistence of chromosomal breaks in actively dividing ATM-deficient peripheral lymphocytes [141] suggesting a role for ATM in cell-cycle control in addition to facilitating DNA repair. However, the mechanism behind the involvement of ATM in the cell-cycle checkpoint during V(D)J recombination, along with the functions of ATM downstream targets responsible for cell-cycle control, has yet to be determined.

AT patients exhibit a wide range of cellular and humoral immune system abnormalities, resulting in variable lymphopenia [142] The most common abnormalities are the absence or marked reduction of IgA, IgG subclasses and IgE [75, 142]. Moreover, the peripheral T-cell population of both AT patients and Atm–/– mice is characterized by a bias toward terminally differentiated effector cells, reflected by an extremely low ratio of naıve to memory T cells (reviewed in [75]).

As a consequence immunodeficiency is very frequent in A-T and A-T patients display a high predisposition to sinopulmonary infections and bacterial pneumonia and chronic lung disease are a major cause of mortality in these patients. (reviewed in [75]).

Another important abnormality of the immune system linked to A-T pathology is the higher incidence of leukaemia and lymphoma development observed both in mice and in humans deficient for ATM gene expression. The risk of developing a lymphoid neoplasm is increased approximately 200-fold in AT patients compared with the normal population. The vast majority of lymphoid tumors that develop in A-T children are T-cell ALL/lymphoma (reviewed in [75]). Consistently, Atm–/– mice generally succumb to pre-T-ALL between 3 and 6 months of age [103-105]. A-T patients display characteristic cytogenetic abnormalities involving chromosomes 7 and 14 that result in disruption of antigen receptor loci [74]. Some of these chromosomal translocations may lead to the juxtaposition of a TCR locus and a proto-oncogene like TCL1 or MTCP1 (chromosomes 14 and X, respectively). T cells harboring these translocations clonally expand, accumulate additional cytogenetic abnormalities, and eventually develop into leukemias/lymphomas. In addition, ATM is frequently inactivated in sporadic cancers, particularly lymphoid malignancies. Loss of 11q22-23 (the location of the human ATM gene) is often observed in leukemias/ lymphomas [73, 111].

A recent study found a surprising role for ATM in promoting the self-renewal capacity of hematopoietic stem cells (HSCs) [108]. The mechanism for HSC depletion in the absence of ATM appears to be increased oxidative stress, suggesting that indeed abnormalities in the oxidative stress response may also contribute to the immune system phenotype in addition to the DDR deficiency [32, 33].

9. Functional links between ATM kinase, neurodegeneration and other neurological features

The neurodegenerative phenotype of A-T is the cardinal aspect of the disease. In A-T, the neurodegeneration is progressive and spinocerebellar in nature, and it usually becomes apparent between 6 and 18 months of age. Patients with A-T manifest hallmarks of cerebellar dysfunction such as dyssynergia, muscle hypotonia, truncal swaying while sitting or standing, and sudden falls [1, 21]. Atrophy of the cerebellum, particularly is a key feature of A-T and is evident upon magnetic resonance imaging and computed tomography imaging [21]. Purkinje cell loss is a hallmark feature of A-T and Purkinje cells have less complex arborizations and are often localized ectopically in the molecular layer of the cerebellum [143].

Although extensive effort has been made to understand how ATM deficiency could result in neuronal degeneration, the mechanisms behind neuronal degeneration of A–T are still poorly understood. It has been speculated that defective responses of ATM to DNA damage could be the cause of neuronal degeneration in A–T. However, Atm$^{-/-}$ mice show compromised function in DNA repair but fail to develop significant neuronal degeneration or exhibit symptoms of ataxia, suggesting a lack of correlation between dysfunction in DNA repair and neuronal degeneration of the A–T disease [103].

Importantly, a substantial amount of ATM resides in the cytoplasm in human and mouse brain, a sub-cellular localization incongruous for a mediator of DDR [Barlow, 2000 #283; Boehrs, 2007 #798; Li, 2012 #820]. In the cytoplasm ATM appears to be involved in the homeostasis of lysosomes [144], in the spontaneous release of synaptic vesicles and in establishment and maintenance of long-term potentiation (LTP) [145].

In contrast with these data, Biton and colleagues showed that ATM is predominantly nuclear in human neuronal-like cells, and that the ATM-mediated response is as robust as in proliferating cells. Knockdown of ATM abolished that response [146]. Similar observations have been obtained from studies in murine cerebellar neurons, in which ATM seems to lacalize essentially in the nucleus and ATM activation measured by autophosphorylation and downstream signaling is comparable with that in other cell lines. This is supported by genetic evidence showing that MRE11 facilitates the activation of ATM at DNA DSBs, and that patients that are hypomorphic for mutations in *MRE11* (patients with ATLD) have a neuronal phenotype that is similar to that in A-T [12].

Recently, the finding that oxidation can directly activate ATM [30], strongly suggests that the enrolment of ATM in the oxidative stress response may provide a molecular base for some features of neurodegeneration observed in A-T patients, which cannot be explained by the classical ATM function in the DDR. Neurons are cells particularly vulnerable to oxidative stress as shown by the fact that oxidative injury is a key feature of both acute brain pathologies such as stroke and traumatic brain injury and neurodegenerative diseases such as Alzheimer's disease, Parkinson's disease, Huntington's disease and amyotropic lateral sclerosis [147]. Neurons have a high energy demand, principally to maintain ion gradients necessary for neuronal signal transmission as well as for the synthesis, the uptake and the recycling of neurotransmitters. To fulfil this requirement neurons depend principally on oxidative phosphorylation, a process that necessarily generates a certain amount of ROS as a byproduct. At the same time neurons are relatively poor in antioxidant defenses as compared, for instance, to astrocytes [147]. Indeed, loss of ATM enhances intracellular ROS levels, and their aberrant excess, may contribute to the neurodegeneration described in A-T [148] Although mouse mutants of ATM do not recapitulate the cerebellar degeneration, ATM deficiency has been shown to be associated with increased levels of reactive oxygen species in Purkinje cells [27, 149]. Furthermore, an age-dependent reduction in the number of dopaminergic neurons present in the substantia nigra and striatum has been observed in $ATM^{-/-}$ mice, which was accompanied by severe gliosis [150] suggesting that ATM-deficient mice may model some of the neurological defects observed in A-T. Persistent oxidative stress in the ATM-deficient brain disturbs intracellular antioxidant defence systems and redox homeostasis, thereby activating downstream signaling pathways, including those involving p38 and ERK1/2 [149]. Overall these observations suggest that, in A-T, neuronal degeneration and ataxia do not only depend from a defective DDR but are also a consequence of the inability to mount an efficient antioxidant response because of a defective ATM signaling. In light of this information, it is not surprising that treatment with antioxidants prevents Purkinje cell loss [151] and partially corrects neurobehavioral deficits of $Atm^{-/-}$ mice [152].

In conclusion, defective DNA damage response associated with ATM deficiency might be sufficient to induce the neurological pathology associated with A-T, but the compounded oxidative stress and DNA repair defects in A-T patients would potentially increase the rate and severity of neurodegeneration.

9.1. ATM and neuronal stem cells

In the normal brain, the number of neuronal stem cells (NSCs) is the result of a tightly controlled balance between self-renewal, differentiation, and death [153]. This means that control of proliferation of the neural stem cells/precursor cells plays a critical role in determining the number of neurons, astrocytes, and oligodendrocytes in the brain. Importantly, ATM expression is abundant in neural stem cells (NSCs), but it is gradually reduced as the cell differentiates [152], suggesting that ATM may play an essential role in NSC survival and function. Paul K. Wang's laboratory reported that ATM is required to maintain normal self-renewal and proliferation of NSCs, due to its role in controlling the redox status. Loss of ATM impairs proliferation of neural stem cells through oxidative stress-mediated p38 MAPK signaling [149, 154].

In addition, it is increasingly apparent that stem cell proliferation and maturation require supportive microenvironment including astrocytes. Astrocytes have well-established roles in regulating the microenvironment in the central nervous system, including redox homeostasis. Astrocytes also support stem cell proliferation and maintenance [155-157]. Abnormal neuronal and astrocytic development was reported in ATM knockout mice [151, 152], which could be the result of abnormal differentiation of NSCs. Interestingly, ATM is also required to maintain survival and proliferation of astrocytes by controlling the redox status of these cells [149].

Recently, Carlessi and colleagues, used a human neural stem cell line model (ihNSCs) to get more insight into the mechanisms of neuronal degeneration in A-T. They could show that ATM plays a central role in terminal differentiation of ihNSCs through its function in DDR [158]. All these data support a role of ATM in the control of neuronal differentiation though its DDR dependent functions and oxidative stress dependent functions and suggest that defective proliferation of NSC could be in part responsible of the neurodegenerative phenotype in $Atm^{-/-}$ mice and A-T patients.

10. General conclusions, remarks and future perspectives

The loss of ATM kinase function leads to A-T, a multisystemic disorder. Contribution from several laboratories allowed, in the recent years, to significantly improve the knowledge on the signalling networks involving ATM kinase. The emerging picture clearly points to ATM as a central player of several cellular functions in addition to the well-established role as master regulator o the DDR.

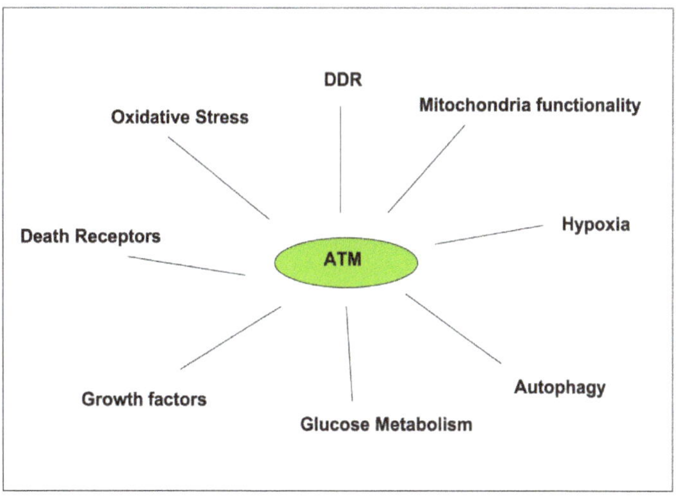

Figure 1. Schematic summary of the signalling pathways in which ATM kinase activity has been described as an important player. ATM activity is modulated by the indicated factors. The molecular mechanisms underneath its modulation and its function deserve further elucidation, as well as the contribution of the individual loss of each function to the development of A-T pathology.

At present there is no therapy to prevent or cure the progression of A-T. It is possible to alleviate some of the symptoms linked to immunodeficiency and deficient lung function, but neither the cancer predisposition, nor the progressive neurodegeneration, can be prevented. In this regard, the identification of cytoplasmic functions of ATM, and in particular its connection with glucose metabolism and with oxidative stress, provided novel hints for the comprehension of the development of this disorder and suggest possible alternative therapeutic strategies. Treatments with antioxidants and phytonutrients have been suggested as potential treatment strategies. Additional approaches include the employment of read-through drugs to allow the production of ATM kinase in those patients with truncating mutations, and the development of stem cell based therapies (reviewed in [2]). The large amount of information produced by high throughput approaches such as the proteomic studies will deserve further attention and implementation to allow a further step into the elucidation of the networks in which ATM is implicated and of the contribution of each interactor, modulator and substrate of ATM to their functionality.

Acknowledgements

We apologize to our colleagues whose data have not been cited due to space limitations. This work has been supported by research grants from Italian Telethon Foundation "Comitato Telethon Fondazione Onlus" (GGP07252) and by AIRC (IG10590) to D.B, S.S: has been supported by Fondazione Santa Lucia.

Author details

Venturina Stagni[1,2], Simonetta Santini[1,2] and Daniela Barilà[1,2]

1 Department of Biology, University of Rome "Tor Vergata", Rome, Italy

2 Laboratory of Cell Signaling, Fondazione Santa Lucia, IRCCS, Rome, Italy

References

[1] Sedgwick RP, Boder E. Ataxia-telangiectasia. In De Jong JMBV (ed) Handbook of Clinical Neurology (Vol 16) Hereditary Neuropathies and Spinocerebellar Atrophies. Amsterdam: Elsevier, 347–423. 1991.

[2] Lavin MF, Gueven N, Bottle S, Gatti RA. Current and potential therapeutic strategies for the treatment of ataxia-telangiectasia. Br Med Bull. 2007;81-82:129-47.

[3] Savitsky K, Bar-Shira A, Gilad S, Rotman G, Ziv Y, Vanagaite L, et al. A single ataxia telangiectasia gene with a product similar to PI-3 kinase. Science. 1995;268:1749-53.

[4] Zhang N, Chen P, Khanna KK, Scott S, Gatei M, Kozlov S, et al. Isolation of full-length ATM cDNA and correction of the ataxia-telangiectasia cellular phenotype. Proc Natl Acad Sci U S A. 1997;94:8021-6.

[5] Rivera-Calzada A, Maman JD, Spagnolo L, Pearl LH, Llorca O. Three-dimensional structure and regulation of the DNAdependent protein kinase catalytic subunit (DNA-PKcs). Structure. 2005;13:243-5.

[6] Bakkenist CJ, Kastan MB. DNA damage activates ATM through intermolecular autophosphorylation and dimer dissociation. Nature. 2003;421:499-506.

[7] Sun Y, Jiang X, Chen S, Fernandes N, Price BD. A role for the Tip60 histone acetyltransferase in the acetylation and activation of ATM. Proc Natl Acad Sci U S A. 2005 Sep 13;102(37):13182-7.

[8] Perry J, Kleckner N. The ATRs, ATMs, and TORs are giant HEAT repeat proteins. Cell. 2003;112:151-5.

[9] Bhatti S, Kozlov S, Farooqi AA, Naqui A, Lavin MF, Khanna KK. ATM protein kinase: the linchpin of cellular defenses to stress. Cell Mol Life Sci. 2011;68:2977-3006.

[10] Ditch S, Paull TT. The ATM protein kinase and cellular redox signaling: beyond the DNA damage response. trends Biochem Sci. 2012;37:15-22.

[11] Shiloh Y. ATM and related protein kinases: safeguarding genome integrity. Nat Rev Cancer. 2003;3:155-67.

[12] Lavin MF. Ataxia-telangiectasia: from a rare disorder to a paradigm for cell signalling and cancer. Nat Rev Mol Cell Biol. 2008;9:759-69.

[13] Ciccia A, Elledge SJ. The DNA damage response: making it safe to play with knives. Mol Cell. 2010;40:179-204.

[14] Bensimon A, Aebersold R, Shiloh Y. Beyond ATM: the protein kinase landscape of the DNA damage response. FEBS Lett. 2011;585:1625-39.

[15] Kim ST, Lim DS, Canman CE, Kastan MB. Substrate specificities and identification of putative substrates of ATM kinase family members. J Biol Chem. 1999 Dec 31;274(53):37538-43.

[16] Matsuoka S, Ballif B, Smogorzewska A, McDonald Er, Hurov K, Luo JL, et al. ATM and ATR substrate analysis reveals extensive protein networks responsive to DNA damage. Science. 2007;316:1160-6.

[17] Mu J-J, Wang Y, Leng M, Zhang J, Yang T, Besusso D, et al. A proteomic analysis of Ataxia Telangiectasia-mutated (ATM/ATM-Rad3-related (ATR) substrates identifies the ubiquitin-proteasome system as a regulator for DNA damage checkpoints. J Biol Chem. 2007;282:17330-4.

[18] Bensimon A, Schmidt A, Ziv Y, Elkon R, Wang SY, Chen DJ, et al. ATM-dependent and -independent dynamics of the nuclear phosphoproteome after DNA damage. Sci Signal. 2010;3:rs3.

[19] Bennetzen MV, Larsen DH, Bunkenborg J, Bartek J, Lukas J, Andersen JS. Site-specific phosphorylation dynamics of the nuclear proteome during the DNA damage response. Mol Cell Proteomics. 2010;9:1314-23.

[20] Marzano V, Santini S, Rossi C, Zucchelli M, D'Alessandro A, Marchetti C, et al. Proteomic profiling of ATM kinase proficient and deficient cell lines upon blockage of proteasome activity. J Proteomics. 2012;75:4632-46.

[21] McKinnon PJ. ATM and the molecular pathogenesis of ataxia telangiectasia. Annu Rev Pathol. 2012;7:303-21.

[22] Schalch DS, McFarlin DE, Barlow MH. An unusual form of diabetes mellitus in ataxia telangiectasia. N Engl J Med. 1970;282:1396-402.

[23] Bar RS, Levis WR, Rechler MM, Harrison LC, Siebert C, Podskalny J, et al. Extreme insulin resistance in ataxia telangiectasia: defect in affinity of insulin receptors. N Engl J Med. 1978;298:1164-71.

[24] Yang DQ, Halaby MJ, Li Y, Hibma JC, Burn P. Cytoplasmic ATM protein kinase: an emerging therapeutic target for diabetes, cancer and neuronal degeneration. Drug Discov Today. 2011;16:332-8.

[25] Lim DS, Kirsch DG, Canman CE, Ahn JH, Ziv Y, Newman LS, et al. ATM binds to beta-adaptin in cytoplasmic vesicles. Proc Natl Acad Sci U S A. 1998 Aug 18;95(17):10146-51.

[26] Watters D, Kedar P, Spring K, Bjorkman J, Chen P, Gatei M, et al. Localization of a portion of extranuclear ATM to peroxisomes. J Biol Chem. 1999 J Biol Chem; 274:34277-82.

[27] Barlow C, Dennery PA, Shigenaga MK, Smith MA, Morrow JD, Roberts LJn, et al. Loss of the ataxia-telangiectasia gene product causes oxidative damage in target organs. Proc Natl Acad Sci U S A. 1999;96:9915-9.

[28] Boehrs JK, He J, Halaby MJ, Yang DQ. Constitutive expression and cytoplasmic compartmentalization of ATM protein in differentiated human neuron-like SH-SY5Y cells. J Neurochem. 2007;100:337-45.

[29] Yang D-Q, Kastan MB. Partecipation of ATM in insulin signalling through phosphorylation of eIF-4E-binding protein 1. Nat Cell Biol. 2000;2:893-8.

[30] Guo Z, Kozlov S, Lavin MF, Person MD, Paull TT. ATM activation by oxidative stress. Science. 2010;330:517-21.

[31] Barzilai A, Rotman G, Shiloh Y. ATM deficiency and oxidative stress: a new dimension of defective response to DNA damage. DNA Repair (Amst). 2002 3-25:1.

[32] Ito K, Hirao A, Arai F, Matsuoka S, Takubo K, Hamaguchi I, et al. Regulation of oxidative stress by ATM is required for self-renewal of haematopoietic stem cells. Nature. 2004;431:997-1002.

[33] Ito K, Hirao A, Arai F, Takubo K, Matsuoka S, Miyamoto K, et al. Reactive oxygen species act through p38 MAPK to limit the lifespan of hematopoietic stem cells. Nat Med. 2006;12:446-51.

[34] Schubert R, Erker L, Barlow C, Yakushiji H, Larson D, Russo A, et al. Cancer chemoprevention by the antioxidant tempol in Atm-deficient mice. Hum Mol Genet. 2004;13:1793-802.

[35] Erker L, Schubert R, Elchuri S, Huang TT, Tarin D, Mueller K, et al. Effect of the reduction of superoxide dismutase 1 and 2 or treatment with alpha-tocopherol on tumorigenesis in Atm-deficient mice. Free Radic Biol Med. 2006;41:590-600.

[36] Kamsler A, Daily D, Hochman A, Stern N, Shiloh Y, Rotman G, et al. Increased oxidative stress in ataxia telangiectasia evidenced by alterations in redox state of brains from Atm-deficient mice. Cancer Res. 2001;61:1849-54.

[37] Liu N, Stoica G, Yan M, Scofield VL, Qiang W, Lynn WS, et al. ATM deficiency induces oxidative stress and endoplasmic reticulum stress in astrocytes. Lab Invest. 2005;85:1471-80.

[38] Cosentino C, Grieco D, Costanzo A. ATM activates the pentose phosphate pathway promoting anti-oxidant defence and DNA repair. EMBO J. 2011;30:546-55.

[39] Guo Z, Deshpande R, Paull TT. ATM activation in the presence of oxidative stress. Cell Cycle. 2010;9:4805-11.

[40] Perry JJ, Tainer JA. All stressed out without ATM kinase. Sci Signal. 2011;4:pe18.

[41] Okuno Y, Nakamura-Ishizu A, Otsu K, Suda T, Kubota Y. Pathological neoangiogenesis depends on oxidative stress regulation by ATM. Nat Med. 2012;18:1208-16.

[42] Taylor RW, Turnbull DM. Mitochondrial DNA mutations in human disease. Nat Rev Genet. 2005;6:389-402.

[43] Schon EA, Manfredi G. Neuronal degeneration and mitochondrial dysfunction. J Clin Invest. 2003;111:303-12.

[44] Eaton JS, Lin ZP, Sartorelli AC, Bonawitz ND, Shadel GS. Ataxia-telangiectasia mutated kinase regulates ribonucleotide reductase and mitochondrial homeostasis. J Clin Invest. 2007;117:2723-34.

[45] Ambrose M, Goldstine JV, Gatti RA. Intrinsic mitochondrial dysfunction in ATM-deficient lymphoblastoid cells. Hum Mol Genet. 2007;16:2154-64.

[46] Scarpulla RC. Nuclear control of respiratory gene expression in mammalian cells. J Cell Biochem. 2006;97:673-83.

[47] Reznick RM, Shulman GI. The role of AMP-activated protein kinase in mitochondrial biogenesis. J Physiol. 2006;574:33-9.

[48] Fu X, Wan S, Lyu YL, Liu LF, Qi H. Etoposide induces ATM-dependent mitochondrial biogenesis through AMPK activation. PLoS One. 2008;3:e2009.

[49] Luo L, Huang W, Tao R, Hu N, Xiao ZX, Luo Z. ATM and LKB1 dependent activation of AMPK sensitizes cancer cells to etoposide-induced apoptosis. Cancer Lett. 2012;Sep 5.

[50] Patel AY, McDonald TM, Spears LD, Ching JK, Fisher JS. Ataxia telangiectasia mutated influences cytochrome c oxidase activity. Biochem Biophys Res Commun. 2011;405:599-03.

[51] Valentin-Vega YA, MacLean KH, Tait-Mulder J, Milasta S, Steeves M, Dorsey FC, et al. Mitochondrial dysfunction in ataxia-telangiectasia. Blood. 2012;119:1490-500.

[52] Greer SN, Metcalf JL, Wang Y, Ohh M. The updated biology of hypoxia-inducible factor. EMBO J. 2012;31:2448-60.

[53] Semenza GL. Hypoxia-inducible factors: mediators of cancer progression and targets for cancer therapy. Trends Pharmacol Sci. 2012;33:207-14.

[54] Hammond EM, Denko NC, Dorie MJ, Abraham RT, Giaccia AJ. Hypoxia links ATR and p53 through replication arrest. Mol Cell Biol. 2002;22:1834-43.

[55] Bencokova Z, Kaufmann MR, Pires IM, Lecane PS, Giaccia AJ, Hammond EM. ATM activation and signaling under hypoxic conditions. Mol Cell Biol. 2009;29:526-37.

[56] Chandel NS, McClintock DS, Feliciano CE, Wood TM, Melendez JA, Rodriguez AM, et al. Reactive oxygen species generated at mitochondrial complex III stabilize hypoxia-inducible factor-1alpha during hypoxia: a mechanism of O2 sensing. J Biol Chem. 2000;275:25130-8.

[57] Mongiardi P, Stagni V, Natoli M, Giaccari D, D'Agnano I, Falchetti M, et al. Oxygen sensing is impaired in ATM defective cells. Cell Cycle. 2011;10(24): 4311-20.

[58] Cam H, Easton J, High A, Houghton P. mTORC1 signaling under hypoxic conditions is controlled by ATM-dependent phosphorylation of HIF-1α. Mol Cell. 2010;40:509-20.

[59] Shintani T, Klionsky DJ. Autophagy in health and disease: a double-edged sword. Science. 2004;306:990-5.

[60] Alexander A, Cai S-L, Kim J, Nanez A, Sahin M, MacLean KH, et al. ATM signals to TSC2 in the cytoplasm to regulate mTORC1 in response to ROS. Proc Natl Acad Sci U S A. 2010;107:4153-8.

[61] Onat A. Metabolic syndrome: nature, therapeutic solutions and options. Expert Opin Pharmacother. 2011;12:1887-90.

[62] Halaby MJ, Hibma JC, He J, Yang DQ. ATM protein kinase mediates full activation of Akt and regulates glucose transporter 4 translocation by insulin in muscle cells. Cell Signal. 2008;20:1555-63.

[63] Armata HL, Golebiowski D, Jung DY, Ko HJ, Kim JK, Sluss HK. Requirement of the ATM/p53 tumor suppressor pathway for glucose homeostasis. Mol Cell Biol. 2010;30:5787-94.

[64] Schneider JG, Finck BN, Ren J, Standley KN, Takagi M, MacLean KH, et al. ATM-dependent suppression of stress signaling reduces vascular disease in metabolic syndrome. Cell Metab. 2006;4:377-89.

[65] GoDARTS and UKPDS Diabetes Pharmacogenetics Study Group, Wellcome Trust Case Control Consortium 2, Zhou K, Bellenguez C, Spencer CC, Bennett AJ, et al. Common variants near ATM are associated with glycemic response to metformin in type 2 diabetes. 2011.

[66] Menendez JA, Cufí S, Oliveras-Ferraros C, Martin-Castillo B, Joven J, Vellon L, et al. Metformin and the ATM DNA damage response (DDR): accelerating the onset of stress-induced senescence to boost protection against cancer. Aging. 2011;3:1063-77.

[67] Yarden Y, Ullrich A. Growth factor receptor tyrosine kinases. Annu Rev Biochem. 1988;57:443-78.

[68] Golding SE, Rosenberg E, Valerie N, Hussaini I, Frigerio M, Cockcroft XF, et al. Improved ATM kinase inhibitor KU-60019 radiosensitizes glioma cells, compromises insulin, AKT and ERK prosurvival signaling, and inhibits migration and invasion. Mol Cancer Ther. 2009;10:2894-902.

[69] Li Y, Yang D-Q. The ATM inhibitor KU-55933 suppresses cell proliferation and induces apoptosis by blocking Akt in cancer cells with overactivated Akt. Mol Cancer Ther. 2010;1:113-25.

[70] Reddy JP, Peddibhotia S, Bu W, Zhao J, Haricharan S, Du Y-CN, et al. Defining the ATM-mediated barrier to tumorigenesis in somatic mammary cells following ErbB2 activation. Proc Natl Acad Sci U S A. 2010.

[71] Peretz S, Jensen R, Baserga R, Glazer PM. ATM-dependent expression of the insulin-like growth factor-I receptor in a pathway regulating radiation response. Proc Natl Acad Sci U S A. 2001;98:1676-81.

[72] De Bacco F, Luraghi P, Medico E, Reato G, Girolami F, Perera T, et al. Induction of MET by Ionizing Radiation and Its Role in Radioresistance and Invasive Growth of Cancer. J Natl Cancer Inst. 2011;103:645-61.

[73] Gumy-Pause F, Wacker P, Sappino AP. ATM gene and lymphoid malignancies. Leukemia. 2004 Feb;18(2):238-42.

[74] Taylor AM, Metcalfe JA, Thick J, Mak YF. Leukemia and lymphoma in ataxia telangiectasia. Blood. 1996 Jan 15;87(2):423-38.

[75] Matei IR, Guidos CJ, Danska JS. ATM-dependent DNA damage surveillance in T-cell development and leukemogenesis: the DSB connection. Immunol Rev. 2006 Feb;209:142-58.

[76] Krammer PH. CD95's deadly mission in the immune system. Nature. 2000 Oct 12;407(6805):789-95.

[77] Takahashi Y, Ohta H, Takemori T. Fas is required for clonal selection in germinal centers and the subsequent establishment of the memory B cell repertoire. Immunity. 2001 Feb;14(2):181-92.

[78] Siegel RM, Chan FK, Chun HJ, Lenardo MJ. The multifaceted role of Fas signaling in immune cell homeostasis and autoimmunity. Nat Immunol. 2000 Dec;1(6): 469-74.

[79] Adachi M, Suematsu S, Kondo T, Ogasawara J, Tanaka T, Yoshida N, et al. Targeted mutation in the Fas gene causes hyperplasia in peripheral lymphoid organs and liver. Nat Genet. 1995 Nov;11(3):294-300.

[80] Davidson WF, Giese T, Fredrickson TN. Spontaneous development of plasmacytoid tumors in mice with defective Fas-Fas ligand interactions. J Exp Med. 1998 Jun 1;187(11):1825-38.

[81] Fleisher TA, Puck JM, Strober W, Dale JK, Lenardo MJ, Siegel RM, et al. The autoimmune lymphoproliferative syndrome. A disorder of human lymphocyte apoptosis. Clin Rev Allergy Immunol. 2001 Feb;20(1):109-20.

[82] Straus SE, Jaffe ES, Puck JM, Dale JK, Elkon KB, Rosen-Wolff A, et al. The development of lymphomas in families with autoimmune lymphoproliferative syndrome with germline Fas mutations and defective lymphocyte apoptosis. Blood. 2001 Jul 1;98(1):194-200.

[83] Muschen M, Rajewsky K, Kronke M, Kuppers R. The origin of CD95-gene mutations in B-cell lymphoma. Trends Immunol. 2002 Feb;23(2):75-80.

[84] Wallach D, Varfolomeev EE, Malinin NL, Goltsev YV, Kovalenko AV, Boldin MP. Tumor necrosis factor receptor and Fas signaling mechanisms. Annu Rev Immunol. 1999;17:331-67.

[85] Peter ME. The flip side of FLIP. Biochem J. 2004 Sep 1;382(Pt 2):e1-3.

[86] Stagni V, di Bari MG, Condò I, Cursi S, Testi R, Larenthal Y, et al. ATM kinase activity modulates Fas sensitivity through the regulation of FLIP in lymphoid cells. Blood. 2008;111:829-37.

[87] Stagni V, Mingardi M, Santini S, Giaccari D, Barilà D. ATM kinase activity modulates cFLIP protein levels: potential interplay between DNA damage signalling and TRAIL-induced apoptosis. Carcinogenesis. 2010;31:1956-63.

[88] Solier S, Sordet O, Kohn KW, Pommier Y. Death receptor-induced activation of the Chk2- and histone H2AX-associated DNA damage response pathways. Mol Cel Biol. 2009;29:68-82.

[89] Stagni V, Santini S, Barilà D. A New Player in the Development of TRAIL Based Therapies for Hepatocarcinoma Treatment: ATM Kinase. Cancers. 2012;4:354378.

[90] Lee JH, Paull TT. ATM activation by DNA double-strand breaks through the Mre11–Rad50–Nbs1 complex. science. 2005;308:551-54.

[91] Kozlov SV, Graham ME, Jakob B, Tobias F, Kijas AW, Tanuji M, et al. Autophosphorylation and ATM activation: additional sites add to the complexity. J Biol Chem. 2011;286:9107-19.

[92] Kozlov SV, Graham ME, Peng C, Chen P, Robinson PJ, Lavin MF. Involvement of novel autophosphorylation sites in ATM activation. EMBO J. 2006;25:3504-14.

[93] Pellegrini M CA, Difilippantonio S, Guo R, Wang W, Feigenbaum L, Nussenzweig A. Autophosphorylation at serine 1987 is dispensable for murine Atm activation in vivo. Nature. 2006;443:222-5.

[94] Daniel JA, Pellegrini M, Lee JH, Paull TT, Feigenbaum L, Nussenzweig A. Multiple autophosphorylation sites are dispensable for murine ATM activation in vivo. J Cell Biol. 2008;183:777-83.

[95] Goodarzi AA, Jonnalagadda JC, Douglas P, Young D, Ye R, Moorhead GB, et al. Autophosphorylation of ataxia-telangiectasia mutated is regulated by protein phosphatase 2A. EMBO J. 2004;23:4451-61.

[96] Ali A, Zhang J, Bao S, Liu I, Otterness D, Dean NM, et al. Requirement of protein phosphatase 5 in DNA-damage-induced ATM activation. Genes Dev. 2004;18:249-54.

[97] Shreeram S, Demidov ON, Hee WK, Yamaguchi H, Onishi N, Kek C, et al. Wip1 phosphatase modulates ATM-dependent signaling pathways. Mol Cell. 2006;23:757-64.

[98] Tian B, Yang Q, Mao Z. Phosphorylation of ATM by Cdk5 mediates DNA damage signaling and regulates neuronal death. Nat Cell Biol. 2009;11:211-18.

[99] Baskaran R, Wood LD, Whitaker LL, Canman CE, Morgan SE, Xu Y, et al. Ataxia telangectasia mutant protein activates c-Abl tyrosine kinase in response to ionizing radiation. Nature. 1997;387:516-9.

[100] Shafman T, Khanna KK, Kedar P, Spring K, Kozlov S, Yen T, et al. Interaction between ATM protein and c-Abl in response to DNA damage. Nature. 1997;387:520-3.

[101] Wang X, Zeng L, Wang J, Chau JF, Lai KP, Jia D, et al. A positive role for c-Abl in Atm and Atr activation in DNA damage response. Cell Deah Differ. 2011;18:5-15.

[102] Sun Y, Xu Y, Roy K, Price BD. DNA damage-induced acetylation of lysine 3016 of ATM activates ATM kinase activity. Mol Cell Biol. 2007;27:8502-9.

[103] Barlow C, Hirotsune S, Paylor R, Liyanage M, Eckhaus M, Collins F, et al. Atm-Deficient mice: a paradigm of Ataxia Telangiectasia. Cell. 1996;86:159-71.

[104] Xu Y, Ashley T, Brainerd E, Bronson RT, Meyn MS, Baltimore D. Targeted disruption of ATM leads to growth retardation, chromosomal fragmentation during meiosis, immune defects, and thymic lymphoma. Genes Dev. 1996;10:2411-22.

[105] Elson A, Wang Y, Daugherty CJ, Morton CC, Zhou F, Campos-Torres J, et al. Pleiotropic defects in ataxia-telangiectasia protein-deficient mice. Proc Natl Acad Sci U S A. 1996;93:13084-9.

[106] Ahmed M, Rahman N. ATM and breast cancer susceptibility. Oncogene. 2006;25:5906-11.

[107] Swift M, Reitnauer pJ, Morrell D, Chase CL. Breast and other cancers in families with ataxia telangiectasia. New Engl J Med 1987;316:1289-94.

[108] Easton DF. Cancer risks in A-T heterozygotes. Int J Radiat Biol. 1994;66:S177-82.

[109] Thompson D, Duedal S, Kirner J, McGuffog L, Last JI, Reiman A, et al. Cancer risks and mortality in heterozygous ATM mutation carriers. J Natl Cancer Inst. 2005;97:813-22.

[110] Goldgar DE, Healey S, Dowty JG, Da Silva L, Chen X, Spurdle AB, et al. Rare variants in the ATM gene and risk of breast cancer. Breast Cancer Res. 2011(13):R73.

[111] Boultwood J. Ataxia telangiectasia gene mutations in leukaemia and lymphoma. J Clin Pathol. 2001 Jul;54(7):512-6.

[112] Starczynski J, Simmons W, Flavell JR, Byrd PJ, Stewart GS, Kullar HS, et al. Variations in ATM protein expression during normal lymphoid differentiation and among B-cell-derived neoplasias. Am J Pathol. 2003 Aug;163(2):423-32.

[113] Greiner TC, Dasgupta C, Ho VV, Weisenburger DD, Smith LM, Lynch JC, et al. Mutation and genomic deletion status of ataxia telangiectasia mutated (ATM) and p53 confer specific gene expression profiles in mantle cell lymphoma. Proc Natl Acad Sci U S A. 2006 Feb 14;103(7):2352-7.

[114] Tommiska J, Bartkova J, Heinonen M, Hautala L, Kilpivaara O, Eerola H, et al. The DNA damage signalling kinase ATM is aberrantly reduced or lost in BRCA1/ BRCA2-deficient and ER/PR/ERBB2-triple-negative breast cancer. Oncogene. 2008;27:2501-6.

[115] Salimi M, Mozdarani H, Majidzadeh K. Expression pattern of ATM and cyclin D1 in ductal carcinoma, normal adjacent and normal breast tissues of Iranian breast cancer patients. Med Oncol. 2012;29:1502-9.

[116] Hu H, Du L, Nagabayashi G, Seeger RC, Gatti RA. ATM is down-regulated by N-Myc-regulated microRNA-421. Proc Natl Acad Sci U S A. 2010;107:1506-11.

[117] Ng WL, Yan D, Zhang X, Mo YY, Wang Y. Over-expression of miR-100 is responsible for the low-expression of ATM in the human glioma cell line: M059J. DNA Repair (Amst). 2010;9:1170-5.

[118] Song L, Lin C, Wu Z, Gong H, Zeng Y, Wu J, et al. miR-18a impairs DNA damage response through downregulation of ataxia telangiectasia mutated (ATM) kinase. PLoS One. 2011;6:e25454.

[119] Vo QN, Kim WJ, Cvitanovic L, Boudreau DA, Ginzinger DG, Brown KD. The ATM gene is a target for epigenetic silencing in locally advanced breast cancer. Oncogene. 2004;23:9432-7.

[120] Kim WJ, Vo QN, Shrivastav M, Lataxes TA, Brown KD. Aberrant methylation of the ATM promoter correlates with increased radiosensitivity in a human colorectal tumor cell line. Oncogene. 2002;21:3864-71.

[121] Roy K, Wang L, Makrigiorgos GM, Price BD. Methylation of the ATM promoter in glioma cells alters ionizing radiation sensitivity. Biochem Biophys Res Commun. 2006;344:821-6.

[122] Bartek J, Bartkova J, Lukas J. DNA damage signalling guards against activated oncogenes and tumour progression. Oncogene. 2007;26:7773-9.

[123] DiTullio RAJ, Mochan TA, Venere M, Bartkova J, Sehested M, Bartek J, et al. 53BP1 functions in an ATM-dependent checkpoint pathway that is constitutively activated in human cancer. Nat Cell Biol. 2002;4:998-1002.

[124] Bartkova J, Horejsi Z, Koed K, Kramer A, Tort F, Ziegert K, et al. DNA damage response as a candidate anti-cancer barrier in early human tumorigenesis. Nature. 2005;434:864-70.

[125] Gorgoulis VG, Vassiliou LV, Karakaidos P, Zacharatos P, Kotsinas A, Liloglou T, et al. Activation of the DNA damage checkpoint and genomic instability in human precancerous lesions. Nature. 2005;434:907-13.

[126] Bartkova J, Rezaei N, Liontos M, Karakaidos P, Kletsas D, Issaeva N, et al. Oncogene-induced senescence is part of the tumorigenesis barrier imposed by DNA damage checkpoints. Nature. 2006;444:633-7.

[127] Di Micco R, Fumagalli M, Cicalese A, Piccinin S, Gasparini P, Luise C, et al. Oncogene-induced senescence is a DNA damage response triggered by DNA hyper-replication. Nature. 2006;444:638-42.

[128] d'Adda di Fagagna F. Living on a break: cellular senescence as a DNA-damage response. Nat Rev Cancer. 2008;8:512-22.

[129] Sarkaria JN, Busby EC, Tibbetts RS, Roos P, Taya Y, Karnitz LM, et al. Inhibition of ATM and ATR kinase activities by the radiosensitizing agent, caffeine. Cancer Res. 1999;59:4375-82.

[130] Blasina A, Price BD, Turenne GA, McGowan CH. Caffeine inhibits the checkpoint kinase ATM. Curr Biol. 1999;9:1135-8.

[131] Hickson I, Zhao Y, Richardson CJ, Green SJ, Martin NM, Orr AI, et al. Identification and characterization of a novel and specific inhibitor of the ataxia-telangiectasia mutated kinase ATM. Cancer Res. 2004 Dec 15;64(24):9152-9.

[132] Rainery MD, Charlton ME, Sytanton RV, Kastan MB. Transient inhibition of ATM kinase is sufficient to enhance cellular sensitivity to ionizing radiation. Cancer Res. 2008;68:7466-74.

[133] Viniegra JG, Martínez N, Modirassari P, Hernández Losa J, Parada Cobo C, Sánchez-Arévalo Lobo VJ, et al. Full activation of PKB/Akt in response to insulin or ionizing radiation is mediated through ATM. J Biol Chem. 2005;280:4029-36.

[134] Macaulay VM, Salisbury AJ, Bohula EA, Playford MP, Smorodinsky NI, Shiloh Y. Downregulation of the type 1 insulin-like growth factor receptor in mouse melanoma cells is associated with enhanced radiosensitivity and impaired activation of Atm kinase. Oncogene. 2001;20:4029-40.

[135] Fraser M, Harding SM, Zhao H, Coackley C, Durocher D, Bristow RG. MRE11 promotes AKT phosphorylation in direct response to DNA double-strand breaks. Cell Cycle. 2011;10:2218-32.

[136] Golding SE, Valerie K. MRE11 and ATM AKTivate pro-survival signaling. Cell Cycle. 2011;10:3227.

[137] Jiang H, Reinhardt HC, Bartkova J, Tommiska J, Blomqvist C, Nevanlinna H, et al. The combined status of ATM and p53 link tumor development with therapeutic response. Genes Dev. 2009;23:1895-909.

[138] Lumsden JM, McCarty T, Petiniot LK, Shen R, Barlow C, Wynn TA, et al. Immunoglobulin class switch recombination is impaired in Atm-deficient mice. J Exp Med. 2004;200:1111-21.

[139] Bredemeyer AL, Sharma GG, Huang CY, Helmink BA, Walker LM, Khor KC, et al. ATM stabilizes DNA double-strand-break complexes during V(D)J recombination. Nature. 2006;442:466-70.

[140] Bredemeyer AL, Huang CY, Walker LM, Bassing CH, Sleckman BP. Aberrant V(D)J recombination in ataxia telangiectasia mutated-deficient lymphocytes is dependent on nonhomologous DNA end joining. . J Immunol. 2008 181:2620–5.

[141] Callén E, Jankovic M, Difilippantonio S, Daniel JA, Chen HT, Celeste A, et al. ATM prevents the persistence and propagation of chromosome breaks in lymphocytes. Cell. 2007;130:63-75.

[142] Waldmann TA, Broder S, Goldman CK, Frost K, Korsmeyer SJ, Medici MA. Disorders of B cells and helper T cells in the pathogenesis of the immunoglobulin deficiency of patients with ataxia telangiectasia. J Clin Invest. 1983;71:282-95.

[143] Gatti RA, Vinters HV. Cerebellar pathology in ataxia-telangiectasia: the significance of basket cells. Kroc Found Ser. 1985;19:225-32.

[144] Barlow C, Ribaut-Barassin C, Zwingman TA, Pope AJ, Brown KD, Owens JW, et al. ATM is a cytoplasmic protein in mouse brain required to prevent lysosomal accumulation. Proc Natl Acad Sci U S A. 2000 Jan 18;97(2):871-6.

[145] Li J, Han YR, Plummer MR, Herrup K. Cytoplasmic ATM in neurons modulates synaptic function. Curr Biol. 2009;19:2091-6.

[146] Biton S, Dar I, Mittelman L, Pereg Y, Barzilai A, Shiloh Y. Nuclear ataxia-telangiectasia mutated (ATM) mediates the cellular response to DNA double strand breaks in human neuron-like cells. J Biol Chem. 2006 Jun 23;281(25): 17482-91.

[147] Uttara B, Singh AV, Zamboni P, Mahajan RT. Oxidative stress and neurodegenerative diseases: a review of upstream and downstream antioxidant therapeutic options. Curr Nuropharmacol. 2009;7:65-74.

[148] Ray PD, Huang BW, Tsuji Y. Reactive oxygen species (ROS) homeostasis and redox regulation in cellular signaling. Cell Signal. 2012;24:981-90.

[149] Kim J, Wong PK. Loss of ATM impairs proliferation of neural stem cells through oxidative stress-mediated p38 MAPK signaling. J Biol Chem. 2009;284:14396-404.

[150] Eilam R, Peter Y, Groner Y, Segal M. Late degeneration of nigro-striatal neurons in ATM-/- mice. . Neuroscience. 2003;121:83-98.

[151] Chen P, Peng C, Luff J, Spring K, Watters D, Bottle S, et al. Oxidative stress is responsible for deficient survival and dendritogenesis in purkinje neurons from ataxia-telangiectasia mutated mutant mice. . J Neuroscience. 2003;11:11453–460.

[152] Allen DM, van Praag H, Ray J, Weaver Z, Winrow CJ, Carter TA, et al. Ataxia telangiectasia mutated is essential during adult neurogenesis. Genes Dev. 2001 Mar 1;15(5):554-66.

[153] Wu Q, Wang X. Neuronal stem cells in the central nervous system and in human diseases. Protein Cell. 2012;3:262-70.

[154] Kim J, Hwangbo J, Wong PK. p38 MAPK-Mediated Bmi-1 down-regulation and defective proliferation in ATM-deficient neural stem cells can be restored by Akt activation. PLoS One. 2011;6:e16615.

[155] Lim DA, Alvarez-Buylla A. Interaction between astrocytes and adult subventricular zone precursors stimulates neurogenesis. Proc Natl Acad Sci U S A. 1999;96:7526-31.

[156] Song HJ, Stevens CF, Gage FH. Neural stem cells from adult hippocampus develop essential properties of functional CNS neurons. . Nat Neurosci. 2002;5:438-45.

[157] Wang Y, Imitola J, Rasmussen S, O'Connor KC, Khoury SJ. Paradoxical dysregulation of the neural stem cell pathway sonic hedgehog-Gli1 in autoimmune encephalomyelitis and multiple sclerosis. Ann Neurol. 2008;64:417-27.

[158] Carlessi L, De Filippis L, Lecis D, Vescovi A, Delia D. DNA-damage response, survival and differentiation in vitro of a human neural stem cell line in relation to ATM expression. Cell Deah Differ. 2009;16:795-806.

Chapter 9

Rett Syndrome: A Model of Genetic Neurodevelopmental Disorders

Christopher A. Chapleau, Jane Lane,
Lucas Pozzo-Miller and Alan K. Percy

Additional information is available at the end of the chapter

1. Introduction

Neurodevelopmental disorders, sometimes referred to as disorders of intellectual disability (ID), are a large family of conditions of genetic, acquired, or environmental origin that are characterized by deficiencies in cognitive and behavioral functions. While many of these disorders share similar behavioral phenotypes, they are often accompanied with other features specific to each disorder. One disorder with a unique progression is Rett Syndrome (RTT; Online Mendelian Inheritance in Man #312750; http://www.ncbi.nlm.nih.gov/omim/). RTT is the leading cause of severe ID in females, with approximately 1:10,000 females worldwide affected by this disorder. Mutations in the gene encoding the transcriptional regulator, methyl-CpG-binding protein 2 (MeCP2), located on the X chromosome (Xq28), have been confirmed in more than 95% of individuals meeting diagnostic criteria for RTT. RTT is characterized by an uneventful early infancy followed by stagnation and regression of growth, motor, language, and social skills later in development.

RTT was first described by Dr. Andreas Rett, an Austrian developmental pediatrician in the 1960's, and was also recognized about the same time by Dr. Bengt Hagberg, a Swedish child neurologist. Dr. Rett was the first to publish initial cases on a number of girls that he was following in his practice that had the same repetitive hand-washing motion with a similar neurodevelopmental phenotype (Rett 1966). Dr. Rett initially described this disorder as an association with increased ammonia levels, but it was latter discovered that this characterization was incorrect due to an improperly calibrated measurement system. These observations and subsequent characterization by Dr. Rett would go unnoticed by the broader medical community in large part related to the publication of the manuscript in a German-language medical journal. A chance meeting of Hagberg and Rett in 1981 in Toronto led to the first widely read

English language publication by Hagberg and colleagues from France and Portugal that attributed the disorder to Rett's early work. Thus, it was not until 1983, in an English-language medical journal, that Bengt Hagberg and colleagues reported 35 females that had a similar disease progression; onset around 7 to 18 months of age, with developmental stagnation followed by rapid worsening of numerous neurological functions (Hagberg, Aicardi et al. 1983).

RTT is typically diagnosed early in the life of a female and based on strict diagnostic criteria that have been extensively established (Neul, Kaufmann et al. 2010); (Percy, Neul et al. 2010). These criteria are based on the unique disease progression, which begins with stalled developmental progress after an apparently normal pregnancy and an uneventful first 6–18 months of life. After development becomes abruptly stagnated, frank regression occurs in growth, motor, language, and social skills that leads to either partial or complete loss of these skills. The next period of RTT consists of stabilization and recovery of socialization skills by age four to five that persist into adulthood. While the research into pathology and genetics of RTT has made great strides from Dr. Rett's initially characterization, a number of things have stayed constant. First, RTT is still an observational disorder; certain hallmark features that differentiate this disorder from other neurodevelopmental disorders. Second, RTT has no cure at present and treatment is based on health issues that are specific for each person.

2. Clinical features

The general overview of this disorder from a clinical perspective is a disease associated with phenotypes that vary depending on the age of the child. The developmental profile is a distinct feature of RTT that includes three unique stages. The first stage is an apparently normal gestational period and a generally ordinary period of development typically occuring until approximately 6-18 months of age. The next developmental period may last up to 4 years of age, characterized first by the stagnation of development and then the frank regression in growth, motor, language, and social skills (Percy 2002). This is the most detrimental period in the progression of the disorder with the prominent loss, partial or complete, of cognitive, social, and motor skills. The last period of RTT consists of stabilization and recovery of socialization skills by age four to five with persistence into adulthood. Due in part to better clinical understanding and immense effort that has been put forth to study this disorder, recent projections predict that individuals with RTT will live into adult life with average survival just over age 50 (Kirby, Lane et al. 2010).

In most individuals with RTT, the single, most observable and characteristic feature consists of stereotypic hand movements. These stereotypies, of yet unknown neurological origin, may consist of hand washing, wringing, squeezing, clapping, tapping, or rubbing and are evident in approximately 94% of individuals (figure 1) (Percy and Lane 2005), (Carter, Downs et al. 2010). Furthermore, they are continuous during waking hours; only subsiding when the individual falls asleep. Another motor difficulty that these individuals display is difficulty maintaining balance and ambulation. Most girls walk at some point in their life (~80%), however gait and balance issues arise, presumably from poor motor control and significant anxiety, such that about 25% lose this ability.

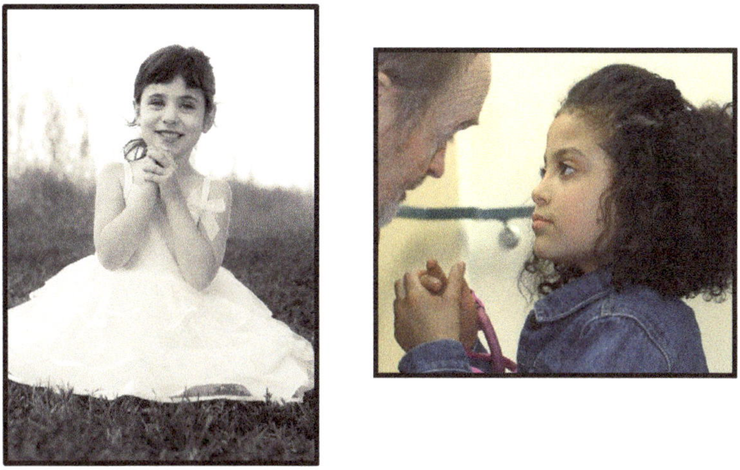

Figure 1. Image of two females with Rett Syndrome, displaying stereotypical hand behavior

Behavioral issues, in addition to cognitive and social regression, are another hallmark of RTT. Heightened anxiety and mood disturbances are well-known features in many girls with RTT, and demonstrated by behaviors including difficulties maintaining posture and breathing irregularities (Mount, Charman et al. 2002; Robertson, Hall et al. 2006). RTT is considered an Autism Spectrum Disorder (ASD) due in part to the girls being withdrawn from social contact, thus demonstrating communication dysfunction (Percy 2011). It is during this period of regression that features consistent with autism emerge. They often lack the ability to respond to commands and lose the ability for verbal communication. For this reason, RTT is commonly compared to autism. However, the autistic features are generally transient in RTT, typically subsiding after the age of three-four years. At this time point, while language acquisition might not ever occur, eye gaze returns and becomes the primary form of communication with the outside world. It is believed that the description of RTT as an autistic disorder and the ability to develop non-verbal communication could be used as a diagnostic sign.

3. Diagnostic criteria

RTT is diagnosed based on observable criteria. While MeCP2 mutation occurs in an overwhelming majority of individuals diagnosed with RTT, positive mutations of the gene are not part of the diagnostic checklist, but as a supporting piece of information. In 2009 investigators from the RettSearch Consortium, an international group of clinicians and researchers revised the diagnostic criteria in order to clarify and simplify the diagnosis of classic (typical) and variant (atypical) forms (Neul, Kaufmann et al. 2010). Listed in table 1 is the set of definitive diagnostic criteria for classic RTT.

Inclusion and exclusion criteria for diagnosis of classic RTT
Period of developmental regression
Period of recovery or stabilization
Evidence of all main criteria
1. Partial or complete loss of acquired purposeful hand skills
2. Partial or complete loss of spoken language
3. Gait Abnormalities
4. Stereotypic hand movements
5. Exclusion of brain injury secondary to trauma or grossly abnormal psychomotor development in first 6 months of life

Table 1. Consensus criteria for the diagnosis of classic RTT

Additionally analysis of the RTT population through the many years of following these individuals in clinics throughout the world have noted a wide variability in severity where individuals might present with some, but not all clinical features that would signify a diagnosis of classical RTT. For this reason, a number of recognized atypical forms have been characterized and documented based on unique characteristics (Neul, Kaufmann et al. 2010). The atypical forms that have been established consist of preserved speech, early seizure, and congenital variants (Hagberg and Skjeldal 1994). The RettSearch Consortium provided consensus criteria and core features essential for diagnosis of atypical forms of RTT (table 2).

Diagnosis of atypical forms of RTT
Period of developmental regression followed by period of stabilization
Meet at least 2 of 4 phenotypes from the main criteria
Meet at least 5 of 11 supportive criteria
Supportive Criteria
1. Abnormal muscle tone
2. Breathing disturbances when awake
3. Bruxism
4. Diminished response to pain
5. Growth retardation
6. Impaired sleep pattern
7. Inappropriate laughing or screaming spells
8. Intense eye communication
9.Peripheral vasomotor disturbances
10. Scoliosis/kyphosis
11. Small/cold hand and feet

Table 2. Consensus criteria and core features essential for diagnosis of atypical forms of RTT; preserved speech, early seizure, and congenital variants

4. Physical features and pathophysiology

From an initial observation, individuals with RTT tend to be very small in terms of height for their age, nearly 2-3 standard deviations from normal (Hagberg, Stenbom et al. 2001). Furthermore, a deceleration of the rate of height and weight is also a characteristic of this disease (Schultz, Glaze et al. 1993). Given that individuals with RTT tend to be very small, it is no surprise that their feet and hand growth are also often stunted.

Many studies have been conducted that have examined head size and brain growth. Head circumference in RTT individuals is also very small for their age and head growth deceleration occurs as early as 1.5 months of age (Tarquinio, Motil et al. 2012 *in press*). Similar to body height, head circumference was also found to be 2-3 standard deviations below values estimated in healthly individuals (Hagberg, Stenbom et al. 2001). Furthermore, RTT brains typically weigh less than those from unaffected individuals (Armstrong 2005). Microscopic studies of brains from autopsy samples have demonstrated that neurons from numerous cortical areas, including the hippocampus and thalamus, are smaller in size and densely packed, without evidence of neurodegeneration or gliosis (Bauman, Kemper et al. 1995; (Armstrong 2005).

It has long been suggested that disorders related to ID have been associated with structural irregularities in neuronal connectivity (Fiala, Spacek et al. 2002) (Kaufmann and Moser 2000). This well supported notion was developed from pioneering studies in the 1970's that described striking abnormalities in the dendritic morphology of cortical neurons obtained from postmortem brain samples from individuals with a number of different disorders associated with ID (Huttenlocher 1970; Marin-Padilla 1972; Huttenlocher 1974; Purpura 1974). From this standpoint, a number of studies have been conducted that provide evidence to suggest that reduced or altered neuronal connectivity at synapses is a characteristic of RTT. To support this notion, magnetic resonance imaging demonstrated a reduction in gray matter volume in the parietal lobe in addition to reductions in cortical white matter (Bauman, Kemper et al. 1995; Carter, Lanham et al. 2008). Consistent with these findings, dendritic growth and arborization are reduced in RTT (Belichenko, Oldfors et al. 1994; Armstrong, Dunn et al. 1995; Chapleau, Calfa et al. 2009).

Another fascinating discovery that was uncovered during these series of observations from the 1970's was the description of alterations in dendritic spines on the postsynaptic side of excitatory synapses. Postmortem observations described reductions in dendritic spine densities in addition to changes in their shape, commonly referred to as "spine dysgenesis" (Purpura 1974). Confocal imaging studies using postmortem brains from individuals diagnosed with RTT or control individuals, have demonstrated a decrease in the density of dendritic spines in several areas of the brains including the somatosensory cortex and hippocampus (Belichenko, Oldfors et al. 1994; Armstrong, Dunn et al. 1995; Chapleau, Calfa et al. 2009). Molecular analysis of postmortem brains further supports this notion, as studies have found that the expression of microtubule-associated protein (MAP-2), a protein involved in microtubule stabilization and a key cytoskeletal component of dendrites, is reduced in the cortex of RTT individuals (Kaufmann, Naidu et al. 1995; Kaufmann, Taylor et al. 1997). Furthermore, expression levels of cyclooxygenase, a protein enriched in dendritic spines is also reduced in RTT cortex (Kaufmann and Moser 2000). With regard to density of synapses, reduced levels of the synaptic vesicle protein, synaptophysin, were detected in the motor, frontal and temporal cortices by immunofluorescence (Belichenko, Hagberg et al. 1997). Intriguingly, glutamate receptor density has a differential distribution during RTT development, where younger individuals with RTT have a higher density compared to controls, while older individuals have a lower density compared to controls (Blue, Naidu et al. 1999). These results suggest that an increase in glutamate receptor density may be a compensation for the reduction in dendritic spines.

In addition to these various anatomical brain findings, a number of alterations have been discovered in its neurochemistry. Specific areas of the brain including the midbrain and caudate, which produce a number of neurotransmitters, have been shown to have reduced volume compared to healthy individuals (Reiss, Faruque et al. 1993). In support of this finding, tyrosine hydroxylase staining was reduced in the substantia nigra, an important region for dopamine production (Jellinger, Armstrong et al. 1988). Furthermore, cerebrospinal fluid (CSF) measurements of RTT individuals, demonstrated a reduction in the dopamine metabolite, homovanillic acid, and the serotonin metabolite, 5-hydroxyindoleacetic acid (Samaco, Mandel-Brehm et al. 2009).

A number of other structural and physical abnormities have been demonstrated. One striking physical finding can be made upon observation and by touching an individual's feet. In many individuals with RTT, feet are not only cold to touch, but may appear blue or purplish in color. It is assumed that defective autonomic function is the pathological culprit; however the exact mechanism for this has yet to be determined. Another finding that might relate to dysfunction in autonomic signaling is abnormal cardiac conduction. A feature that has been observed in a number of individuals diagnosed with RTT is a prolonged QT interval, where the timing between ventricle depolarization and repolarization is delayed, which is estimated to occur in approximately 20% of individuals (McCauley, Wang et al. 2011) (Sekul, Moak et al. 1994). For this reason, at the time of the diagnosis of RTT (and every one to two years thereafter), one of the first tests to be ordered is an electrocardiogram (EKG), in order to guard against the sudden death risk with prolonged QT intervals.

Another condition that arises in the RTT population, presumably because of altered metabolic requirements, lack of physical mobility, and their small stature, is osteopenia, a condition characterized by reduced bone mineralization and increased likelihood of fractures (Haas, Dixon et al. 1997). Reduced bone size and lower bone mass have been detected in the RTT population (Roende, Ravn et al. 2011). Lastly, irregularities in the motility of the gastric region and esophageal tract lead to the development of gastroesophageal reflux, which is a major cause of pain and discomfort (Motil, Schultz et al. 1999). Abnormalities in gallbladder function, in addition to the accumulation of gallstones, have been identified as a serious concern in the RTT population and may require surgical assessment (Percy and Lane 2005).

5. Genetics and MeCP2

A number of clinical observations linked this disorder to a genetic mutation of *de novo* origin. First, RTT predominantly affected female individuals; second, RTT rarely recurred in the same family, and third, RTT was a worldwide disorder that affected all racial and ethnic groups, not commonly associated with a pattern of inheritance. In the 1990's after much early speculation, numerous studies determined that RTT was indeed caused by a genetic mutation. First, mapping studies using RTT families mapped the mutation to the X chromosome with subsequent analyses localizing the likely gene at Xq28, confirming an X-linked dominant pattern of inheritance (Archidiacono, Lerone et al. 1991; Ellison, Fill et al. 1992; Sirianni, Naidu et al. 1998). After this lengthy study of the X chromosome, a hallmark paper was published in 1999 identifying the gene encoding methyl-CpG-binding protein 2 (*MECP2*) (Amir, Van den Veyver et al. 1999).

More than 95% of individuals with classic RTT carry a *de novo* mutation in the gene encoding *MECP2*. To date, more than 250 different mutations of *MECP2* have been identified in the RTT population, with about 60% of the mutations coming from 8 specific point mutations involving the following amino acid changes (R106W, R133C, T158M, R168X, R255X, R270X, R294X, R306C) (Williamson and Christodoulou 2006). Interestingly, mutations on *MECP2* have only been identified in approximately ~75% of atypical or variant RTT (Percy, Lane et al. 2007). Characterizations of *MECP2* mutations through genetic testing provide molecular confirmation of the diagnosis of RTT but should not be used as the sole diagnostic factor, as roughly 5% of the classical RTT population do not have defined mutations of MeCP2, but meet the clinical criteria (Neul, Fang et al. 2008). While the reason that the *MECP2* gene is susceptible to mutations is not understood, the overwhelming majority of RTT cases are a result of spontaneous *de novo MECP2* mutations in the paternal X chromosome germlines (Trappe, Laccone et al. 2001). However, some families do exist where *MECP2* mutations are present throughout multiple generations (Augenstein, Lane et al. 2009).

MeCP2, a member of the methyl-CpG-binding domain (MBD) family of transcriptional regulator proteins, is encoded by a ~76kb gene located on chromosome Xq28 and constructed from four exons associated with two protein isoforms, MECP2_e1 and MECP2_e2. The MeCP2 protein has two major functional domains; the methyl-binding domain (MBD), consisting of 85 amino acids that binds specifically to DNA at methylated CpG's, and the transitional repressing domain (TRD), consisting of 104 amino acids, that is responsible for recruiting other proteins to form complexes that mediate transcription of various genes (Guy, Cheval et al. 2011). MeCP2 binds specifically to A/T rich sites in close proximity to CpG-methylated DNA sites, working with other proteins in recruiting co-repressors and histone deacetylase complexes, thereby altering the structure of genomic DNA and modifying the transcription of specific target genes (Klose and Bird 2006). Recent studies have demonstrated that MeCP2 has both repressor and activator transcription activities (Chahrour, Jung et al. 2008). MeCP2 has been shown to be tightly bound to DNA at all times and its transcriptional control activity is regulated by post-translational modifications such as phosphorylation and acetylation, that alter the conformational shape of DNA, enabling or repressing transcription of a potential target gene (Skene, Illingworth et al. 2010; Cohen, Gabel et al. 2011). Furthermore, a role of MeCP2 in RNA splicing has also been hypothesized due to its ability to interact with the RNA-binding protein, Y box-binding protein (Young, Hong et al. 2005).

6. MeCP2 function

The precise mechanism of dysfunction of mutated MeCP2 that is responsible for RTT symptomatology remains unknown. MeCP2 is highly expressed in the brain and is critical for the development and maturation of neurons (Akbarian, Chen et al. 2001);,(Jung, Jugloff et al. 2003);,(Mullaney, Johnston et al. 2004). Recent reports suggest that the MeCP2 is also expressed in glial cells and altered function of glial cells might be another reason for disease progression (Ballas, Lioy et al. 2009);,(Maezawa, Swanberg et al. 2009);,(Maezawa and Jin 2010). Expression of MeCP2 in humans and mice increases with neuronal development and maturation (Shahbazian et al., 2002). In addition, the expression levels of MeCP2 control the development of excitatory synapses early in postnatal development (Chao, Zoghbi et al. 2007). Since MeCP2 expression in cortical areas increases during neuronal development, it is assumed that MeCP2 is crucial for axonal and dendritic differentiation during the first 6–18 months of age leading to proper synapse formation and maturation. Furthermore, new data suggests that MeCP2 expression is also important in adulthood, as MeCP2 removal during later stages of postnatal/adult development, altered the density of excitatory synapses and the expression of synaptic proteins involved with maintaining synapses (Nguyen, Du et al. 2012).

The functions of MeCP2 have been shown to extend beyond its importance in the development and maintainence of synapses in the brain. It has been shown that MeCP2 regulates the balance between excitatory and inhibitory transmission. It is unknown exactly how MeCP2 governs the balance between glutamate and GABA, but recent studies suggest that altered MeCP2 might also be expressed on non-neuronal brain cells (i.e., oligodendroglia and astrocytes) that regulate the uptake of glutamate (Maezawa and Jin 2010). Astrocytes from mutant *Mecp2* mice co-cultured with wild-type neurons caused significant dendritic damage to the neurons. In support of these findings, recent studies using hippocampal slices from *mecp2* mutant mice demonstrate these tissues to be extremely hyperexcitable (Calfa, Hablitz et al. 2011). Furthermore, studies in null mice demonstrated that GABAergic synaptic transmission is weakened in the ventrolateral medulla region of the brain stem (Chao, Chen et al. 2010).

Another important finding related to MeCP2 function relates to the concept of homeostatic plasticity, a type of plasticity whereby an optimal level of transmission is regulated by modulating the strength of excitatory and inhibitory synapses. Recent evidence has demonstrated that MeCP2 functions in synaptic scaling, a form of homeostatic plasticity that regulates the strength of excitatory synapse currents in response to neuronal activity (Qiu, Sylwestrak et al. 2012). These data suggest that MeCP2 is involved with balancing network excitability. Since glutamate levels tend to be increased in individuals with RTT, in addition to the common occurrence of seizures (Glaze, Percy et al. 2010), mechanisms responsible for modulating glutamate transmission or increasing GABAergic transmission need to be explored as a treatment option.

7. Disease severity

As we discussed previously, wide variability in phenotypic severity is observed in RTT. Since the gene for MeCP2 resides on the X-chromosome, the balance of X-chromosome inactivation (XCI) plays an important factor in disease severity. Studies have shown that individuals with classical RTT have XCI that has a random distribution, whereas nonrandom XCI is associated with milder phenotypes (Amir, Van den Veyver et al. 2000). However, a dramatic example of the importance of XCI in RTT comes from a family in which the same *MECP2* mutation was present in several family members (Augenstein, Lane et al. 2009). The mother, had a 44bp mutation, passed the mutation to a daughter with classical RTT and a son with a progressive neurological disorder. The mother, who had some cognitive deficits, does not have any features of RTT and has an XCI ratio that favors the "good" X-chromosome (89:11).

In addition to XCI, another factor to consider is the genotype-phenotype relationship. Various mutations or types of mutation tend to be associated with different phenotypes. For the most part, nonsense mutations, mutations that cause a premature stop transcription, tend to produce more severe effects than missense mutations. For instance, the R133C mutation is associated with a less severe phenotype compared to the R168X mutation, one of the most severe mutations as individuals tend not to walk, use hands, or speak (Neul, Fang et al. 2008). Furthermore, missense mutations in the TRD tend to have a milder phenotype (Schanen, Houwink et al. 2004).

8. Treatment options

Therapeutic management for these individuals can be quite complicated when taking into account their specific neurodevelopmental phenotype. Research into the clinical management of RTT relies on focusing on present day treatment using FDA approved agents and future research using newly found molecules. Moreover, the present day treatment research focuses on reviewing the entire spectrum of symptoms that relate to RTT, while future treatment options focus on discovering molecules that could cure the entire disorder. Conducting clinical trials in this population is challenging as stratification of participants requires careful planning. Additionally as a result of the difficulty in performing clinical trials in these individuals, few results have come from previous clinical trials that have provided unquestionable therapeutic recommendations. An issue in performing studies in the RTT population is the huge variability in disease severity, which makes comparison between groups an extremely challenging task. Trials using the drug naltrexone to blocked the observed increase in beta-endorphin expression, appeared to diminish motor behavior overall (Budden, Myer et al. 1990) (Percy, Glaze et al. 1994). Other clinical trials have been conducted in the RTT population to examine the potential effectiveness of the vitamin, folate, on disease progression. Results from the study demonstrated no major improvement in objective measurements (Glaze, Percy et al. 2009).

Numerous strategies to cure RTT have been proposed that are based on preclinical evaluation of potential pharmacological agents or based on the proposed mechanism of MeCP2 dysfunction. One issue to address in treatment options is to determine if a specific point in development exists where treatment has to be initiated to rescue function. Studies have shown symptom resolution can be accomplished in MeCP2 null transgenic mice by simply turning on the expression of MeCP2 in adult mice. Using an insertion of the *lox-stop* cassette into the Mecp2 gene of mice, where tamoxifen administration removed the stop cassette causing *Mecp2* expression to be activated fully, symptomatic mice were noted to have markedly diminished severity of RTT-like phenotypes. (Guy, Gan et al. 2007).

These studies suggest that for a potential curative agent, therapy could be initiated at any time point in development and lead to potential benefit. Potential therapies that could be developed stem from these basic properties of MeCP2. The first option revolves around the lifespan of mutant proteins. Transgenic mice were created with a mutation in the methyl binding domain of the MeCP2 protein (T158A), causing a reduction in MeCP2 binding affinity to methylated DNA and reducing the protein's half-life (Goffin, Allen et al. 2011). Thus a potential therapeutic option is to increase either the protein's expression or half-life, granted that mutant MeCP2 proteins do not lead to a gain of function deficit. Another potential therapy relates to the location of the *MECP2* gene and the modulation of XCI. When XCI is randomly distributed in RTT, individuals tend to be more severely affected compared to situations of nonrandom XCI where a greater percentage of cells express the normal allele (Amir, Van den Veyver et al. 2000). By taking advantage of this process, if the normal allele is turned on and the mutate allele is turned off, it is possible that symptom improvement would occur. In an overwhelming majority of instances, *de novo MECP2* mutations have been identified in the paternal X chromosome (Trappe, Laccone et al. 2001). If this is the case, by identifying the locus of the mutation, a practical approach could be developed to turn off the mutant allele and activate the normal allele. This is a technically challenging, but potentially exciting strategy.

Another potential therapy that revolves around modulating the existing genetic environment is by using a molecule that allows read-through of premature STOP codons in mutant genes. Nonsense mutation in *MECP2* resulting in premature transcription termination occurs in approximately 35% of North American RTT patients (Percy, Lane et al. 2007). Aminoglycosides are antibiotics that are used today against resistant gram-negative bacteria, but studies have shown that they also have potential as pharmacological agents to overcome transcriptional termination caused by nonsense mutations (Rowe and Clancy 2009),(Zingman, Park et al. 2007). In various models, the full-length MeCP2 protein was discovered in different cell cultures expressing nonsense mutations after incubation with an aminoglycoside antibiotic. (Brendel, Klahold et al. 2009),(Brendel, Belakhov et al. 2011),(Popescu, Sidorova et al. 2010). From a functional standpoint, iPSC-derived neurons from RTT patients expressing nonsense mutations, when treatment with the aminoglycoside gentamicin was employed, demonstrated increased dendritic spine density (Marchetto, Carromeu et al. 2010). While a potentially useful molecule has yet to be tested in transgenic mouse expressing a nonsense MeCP2 protein, this particular approach might be of great promise for this subset of the RTT population.

Another option revolves around the use of the growth factor, BDNF, a member of the neurotrophin family of growth factors that have essential roles in neuronal survival and differentiation in early development and a strong modulator of synaptic transmission and plasticity in the mature brain (Amaral, Chapleau et al. 2007). BDNF protein levels measured by ELISA were found to be lower in brain samples of *Mecp2* mutant mice (Chang, Khare et al. 2006). Intriguingly, crossbreeding *Bdnf* heterozygous mice with *Mecp2* mutant mice exacerbated the onset of the RTT-associated phenotypes.(Chang, Khare et al. 2006) More importantly, BDNF mRNA levels are lower in brain samples from RTT patients, similar to the finding described in MeCP2 mutant mice (Deng, Matagne et al. 2007).

Promising work has shown that the genetic overexpression of BDNF can rescue some of the deleterious consequences of MeCP2 dysfunction. For example, crossbreeding *Bdnf* overexpressing mice with *Mecp2* mutants alleviated numerous phenotypes, including motor hypoactivity, reduced activity of cortical neurons, in addition to extending their lifespan (Chang, Khare et al. 2006) Consistently, *BDNF* overexpression in neurons transfected with RTT-associated *MECP2* mutations or with *Mecp2* shRNA to knockdown its expression reversed dendritic atrophy in primary hippocampal neuron cultures (Larimore, Chapleau et al. 2009). While the genetic overexpression of BDNF is promising in rodent models, the administration of BDNF is not a useful clinical approach due to its short half-life and inability to cross the blood–brain barrier.(Kingwell 2010) However, small molecules that can mimic BDNF's effects or that can increase the levels of endogenous BDNF are attractive potential therapeutic options. Small molecules that act like BDNF, so called "BDNF mimetics," are blood-brain barrier permeable factors and have shown promise to reverse RTT-like features in experimental mouse models. Heterozygous female *mecp2* mutant mice, treated with LM22A-4, rescued breathing abnormalities and increased TrkB phosphorylation in areas of the brain central for respiration, medulla and pons.(Schmid, Yang et al. 2012) 7,8-DHF delayed body mass deficits and improved wheel running and breathing impairments in mutant male mice.(Johnson, Lam et al. 2011) While these agents present limited supporting research, they do offer hope of targeting BDNF without administering the actual protein.

Another potential option that has recently gained much attention as therapeutic treatment of RTT individuals is the pleiotropic growth factor insulin-like growth factor-1 (IGF-1). Unlike BDNF, IGF-1 crosses the blood-brain barrier and gains access to the CNS. IGF-1 stimulates proliferation of neural progenitors, neuronal survival, neurite outgrowth, and synapse formation (D'Ercole, Ye et al. 1996),(D'Ercole, Ye et al. 2002). Consistent with these BDNF mimetic actions, daily injections of the active tri-peptide fragment of IGF-1 improved motor function, breathing rhythm and cardiac irregularities, in addition to increased brain weight in *Mecp2* mutant mice (Tropea, Giacometti et al. 2009). The active tri-peptide also improved a number of synaptic features, including dendritic spine density in pyramidal neurons of layer V of the motor cortex. In the same region of the cerebral cortex, IGF-1 restored the motility of dendritic spines, a process crucial for synaptic development and plasticity (Landi, Putignano et al. 2011). Since the full-length IGF-1 is approved by the Food and Drug Administration for the treatment of growth failure in children that were unresponsive to treatment with growth hormone,(Fintini, Brufani et al. 2009) a clinical trial is currently underway to determine if administration of Mecasermin (Increlex®), a synthetic analog of full-length IGF-1 improves the symptoms and health of RTT patients (ClinicalTrials.gov identifier: NCT01253317).

9. Conclusions

It should also be noted that other genes have been linked to variant RTT, including cyclin-dependent kinase-like 5 (CDKL5), FOXG1, and the Netrin G1 genes. Future research examining MeCP2 dysfunction needs to consider the influence of MeCP2 mutations on other disorders.

The greatest challenge at present is to develop translational research that implements unique options developed at the basic science level and moves them efficiently and smoothly to the clinical setting. Furthermore, since many common neurobiological mechanisms exist in the spectrum of neurodevelopmental disorders, understanding the key components might hasten the progress of novel treatment for all these unique and devastating disorders. As the clinical and basic science understanding of RTT has unfolded, key points of interaction have been targeted to approach its understanding and potential management. From the clinical perspective, the array of medical issues includes epilepsy, periodic breathing, altered growth patterns, gastrointestinal dysfunction, and significant orthopedic issues including scoliosis. From the basic science viewpoint, the epigenetic role of *MECP2*, with emphasis on known elements such as brain derived neurotrophic factor and corticotrophin releasing hormone, and the broad impact on neural function have led to exciting opportunities for therapeutic intervention currently receiving intense scrutiny at the translational level at the same time that clinical investigation and intervention, particularly related to augmentative communication strategies are increasing. Future research regarding the treatment of RTT must rely on determining which dysregulated genes contribute to a specific symptom or symptom cluster, and what drug therapy might overcome this dysfunction.

List of abbreviations

ASD autism spectrum disorder

CDKL5 cyclin-dependent kinase like 5

CSF cerebrospinal fluid

ID Intellectual disability

MAP-2 Microtubule-associated protein-2

MBD methyl binding domain

MeCP2 methyl-CpG-binding protein 2

Human gene: MECP2

Human protein: MeCP2

Mouse gene: Mecp2

Mouse protein: Mecp2

RTT Rett syndrome

TRD Transitional Repressor Domain

XCI X chromosome inactivation

Author details

Christopher A. Chapleau[1], Jane Lane[2], Lucas Pozzo-Miller[1] and Alan K. Percy[2]

*Address all correspondence to: apercy@uab.edu

1 Department of Neurobiology, Civitan International Research Center, The University of Alabama at Birmingham, USA

2 Department of Pediatrics, Civitan International Research Center, UAB Rett Syndrome Clinic, The University of Alabama at Birmingham, USA

References

[1] Akbarian, S., Chen, R. Z., et al. (2001). Expression pattern of the Rett syndrome gene MeCP2 in primate prefrontal cortex. *Neurobiology of disease*, 8(5), 784-791.

[2] Amaral, M. D., Chapleau, C. A., et al. (2007). Transient receptor potential channels as novel effectors of brain-derived neurotrophic factor signaling: potential implications for Rett syndrome. *Pharmacology & therapeutics*, 113(2), 394-409.

[3] Amir, R. E., Van den, I. B., Veyver, et., & al, . (2000). Influence of mutation type and X chromosome inactivation on Rett syndrome phenotypes. *Annals of neurology*, 47(5), 670-679.

[4] Amir, R. E., Van den, I. B., Veyver, et., & al, . (1999). Rett syndrome is caused by mutations in X-linked MECP2, encoding methyl-CpG-binding protein 2. *Nature genetics*, 23(2), 185-188.

[5] Archidiacono, N., Lerone, M., et al. (1991). Rett syndrome: exclusion mapping following the hypothesis of germinal mosaicism for new X-linked mutations. *Human genetics*, 86(6), 604-606.

[6] Armstrong, D., Dunn, J. K., et al. (1995). Selective dendritic alterations in the cortex of Rett syndrome. *Journal of neuropathology and experimental neurology*, 54(2), 195-201.

[7] Armstrong, D. D. (2005). Neuropathology of Rett syndrome. Journal of child neurology , 20(9), 747-753.

[8] Augenstein, K., Lane, J. B., et al. (2009). Variable phenotypic expression of a MECP2 mutation in a family. *Journal of neurodevelopmental disorders*, 313 EOF.

[9] Ballas, N., Lioy, D. T., et al. (2009). Non-cell autonomous influence of MeCP2-deficient glia on neuronal dendritic morphology. *Nature neuroscience*, 12(3), 311-317.

[10] Bauman, M. L., Kemper, T. L., et al. (1995). Microscopic observations of the brain in Rett syndrome. *Neuropediatrics*, 26(2), 105-108.

[11] Belichenko, P. V., Hagberg, B., et al. (1997). Morphological study of neocortical areas in Rett syndrome. *Acta neuropathologica*, 93(1), 50-61.

[12] Belichenko, P. V., Oldfors, A., et al. (1994). Rett syndrome: 3-D confocal microscopy of cortical pyramidal dendrites and afferents. *Neuroreport*, 5(12), 1509-1513.

[13] Blue, M. E., Naidu, S., et al. (1999). Development of amino acid receptors in frontal cortex from girls with Rett syndrome. *Annals of neurology*, 45(4), 541-545.

[14] Brendel, C., Belakhov, V., et al. (2011). Readthrough of nonsense mutations in Rett syndrome: evaluation of novel aminoglycosides and generation of a new mouse model. *Journal of molecular medicine*, 89(4), 389-398.

[15] Brendel, C., Klahold, E., et al. (2009). Suppression of nonsense mutations in Rett syndrome by aminoglycoside antibiotics. *Pediatric research*, 65(5), 520-523.

[16] Budden, S. S., Myer, E. C., et al. (1990). Cerebrospinal fluid studies in the Rett syndrome: biogenic amines and beta-endorphins. *Brain & development*, 12(1), 81-84.

[17] Calfa, G., Hablitz, J. J., et al. (2011). Network hyperexcitability in hippocampal slices from Mecp2 mutant mice revealed by voltage-sensitive dye imaging. Journal of neurophysiology , 105(4), 1768-1784.

[18] Carter, J. C., Lanham, D. C., et al. (2008). Selective cerebral volume reduction in Rett syndrome: a multiple-approach MR imaging study. AJNR. American journal of neuroradiology, 29(3), 436-441.

[19] Carter, P., Downs, J., et al. (2010). Stereotypical hand movements in 144 subjects with Rett syndrome from the population-based Australian database. Movement disorder-sofficial journal of the Movement Disorder Society , 25(3), 282-288.

[20] Chahrour, M., Jung, S. Y., et al. (2008). MeCP2, a key contributor to neurological disease, activates and represses transcription." Science , 320(5880), 1224-1229.

[21] Chang, Q., Khare, G., et al. (2006). The disease progression of Mecp2 mutant mice is affected by the level of BDNF expression. *Neuron*, 49(3), 341-348.

[22] Chao, H. T., Chen, H., et al. (2010). Dysfunction in GABA signalling mediates autism-like stereotypies and Rett syndrome phenotypes. *Nature*, 468(7321), 263-269.

[23] Chao, H. T., Zoghbi, H. Y., et al. (2007). MeCP2 controls excitatory synaptic strength by regulating glutamatergic synapse number. *Neuron*, 56(1), 58-65.

[24] Chapleau, C. A., Calfa, G. D., et al. (2009). Dendritic spine pathologies in hippocampal pyramidal neurons from Rett syndrome brain and after expression of Rett-associated MECP2 mutations. *Neurobiology of disease*, 35(2), 219-233.

[25] Cohen, S., Gabel, H. W., et al. (2011). Genome-Wide Activity-Dependent MeCP2 Phosphorylation Regulates Nervous System Development and Function. *Neuron*, 72(1), 72-85.

[26] D'Ercole, A. J., Ye, P., et al. (1996). The role of the insulin-like growth factors in the central nervous system." Molecular neurobiology , 13(3), 227-255.

[27] D'Ercole, A. J., Ye, P., et al. (2002). Mutant mouse models of insulin-like growth factor actions in the central nervous system." Neuropeptides 36(2-3): 209-220.

[28] Deng, V., Matagne, V., et al. (2007). FXYD1 is an MeCP2 target gene overexpressed in the brains of Rett syndrome patients and Mecp2-null mice." Human molecular genetics , 16(6), 640-650.

[29] Ellison, K. A., Fill, C. P., et al. (1992). Examination of X chromosome markers in Rett syndrome: exclusion mapping with a novel variation on multilocus linkage analysis." American journal of human genetics , 50(2), 278-287.

[30] Fiala, J. C., Spacek, J., et al. (2002). Dendritic spine pathology: cause or consequence of neurological disorders?" Brain research. Brain research reviews , 39(1), 29-54.

[31] Fintini, D., Brufani, C., et al. (2009). Profile of mecasermin for the long-term treatment of growth failure in children and adolescents with severe primary IGF-1 deficiency." Therapeutics and clinical risk management , 5(3), 553-559.

[32] Glaze, D. G., Percy, A. K., et al. (2009). A study of the treatment of Rett syndrome with folate and betaine." Journal of child neurology , 24(5), 551-556.

[33] Glaze, D. G., Percy, A. K., et al. (2010). Epilepsy and the natural history of Rett syndrome." Neurology , 74(11), 909-912.

[34] Goffin, D., Allen, M., et al. (2011). Rett syndrome mutation MeCP2 T158A disrupts DNA binding, protein stability and ERP responses." Nature neuroscience.

[35] Guy, J., Cheval, H., et al. (2011). The role of MeCP2 in the brain." Annual review of cell and developmental biology , 27, 631-652.

[36] Guy, J., Gan, J., et al. (2007). Reversal of neurological defects in a mouse model of Rett syndrome." Science , 315(5815), 1143-1147.

[37] Haas, R. H., Dixon, S. D., et al. (1997). Osteopenia in Rett syndrome." The Journal of pediatrics , 131(5), 771-774.

[38] Hagberg, B., Aicardi, J., et al. (1983). A progressive syndrome of autism, dementia, ataxia, and loss of purposeful hand use in girls: Rett's syndrome: report of 35 cases." Annals of neurology , 14(4), 471-479.

[39] Hagberg, B. A., & Skjeldal, O. H. (1994). Rett variants: a suggested model for inclusion criteria." Pediatric neurology , 11(1), 5-11.

[40] Hagberg, G., Stenbom, Y., et al. (2001). Head growth in Rett syndrome." Brain & development 23 Suppl 1: S, 227-229.

[41] Huttenlocher, P. R. (1970). Dendritic development and mental defect." Neurology 20(4): 381.

[42] Huttenlocher, P. R. (1974). Dendritic development in neocortex of children with mental defect and infantile spasms." Neurology , 24(3), 203-210.

[43] Jellinger, K., Armstrong, D., et al. (1988). Neuropathology of Rett syndrome." Acta neuropathologica , 76(2), 142-158.

[44] Johnson, R. A., Lam, M., et al. (2011). dihydroxyflavone (7,8-DHF) exhibits therapeutic efficacy in a mouse model of Rett syndrome." Journal of applied physiology., 7, 8.

[45] Jung, B. P., Jugloff, D. G., et al. (2003). The expression of methyl CpG binding factor MeCP2 correlates with cellular differentiation in the developing rat brain and in cultured cells." Journal of neurobiology , 55(1), 86-96.

[46] Kaufmann, W. E., & Moser, H. W. (2000). Dendritic anomalies in disorders associated with mental retardation." Cerebral cortex , 10(10), 981-991.

[47] Kaufmann, W. E., Naidu, S., et al. (1995). Abnormal expression of microtubule-associated protein 2 (MAP-2) in neocortex in Rett syndrome." Neuropediatrics , 26(2), 109-113.

[48] Kaufmann, W. E., Taylor, C. V., et al. (1997). Abnormalities in neuronal maturation in Rett syndrome neocortex: preliminary molecular correlates." European child & adolescent psychiatry 6 Suppl , 1, 75-77.

[49] Kingwell, K. (2010). Neurodegenerative disease: BDNF copycats." Nature reviews. Drug discovery 9(6): 433.

[50] Kirby, R. S., Lane, J. B., et al. (2010). Longevity in Rett syndrome: analysis of the North American Database." The Journal of pediatrics e131., 156(1), 135-138.

[51] Klose, R. J., & Bird, A. P. (2006). Genomic DNA methylation: the mark and its mediators." Trends in biochemical sciences , 31(2), 89-97.

[52] Landi, S., Putignano, E., et al. (2011). The short-time structural plasticity of dendritic spines is altered in a model of Rett syndrome." Scientific Reports 1.

[53] Larimore, J. L., Chapleau, C. A., et al. (2009). Bdnf overexpression in hippocampal neurons prevents dendritic atrophy caused by Rett-associated MECP2 mutations." Neurobiology of disease , 34(2), 199-211.

[54] Maezawa, I., & Jin, L. W. (2010). Rett syndrome microglia damage dendrites and synapses by the elevated release of glutamate." The Journal of neuroscience : the official journal of the Society for Neuroscience , 30(15), 5346-5356.

[55] Maezawa, I., Swanberg, S., et al. (2009). Rett syndrome astrocytes are abnormal and spread MeCP2 deficiency through gap junctions." The Journal of neuroscience : the official journal of the Society for Neuroscience , 29(16), 5051-5061.

[56] Marchetto, M. C., Carromeu, C., et al. (2010). A model for neural development and treatment of Rett syndrome using human induced pluripotent stem cells." Cell , 143(4), 527-539.

[57] Marin-Padilla, M. (1972). Structural abnormalities of the cerebral cortex in human chromosomal aberrations: a Golgi study." Brain research , 44(2), 625-629.

[58] Mc Cauley, M. D., Wang, T., et al. (2011). Pathogenesis of lethal cardiac arrhythmias in Mecp2 mutant mice: implication for therapy in Rett syndrome." Science translational medicine 3(113): 113ra125.

[59] Motil, K. J., Schultz, R. J., et al. (1999). Oropharyngeal dysfunction and gastroesophageal dysmotility are present in girls and women with Rett syndrome." Journal of pediatric gastroenterology and nutrition , 29(1), 31-37.

[60] Mount, R. H., Charman, T., et al. (2002). The Rett Syndrome Behaviour Questionnaire (RSBQ): refining the behavioural phenotype of Rett syndrome." Journal of child psychology and psychiatry, and allied disciplines , 43(8), 1099-1110.

[61] Mullaney, B. C., Johnston, M. V., et al. (2004). Developmental expression of methyl-CpG binding protein 2 is dynamically regulated in the rodent brain." Neuroscience , 123(4), 939-949.

[62] Neul, J. L., Fang, P., et al. (2008). Specific mutations in methyl-CpG-binding protein 2 confer different severity in Rett syndrome." Neurology , 70(16), 1313-1321.

[63] Neul, J. L., Kaufmann, W. E., et al. (2010). Rett syndrome: revised diagnostic criteria and nomenclature." Annals of neurology , 68(6), 944-950.

[64] Nguyen, M. V., Du, F., et al. (2012). MeCP2 Is Critical for Maintaining Mature Neuronal Networks and Global Brain Anatomy during Late Stages of Postnatal Brain De-

velopment and in the Mature Adult Brain." The Journal of neuroscience : the official journal of the Society for Neuroscience , 32(29), 10021-10034.

[65] Percy, A. K. (2002). Rett syndrome. Current status and new vistas." Neurologic clinics , 20(4), 1125-1141.

[66] Percy, A. K. (2011). Rett syndrome: exploring the autism link." Archives of neurology , 68(8), 985-989.

[67] Percy, A. K., Glaze, D. G., et al. (1994). Rett syndrome: controlled study of an oral opiate antagonist, naltrexone." Annals of neurology , 35(4), 464-470.

[68] Percy, A. K., & Lane, J. B. (2005). Rett syndrome: model of neurodevelopmental disorders." Journal of child neurology , 20(9), 718-721.

[69] Percy, A. K., Lane, J. B., et al. (2007). Rett syndrome: North American database." Journal of child neurology , 22(12), 1338-1341.

[70] Percy, A. K., Neul, J. L., et al. (2010). Rett syndrome diagnostic criteria: lessons from the Natural History Study." Annals of neurology , 68(6), 951-955.

[71] Popescu, A. C., Sidorova, E., et al. (2010). Aminoglycoside-mediated partial suppression of MECP2 nonsense mutations responsible for Rett syndrome in vitro." Journal of neuroscience research , 88(11), 2316-2324.

[72] Purpura, D. P. (1974). Dendritic spine "dysgenesis" and mental retardation." Science , 186(4169), 1126-1128.

[73] Qiu, Z., Sylwestrak, E. L., et al. (2012). The Rett syndrome protein MeCP2 regulates synaptic scaling." The Journal of neuroscience : the official journal of the Society for Neuroscience , 32(3), 989-994.

[74] Reiss, A. L., Faruque, F., et al. (1993). Neuroanatomy of Rett syndrome: a volumetric imaging study." Annals of neurology , 34(2), 227-234.

[75] Rett, A. (1966). On a unusual brain atrophy syndrome in hyperammonemia in childhood]." Wiener medizinische Wochenschrift , 116(37), 723-726.

[76] Robertson, L., Hall, S. E., et al. (2006). The association between behavior and genotype in Rett syndrome using the Australian Rett Syndrome Database." American journal of medical genetics. Part B, Neuropsychiatric genetics : the official publication of the International Society of Psychiatric Genetics 141B(2): 177-183.

[77] Roende, G., Ravn, K., et al. (2011). DXA measurements in Rett syndrome reveal small bones with low bone mass." Journal of bone and mineral research : the official journal of the American Society for Bone and Mineral Research , 26(9), 2280-2286.

[78] Rowe, S. M., & Clancy, J. P. (2009). Pharmaceuticals targeting nonsense mutations in genetic diseases: progress in development." BioDrugs : clinical immunotherapeutics, biopharmaceuticals and gene therapy , 23(3), 165-174.

[79] Samaco, R. C., Mandel-Brehm, C., et al. (2009). Loss of MeCP2 in aminergic neurons causes cell-autonomous defects in neurotransmitter synthesis and specific behavioral abnormalities." Proceedings of the National Academy of Sciences of the United States of America , 106(51), 21966-21971.

[80] Schanen, C., Houwink, E. J., et al. (2004). Phenotypic manifestations of MECP2 mutations in classical and atypical Rett syndrome." American journal of medical genetics. Part A 126A(2): 129-140.

[81] Schmid, D. A., Yang, T., et al. (2012). A TrkB Small Molecule Partial Agonist Rescues TrkB Phosphorylation Deficits and Improves Respiratory Function in a Mouse Model of Rett Syndrome." The Journal of neuroscience : the official journal of the Society for Neuroscience , 32(5), 1803-1810.

[82] Schultz, R. J., Glaze, D. G., et al. (1993). The pattern of growth failure in Rett syndrome." American journal of diseases of children , 147(6), 633-637.

[83] Sekul, E. A., Moak, J. P., et al. (1994). Electrocardiographic findings in Rett syndrome: an explanation for sudden death?" The Journal of pediatrics , 125(1), 80-82.

[84] Sirianni, N., Naidu, S., et al. (1998). Rett syndrome: confirmation of X-linked dominant inheritance, and localization of the gene to Xq28." American journal of human genetics , 63(5), 1552-1558.

[85] Skene, P. J., Illingworth, R. S., et al. (2010). Neuronal MeCP2 is expressed at near histone-octamer levels and globally alters the chromatin state." Molecular cell , 37(4), 457-468.

[86] Trappe, R., Laccone, F., et al. (2001). MECP2 mutations in sporadic cases of Rett syndrome are almost exclusively of paternal origin." American journal of human genetics , 68(5), 1093-1101.

[87] Tropea, D., Giacometti, E., et al. (2009). Partial reversal of Rett Syndrome-like symptoms in MeCP2 mutant mice." Proceedings of the National Academy of Sciences of the United States of America , 106(6), 2029-2034.

[88] Williamson, S. L., & Christodoulou, J. (2006). Rett syndrome: new clinical and molecular insights." European journal of human genetics : EJHG , 14(8), 896-903.

[89] Young, J. I., Hong, E. P., et al. (2005). Regulation of RNA splicing by the methylation-dependent transcriptional repressor methyl-CpG binding protein 2." Proceedings of the National Academy of Sciences of the United States of America , 102(49), 17551-17558.

[90] Zingman, L. V., Park, S., et al. (2007). Aminoglycoside-induced translational read-through in disease: overcoming nonsense mutations by pharmacogenetic therapy." Clinical pharmacology and therapeutics , 81(1), 99-103.

Chapter 10

Genetic Diseases Associated with Protein Glycosylation Disorders in Mammals

Yoshiaki Nakayama, Naosuke Nakamura,
Daisuke Tsuji, Koji Itoh and Akira Kurosaka

Additional information is available at the end of the chapter

1. Introduction

Protein glycosylation is an important posttranslational modification that confers both structural and functional properties to the molecules [1]. There are several types of glycosylation with various carbohydrate structures, and biosynthesis of each sugar chain, in general, is an elaborate process of addition and processing of carbohydrates in the endoplasmic reticulum (ER) and Golgi, where a number of glycosyltransferases and glycosidases are involved in these reactions. Glycoprotein degradation, on the other hand, requires many hydrolases to act on carbohydrates and involves intracellular transport of both glycosidases and their substrate glycoproteins. Collectively, enzymes that modulate glycoprotein carbohydrates during their biosynthesis and degradation are called glycoenzymes, which play critical roles in maintaining cellular structure and function. Biosynthesis of carbohydrate moieties of glycoproteins, unlike that of DNA, RNA, or proteins, is a template-independent reaction, that is, their structures are not directly encoded by genes. However, they reflect biochemical reactions catalyzed by glycoenzymes expressed in a cell. In other words, structural integrity of carbohydrates is indirectly determined by a large number of genes coding for glycoenzymes. Therefore, mutations in any of these enzymes that affect the structures and functions of glycoproteins will cause deleterious effects on cellular activities.

Glycosylation is categorized into 2 major classes on the basis of the linkage structure between a polypeptide and a carbohydrate chain, i.e., N-linked and O-linked oligosaccharides (Fig. 1). N-Linked glycans, the most extensively studied class, are the ones attached to an asparagine (Asn) residue in the Asn-X-Ser/Thr triplet sequence (X, any amino acid except proline; Ser, serine; Thr, threonine) in a polypeptide chain. Glycans that are attached to a hydroxylamino acid residue are called O-linked oligosaccharides and can be categorized into several subclasses, according to the types of monosaccharides directly attached to the amino acid (Fig. 1). Among them, *O*-GalNAc and *O*-Xyl are the most frequently observed modifications in mucins and proteoglycans, respectively; therefore, the former oligosaccharides are also called mucin-type glycans. In addition, novel types of O-glycosylation, including *O*-Fuc and *O*-Man, were recently identified and suggested to be involved in the regulation of essential proteins, such as notch, dystroglycan, etc. [2,3]. Since these carbohydrate chains have characteristic structures and play critical roles in cellular functions, their alterations have been found to be associated with a number of inherited diseases.

In this article, diseases that are associated with altered protein glycosylation are described. Moreover, to achieve the normal cellular function, glycoenzymes involved in glycosylation processes such as synthesis, processing, and degradation must be under the proper control. Important roles of some of these enzymes are also discussed, with a focus especially on those modulating *N*-Asn-, *O*-Man-, and *O*-GalNAc-type oligosaccharides.

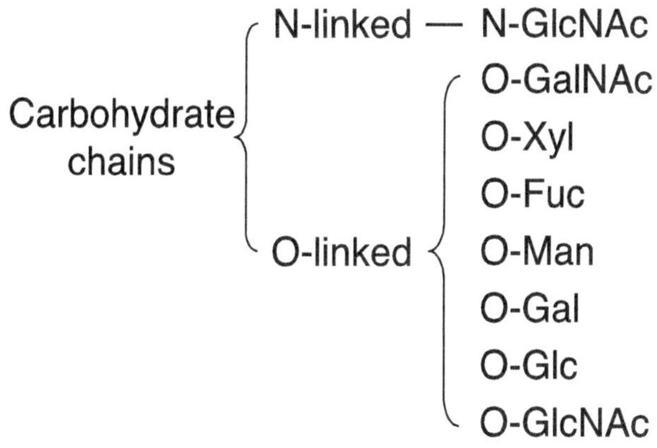

Figure 1. Classification of glycoprotein carbohydrate chains.

2. N-glycan biosynthesis

2.1. Glycoenzymes involved in N-glycan biosynthesis

N-Glycans are characterized by a linkage structure of GlcNAcβ1Asn. Its biosynthesis is distinct from that of other glycans in that a precursor oligosaccharide preassembled on a lipid dolichol (Dol) is *en block* transferred to a polypeptide chain that is being translated in the ER (Fig. 2). Consecutive addition of sugars onto dolichyl-phosphate gives rise to the final precursor product, $Glc_3Man_9GlcNAc_2$-P-P-Dol. The completed glycan is then transferred to a nascent polypeptide with an essential Asn-X-Ser/Thr sequence in the ER lumen, which is catalyzed by an oligosaccharyltransferase. Following transfer to polypeptides, N-glycans are usually processed during intracellular transport of glycoprotein (Fig. 2). In the ER, glucosidases I and II remove the outermost α1,2-linked and 2 inner α1,3-linked glucose residues. The outermost α1,2-linked mannose is then released by ER α-mannosidase to generate $Man_8GlcNAc_2$-Asn. After transit to cis-Golgi, mannosidases remove 3 mannose residues, thereby producing $Man_5GlcNAc_2$-Asn, a substrate for GlcNAc-transferase I that adds a GlcNAc residue to the α1,3-linked Man. Subsequent removal of 2 mannose residues on the α1,6-linked Man occurs, and the second GlcNAc is added on the non-reducing mannose residues. Final addition of galactose and sialic acid residues completes biantennary complex-type N-glycans. It should be noted that additional GlcNAc-transferases can make 5 or more branched complex-type sugar chains. The branched structures in most cases are modified by consecutive addition of galactose and sialic acid residues, such that a variety of N-glycans can be generated by a series of actions of glycosidases and glycosyltransferases. Therefore, mutations of these enzymes would potentially result in production and accumulation of unusual oligosaccharides in the cell.

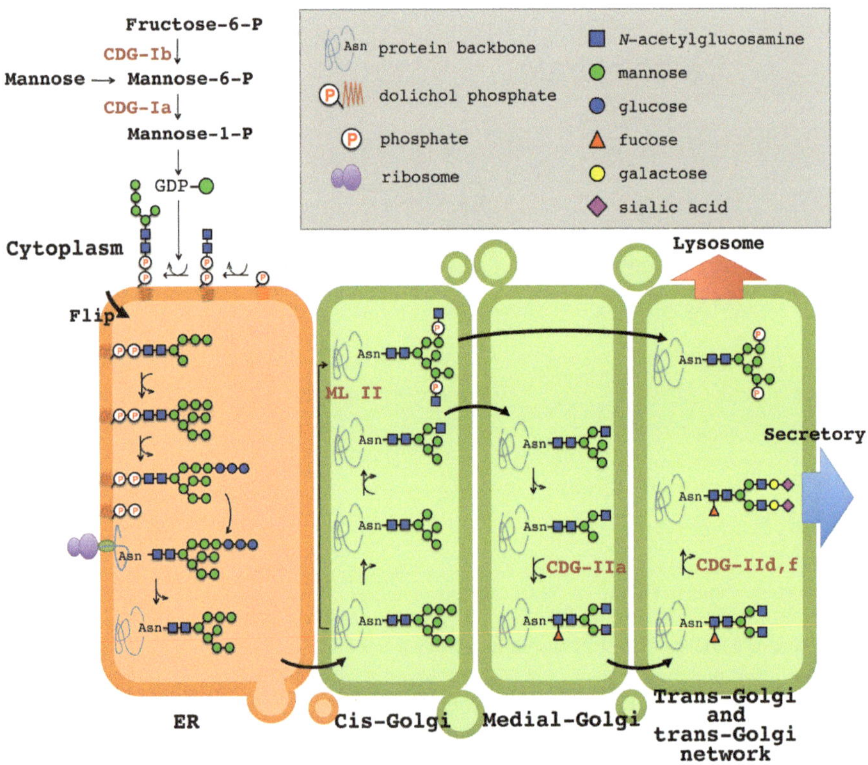

Figure 2. Biosynthesis and processing of N-linked oligosaccharides.

2.2. Disorders in N-glycan biosynthesis: CDG-I and CDG-II

Congenital disorders of glycosylation (CDG), previously known as carbohydrate-deficient glycoprotein syndrome, are a subset of genetic diseases characterized by abnormalities in glycosylation. N-Glycans are physiologically and developmentally important in various tissues, and therefore the complete absence of these oligosaccharides is lethal. Almost all CDGs are autosomal recessive; patients carrying hypomorphic mutant alleles exhibit multiple organ failure, such as neurodevelopmental disorders, hepatopathy, and immunological diseases. Since the biosynthesis of N-glycans consists of 2 distinct processes (i.e., the assembly of precursor oligosaccharides on dolichol and the processing of oligosaccharides after transfer to acceptor proteins), CDGs can be categorized into 2 general types. One type is caused by insufficient assembly of the lipid-linked precursor oligosaccharides in the ER, which is characterized by decreases in the number of N-glycans with normal structures. The other type involves defects in the processing of oligosaccharides that are transferred to proteins, thereby resulting in the production of short and simple sugar chains without affecting the number of glycans. The former type, designated as CDG-I, constitutes defects in the synthesis of dolichol lipid-linked oligosaccharide (LLO) chain as well as its transfer to proteins in the ER. The first report on CDG was made in 1980 [4], and 15 years later, it was proposed that the disease, CDG-Ia, is caused by the deficiency of an enzyme, phosphomannomutase [5]. This enzyme catalyzes the interconversion of mannose 6-phosphate and mannose 1-phosphate (Fig. 2), and its deficiency leads to a shortage of substrates (GDP-Man and Dol-P-Man) that are required for the synthesis of dolichol-oligosaccharides. CDG-Ia is the most common CDG, and its frequency has been estimated as 1 in 20,000 live births. A less common type of CDG, CDG-1b, possesses deficiency in phosphomannose isomerase (Fig. 2) [6,7]. Without this enzyme, the cells fail to convert fructose 6-phosphate to mannose 6-phosphate and, similarly to CDG-Ia, cannot generate LLOs efficiently. Interestingly, it was found that treating patients with CDG-Ib, but not CDG-Ia, with high-mannose diet alleviates the clinical manifestation, since mannose 6-phospahte can be produced by hexokinase from mannose ingested from food [7]. To date, there are several different types of CDG-I, all of which are due to genetic defects in enzymes involved in the generation of LLOs. CDG-II, on the other hand, involves malfunctions in the trimming or processing of the protein-bound chains in the ER and Golgi. For example, CDG-IIa is caused by mutations in *N*-acetylglucosaminyltransferase II (GlcNAc-TII), which adds the second GlcNAc residue to biantennary complex glycans (Fig. 2) [8]. β1,4-Galactosyltransferase, the enzyme that adds galactose after GlcNAc-TII, is mutated in CDG-IId (Fig. 2) [9]. Failure in sialylation of biantennary complex chains (Fig. 2), which results from a defect in the CMP-Sia transporter, is observed in CDG-IIf [10]. CDG-IIa, -IId, and -IIf cannot produce complex-type carbohydrates and exhibit severe phenotypes, such as mental retardation, hypotonia, and neutropenia. In addition to these examples, CDG-II patients also have diverse disorders that result from mutations in other glycosyltransferases and nucleotide sugar transporters. Moreover, there are other types of N-glycosylation disorders, including mucolipidosis II (MLII), alternatively called as I-Cell disease, caused by the lack of mannose 6-phosphate, which serve as a molecular tag to direct transport to lysosomes (Fig. 2) [11].

3. O-glycan biosynthesis

As shown in Fig. 1, there are several subclasses of O-glycosylation, and each subclass has its own biosynthetic process with specific glycosyltransferases. Disorders associated with altered *O*-Man and *O*-GalNAc glycans are described below.

3.1. Deficiency in O-mannosylation: congenital muscular dystrophies and dystroglycopathies

O-Mannosylation is related to congenital muscular dystrophies with neuronal abnormalities, such as lissencephaly and mental retardation. Muscular dystrophies are genetic diseases with degeneration and disruption of muscle fibers, resulting in the progressive wasting of skeletal muscles and atrophy. The dystrophin-glycoprotein complex (DGC) (Fig. 3) plays a critical role in maintaining muscle integrity [12,13]. It contains αDG, βDG, dystrophin, and other components, and αDG and βDG are produced from a single polypeptide called dystrophin-associated glycoprotein or dystroglycan [14] after its proteolytic cleavage. Mutations in the DGC components lead to unstable complex formation, which can be a potential cause of the diseases. In fact, dystrophin has been known to be a causative gene of Duchunne-type muscular dystrophy [15,16]. Moreover, among the DGC components, αDG is a peripheral membrane protein with a mucin-like domain, which is heavily modified with O-mannosylglycans. These sugar chains can bind to extracellular matrix proteins, such as laminin, agrin, and perlecan, through their laminin G domains [17]. The reduced αDG glycosylation was observed in a mouse model of muscular dystrophies, myd, indicating that its hypoglycosylation might be a causal factor for the disorders [18,19]. Several studies demonstrated that αDG also contains mucin-type carbohydrates, suggesting that mucin-type O-glycosylation may be involved in the proper glycosylation of αDG [20]. As described below, other mutations also cause αDG hypoglycosylation with a very wide spectrum of phenotypes [21], and all the diseases caused by the altered αDG glycosylation have been collectively designated as dystroglycanopathies [22].

O-Mannosylation, a recently appreciated glycosylation, is predominantly observed on αDG. Representative structures of O-mannosylglycans are described in the Fig. 3. The addition of a mannose residue to Ser/Thr in the α-configuration is catalyzed by an enzyme complex composed of protein *O*-mannosyltransferases, POMT1 and POMT2, in the ER [23]. GlcNAc is then transferred by a protein *O*-mannose β1,2-*N*-acetylglucosaminyltransferase, POMGnT1, in the Golgi [24]. Mutations in these enzymes result in muscular dystrophies known as Walker–Warburg syndrome (WWS) and Muscle–Eye–Brain disease [24,25]. Moreover, the disaccharide, GlcNAcβ1,2Manα1Ser/Thr, can be extended into a tetrasaccharide Siaα2,3Galβ1,4GlcNAcβ1,2Manα1Ser/Thr [26]. Occurrence of sugar chains linked to the reducing mannose residue through a phosphodiester linkage has been reported [27]. Besides POMT1, POMT2, and POMGnT1, the enzymes responsible for formation of these carbohydrates have yet to be identified. While mutations in a few genes, such as fukutin, fukutin-related protein (FKRP), and LARGE, have been suggested to cause muscular dystrophies with the αDG hypoglycosylation, their functions are still unclear, even though they possess features characteristic of glycosyltransferases [27-30]. Very recently, LARGE has been identified as a bifunctional glycosyltransferase, with both xylosyltransferase and glucuronyltransferase activities to produce repeating units of [-Xylα1,3GlcAβ1,3-], which may be added to the phosphodiester linkages (Fig. 3)[31]. Fukutin has also been reported to be related to the extended structure of αDG, which is essential for the αDG binding to its ligand laminin; however, its catalytic properties are unclear. Interestingly, while other proteins such as CD24, IgG2 light chain, tenascin R, receptor-type protein-tyrosine phosphatase, and neurofascin [32-36] are also modified with *O*-mannosylglycans, αDG is most likely to be the only molecule that is responsible for dystroglycanopathies [37].

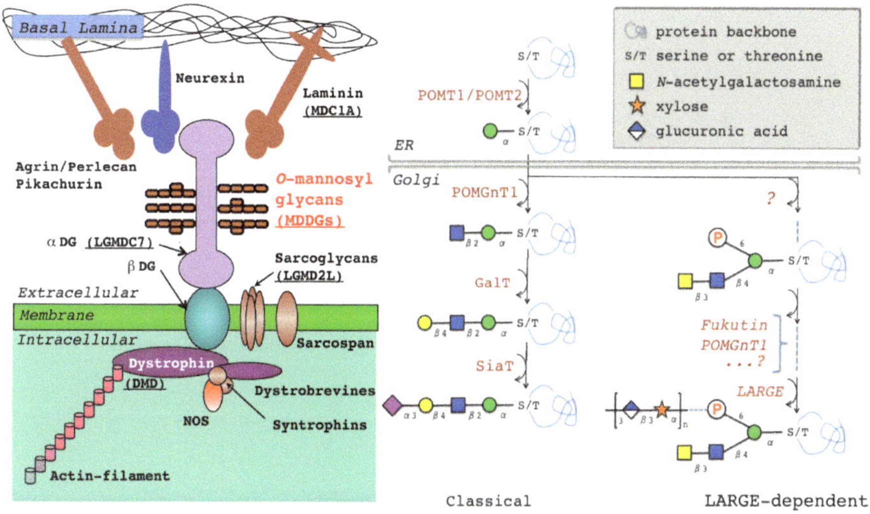

Figure 3. Dystrophin glycoprotein complex (DGC) and representative structure of O-mannosyl glycans of αDG. DGC components and disorders associated with their mutations are illustrated. MDC1A, Muscular dystrophy, congenital merosin-deficient 1A (OMIM; 607855); DMD, Duchenne muscular dystrophy (OMIM; 310200); LGMD2C, Muscular dystrophy, limb-girdle, type 2C (OMIM; 611307); LGMDC7, LGMD type C 7 (OMIM; 613818); MDDGs, Musclar dystrophy-dystroglycanopathies (see ref. [22]); NOS, nitric oxide synthase.

It is important to note that only half of congenital muscular dystrophy can be explained by gene mutations described above, suggesting that other alleles also exert effects on the phenotypes [21,22,38]. The Dol-P-mannose synthase subunit DPM3 is one candidate gene; its mutation was found in muscular dystrophy patients whose αDG glycosylation was impaired [39]. Recently, mutations in the *ISPD* gene, which encodes isoprenoid synthase domain containing, were also observed in WWS patients and are considered the second most common cause of this disorder [40,41]. While the *ISPD* function in mammals is unknown, it is involved in αDG glycosylation in zebrafish. Furthermore, a recent study suggested that glycosyltransferase-like domain containing 2, *GTDC2* or also known as *AGO61,* is a novel causative gene of WWS, based on the data from whole-exome sequencing [42], even though DG hypoglycosylation was not confirmed in patients.

3.2. Deficiency in mucin-type O-glycosylation

3.2.1. Enzymes involved in the biosynthesis of mucin-type O-glycosylation

Biosynthesis of *O*-GalNAc (mucin-type) carbohydrates begins with α-GalNAc transfer from UDP-GalNAc to a Ser/Thr residue in an acceptor polypeptide (Fig. 4). A family of UDP-GalNAc: polypeptide *N*-acetylgalactosaminyltransferases (GalNAc-Ts) catalyzes this reaction predominantly in the Golgi, in contrast to the initiation of other glycosylation occurring in the ER. GalNAc-Ts, the largest family members among glycosyltransferases with 20 isozymes in mammals, are cis-Golgi resident enzymes, with some of which are translocated into the ER upon signal transduction by EGF [43]. The reaction product, GalNAcα1Ser/Thr, is called the Tn-antigen and regarded as a cancer-associated carbohydrate antigen because of its accumulation in cancer cells. Moreover, distinctive core structures (cores 1, 3, 5, 6, 7, and 8) are synthesized depending on glycosyltransferases that act on the Tn-antigen, which also appears to be tissue-specific (Fig.4). Among these core structures, core 1 (Galβ1,3GalNAcα1Ser/Thr), also called the T-antigen, is the most common structure and is generated by T-synthase (C1GalT-1). This enzyme is ubiquitously expressed; however, for the proper folding and export from the ER to Golgi, it requires a specific molecular chaperone, Cosmc. Therefore, defects in either T-synthase or Cosmc would result in deficient synthesis of T-antigens. Furthermore, addition of β1,6-linked GlcNAc to cores 1 and 3 converts them into cores 2 and 4, respectively. Some of these core structures can also be extended into complex O-glycans following modifications with galactose, *N*-acetylglucosamine, fucose, and sialic acid.

3.2.2. Involvement of GalNAc-T family in genetic disorders

3.2.2.1. GalNAc-T3 as a modulator of FGF23 levels

Familial tumoral calcinosis (FTC) is a rare, autosomal recessive metabolic disorder that manifests with hyperphosphatemia and massive calcium deposits in periarticular spaces, soft tissues, and sometimes in bone. The gene underlying FTC was mapped to 2q24-q31 [44] which includes the *GALNT3* gene encoding GalNAc-T3. GalNAc-T3 protects a phosphaturic factor, FGF23, from proteolysis [45], and FGF23 inhibits the reabsorption of phosphates in proximal renal tubule. Gain-of-function mutations in the *FGF23* gene were shown to result in autosomal dominant hypophosphatemic rickets [46,47]. FGF23 secretion also requires addition of GalNAc at Thr173 in a recognition sequence motif of subtilisin-like proprotein convertases, which in turn blocks FGF23 proteolysis before its secretion. Therefore, mutations in GALNT3 would result in the cleavage of intact FGF23 and lead to FTC due to accumulation of fragmented, inactive FGF23 as well as upregulation of phosphate reabsorption.

3.2.2.2. GalNAc-T2 as a regulator of plasma lipid levels

Extensive genomic analyses recently revealed that 1q42 is associated with plasma lipid concentrations [48,49], and the *GALNT2* gene located in 1q42 was later found primarily associated

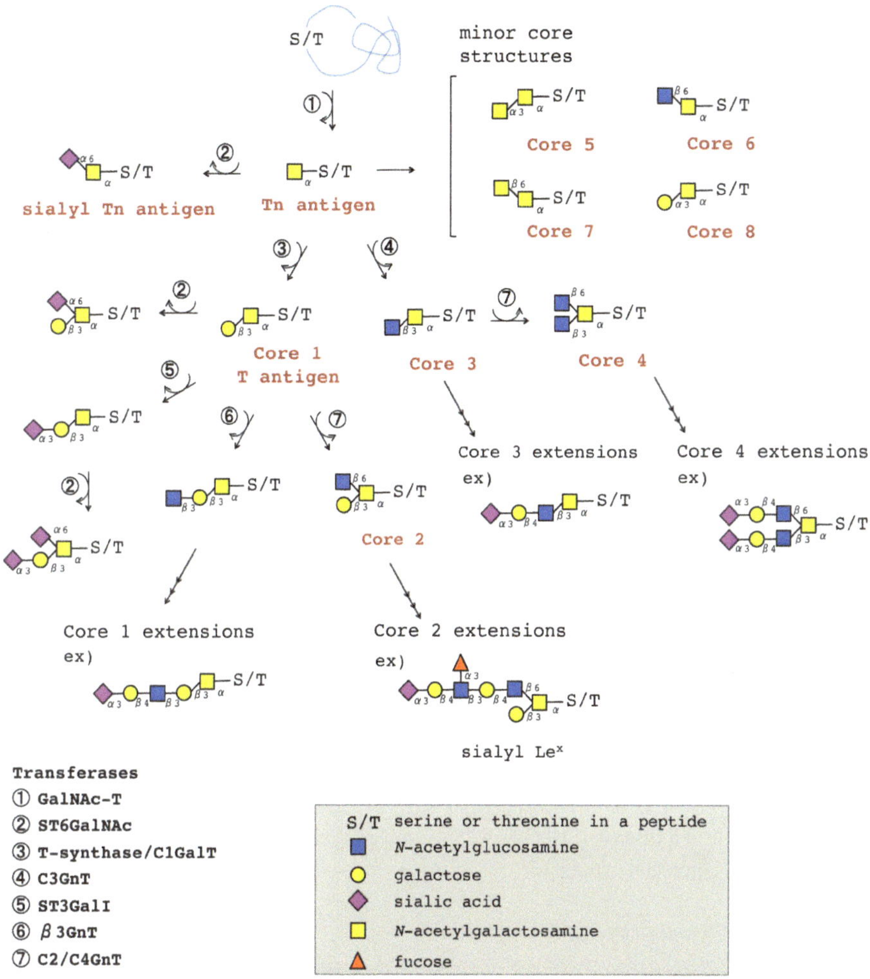

Figure 4. Biosynthetic pathway of mucin-type O-glycosylation.

with the levels of plasma high-density lipoprotein cholesterol (HDL-C). In addition, *Galnt2* overexpression in mouse liver has been shown to downregulate plasma HDL-C, and knock-down of endogenous liver *Galnt2* resulted in the opposite [50]. Moreover, apolipoprotein (apo) C-III, identified as a candidate target protein of GalNAc-T2, inhibits lipoprotein lipase (LPL), a hydrolase that degrades plasma triglycerides [51]. An apoC-III-based peptide is a substrate for GalNAc-T2 while its glycosylation by the enzyme from patient is not observed. Furthermore, neuraminidase treatment of apoC-III decreases its potential to inhibit LPL. These data suggest that GalNAc-T2 is involved in lipid metabolism via apoC-III O-glycosylation.

3.2.2.3. GalNAc-T17 as a candidate gene for Williams–Beuren syndrome and dog domestication

Williams-Beuren syndrome (WBS) is a neurodevelopmental disorder associated with physical, behavioral, and cognitive abnormalities [52] and is caused by haploinsufficiency of multiple genes at 7q11.23. GalNAc-T17, also known as WBS chromosome region 17/WBSCR17 [52], was identified in the flanking region (7q11.22) of the chromosomal deletion in WBS patients' genome. Interestingly, WBSCR17 mRNA is predominantly expressed in the nervous system [53]; therefore, haploinsufficiency of GalNAc-T17 can be expected to be related to characteristic traits of WBS patients, such as hypersociality and impairment in visuospatial processing. In addition, a recent study on the process of dog domestication reported a single SNP located near WBSCR17 in the dog genome and has implicated WBSCR17 in the early domestication of dogs [54]. It is also noted that GalNAc-T17 is a very inert isozyme, in terms of catalytic activity. GalNAc-T17, together with GalNAc-T8, -T9, and -T18, belongs to the Y subfamily, a group defined by Li *et al.* [55]. These Y isozymes contain several conservative substitutions in the catalytic domain and therefore exhibit no or extremely low catalytic activity when tested under the standard assay conditions by using synthetic mucin peptides. GalNAc-T17 in zebrafish, on the other hand, seems to be physiologically important, because its knockdown resulted in embryos that exhibited malformed brain with severe alterations in the hindbrain (ref). GalNAc-T17 has also been shown to negatively modulate macropinocytosis and lamellipodium formation in cultured cells [56].

3.2.2.4. GalNAc-Ts in other genetic diseases

Recent genome-wide studies have successively revealed novel loci associated with numerous genetic diseases. Among them, some GALNT genes have been implicated in diverse disorders or tumor susceptibility: *GALNT1*, epithelial ovarian cancer [57]; *GALNT4*, acute coronary disease [58]; *GALNT11*, congenital heart disease [59]; *GALNT12*, colon cancer [60]; *GALNT13*, sickle cell disease [61]; *GALNT14*, death-receptor mediated cancer cell death [62]; and *GALNT15*, colorectal cancer [63].

3.2.3. Tn syndrome caused by Cosmc mutations

The Tn syndrome is a rare autoimmune disease. In patients, subpopulations of all blood cell lineages carry an incompletely glycosylated membrane glycoprotein, known as the Tn antigen (GalNAcα1Ser/Thr). Since the anti-Tn antibody is present in most normal human adult sera, patients with Tn syndrome display anemia, leucopenia, and thrombocytopenia [64]. It has been suggested that the Tn syndrome is associated with somatic mutations in the *Cosmc* gene on the X chromosome. *Cosmc* encodes a molecular chaperone required for the proper folding and hence full activity of T synthase, which is responsible for adding Gal to the Tn antigen [65]. The sequence analyses of the *T synthase* and *Cosmc* genes in whole blood cells from individuals with Tn syndrome also showed that mutations were only present in the *Cosmc* gene, suggesting that these *Cosmc* mutations lead to T synthase inactivation as well as the autoimmune Tn antigen expression in blood cells of all lineages.

4. Degradation of carbohydrate units of glycoproteins

4.1. Degradation by lysosomal enzymes

Glycoconjugates, including glycoproteins, glycolipids, and proteoglycans, are biosynthesized intracellularly and incorporated extracellularly by endocytic and phagocytic mechanisms; they are transported via intracellular trafficking to lysosomes, where they are then catabolized [66]. Both N- and O-linked oligosaccharides of glycoproteins are ultimately degraded in lysosomes. Lysosomes contain more than 60 distinct acid hydrolases, so-called lysosomal enzymes, as well as their co-factors, including activators and stabilizing proteins. Most lysosomal glycosidases are classified as exo-type enzymes acting sequentially at the non-reducing termini [67] and exhibit their optimal catalytic activity under acidic pH conditions because of the function of vacuolar ATPase [68]. Some of them can also localize in non-lysosomal compartments, including early endosomes and cell membrane [69]. In addition, a group of them interact with other enzymes and activator proteins, thereby enhancing the catalytic efficiency through direct binding or presenting the substrates [70-72].

The biosynthesis of lysosomal enzymes and their co-factors is controlled by gene expression [73], posttranslational modifications, and intracellular trafficking [67,74]. Specifically, soluble matrix enzymes are N-glycosylated in the ER and phosphorylated in the Golgi apparatus at the sixth position of the terminal mannose residues (M6P), via a 2-step reaction catalyzed by Golgi-localized phosphotransferase and uncovering enzyme (*N*-acetylglucosaminidase) necessary to expose terminal M6P residues. The M6P-carrying enzymes then bind the cation-dependent mannose 6-phosphate receptor (CD-M6PR) at physiological pH in the Golgi [67,74]. The enzyme–receptor complex is subsequently transported via late endosomes (where the enzyme dissociates from the receptor at acidic pH) to lysosomes by vesicle fusion, whereas CD-M6PR, serving as a shuttle, traffics back to the Golgi apparatus. A small percentage of lysosomal enzymes are also secreted from the cell. The secreted M6P-carrying enzymes can bind to the cation-independent M6P/IGFII receptor (CI-M6PR) on the plasma membrane [67,74]. The extracellular lysosomal enzymes can then be endocytosed via glycan receptors and delivered to lysosomes, where the captured enzymes exert their normal catabolic functions. Taken together, intracellular and extracellular distributions of lysosomal enzymes are regulated by intracellular trafficking and secretion/capture system.

4.2. Lysosomal multienzyme complex for carbohydrate degradation

A group of lysosomal enzymes form a multienzyme complex to regulate their catalytic activities and turnover for efficient catabolism and stabilization. Lysosomal protective protein/cathepsin A (EC3.4.16.1; CTSA) is a multifunctional glycoprotein that exhibits not only catalytic activities but also protective functions [70,75]. CTSA is synthesized as a 452-amino-acid (54-kDa) precursor zymogen that contains intramolecular disulfide bonds and 2 N-glycans [70,75,76]. In the endosomal/lysosomal compartment, the precursor undergoes endoproteolytic processing and is converted to the enzymatically active mature form composed of 32- and 20-kDa subunits [70,75]. The mature enzyme is active at both acidic and neutral pH and functions as cathepsin A (acid carboxypeptidase)/neutral deamidase/esterase on a subset of bioactive peptides, including tachykinins and endothelin-1 [77-79], suggesting its contribution to a variety of intracellular and extracellular cell processes [80,81]. As for the protective functions of CTSA, it forms a multienzyme complex with lysosomal neuraminidase 1 (EC 3.2.1.18; NEU1) and acid β-galactosidase (EC 3.2.1.23; GLB1) to activate NEU1 and protect GLB1 from physiological proteolysis [70,75] The association of NEU1 with CTSA, which probably serves as a molecular chaperone, is particularly crucial for NEU1 neuramindase activity, since the activity is lost in the absence of CTSA, even though GLB1 retains at least 10–15% of the normal enzymatic activity levels [70,75]. The presence of combined deficiency of these enzymes and the excessive accumulation of sialyloligosaccharides derived from glycoproteins reveal the importance and contribution of the multienzyme complex to the physiological degradation of the N- and O-glycans derived from glycoproteins.

5. Disorders of glycoprotein carbohydrates and therapeutic approach

5.1. Lysosomal storage diseases (LSDs) causing metabolic errors of glycoprotein catabolism

Lysosomal storage diseases (LSDs) are inherited metabolic disorders caused by genetic defects in the lysosomal enzymes and their cofactors. LSDs result in the excessive accumulation in lysosomes of undegraded substrates, including oligosaccharides derived from glycoproteins, glycosphingolipids, and glycosaminoglycans derived from proteoglycans [66,81]. LSDs comprise more than 40 different disorders, and each incidence is about 1 per 100 thousand births, with differences among disorders and races. The clinical manifestations of LSDs are quite heterogeneous, but many of them involve neurological disorders.

LSDs that are associated with the accumulation of oligosaccharides derived from glycoproteins include α-mannosidosis [82-84], β-mannosidosis [82,83], fucosidosis [82-84], sialidosis [82,85-87], galactosialidosis [70,75], etc. (Table 1). In this chapter, we will focus on sialidosis and galactosialidosis, both of which are associated with NEU1 deficiency and characterized by the accumulation of sialylololigosaccharides and lead to heterogeneous clinical manifestations.

Diseases	Responsible enzymes	Responsible genes	References
Fucosidosis	α-Fucosidase	*FUCA1*	[82,83]
α-Mannosidosis	α-Mannosidase	*MAN2B1*	[82,83]
β-Mannosidosis	β-Mannosidase	*MANBA*	[82,83]
Sialidosis	Lysosomal sialidase (Neuraminidase 1)	*NEU1*	[82,85-87]
Galactosialidosis	Protective protein/cathepsinA*	*CTSA*	[70,75,85,88]
Aspartylglucosaminuria	Aspartylglucosaminidase	*AGA*	[66]
Schindler disease / Kanzaki disease	α-*N*-Acetylgalactosaminidase	*NAGA*	[66]

Table 1. Lysosomal storage diseases (LSDs) caused by the defect in glycoprotein catabolism. *The defect of protective protein/cathepsin A causes the combined deficiencies of lysosomal sialidase (NEU1) and acid β-galacosidase (GLB1).

5.1.1. Sialidosis (MIM 256550)

Sialidosis is an autosomal recessive, lysosomal neuraminidase 1 (*NEU1*; 6p21) deficiency [82,89]. NEU1 normally cleaves terminal $\alpha2 \rightarrow 3$ and $\alpha2 \rightarrow 6$ sialyl linkages of several oligosaccharides and glycopeptides and was found increased in tissues and fluids of affected patients. A 1.9-kb cDNA containing an open reading frame of 1,245 nucleotides in size is predicted to code for a protein that is 415 amino acids long. Distinct from other human neuraminidases (including cytoplasmic NEU2, plasma membrane NEU3, and mitochondrial/lysosomal NEU4), NEU1 needs to form a complex with CTSA and GLB1 to be catalytically active, as described above [70,75]. Type I sialidosis, the milder form, is characterized by the development of ocular cherry-red spots and generalized myoclonus in the second or third decade of life. Additional manifestations, reported in more than 50% of patients, include seizures, hyperreflexia, and ataxia [86,87]. Type II sialidosis is distinguished from the Type I milder form by the early onset of a progressive, rather severe [82,86,87] mucopolysaccharidosis-like phenotype with visceromegaly, dysostosis multiplex, and mental retardation. It has also been suggested that the residual NEU1 activities in the affected patients in relation to the kinds of identified missense mutations may be responsible for determining the clinical phenotypes (milder Type I and severe Type II) of the patients [82,86,87].

5.1.2. Galactosialidosis (MIM 256540)

Galactosialidosis is an autosomal recessive deficiency in the *lysosomal protective protein/cathepsin A* gene (*CTSA*; 20q13.2) [75,85]. This disorder is characterized by combined deficiency of its acid carboxypeptidase/neutral deamidase as well as GLB1 and NEU1, due to the defect of multienzyme complex formation. Multiple deficiencies arise because CTSA needs to physiologically associate with NEU1 and GLB1 and form a high-molecular-weight multienzyme complex to activate NEU1 and protect GLB1 from proteolytic degradation, as described above [70,85,88]. All patients exhibit clinical manifestations that are typical of a lysosomal disorder, such as coarse facies, cherry-red spots, vertebral changes, foam cells in the bone marrow, and vacuolated lymphocytes. Three phenotypic subtypes have been recognized. First, the early infantile form is associated with fetal hydrops, edema, ascites, visceromegaly, skeletal dysplasia, and early death. Second, the late infantile type is characterized by hepatosplenomegaly, growth retardation, cardiac involvement, and rare occurrence of neurologic signs. Third, the juvenile/adult form is characterized by myoclonus, ataxia, angiokeratoma, mental retardation, neurologic deterioration, absence of visceromegaly, and long survival. The majority of patients belonging to the juvenile/adult group was reported Japanese origin.

5.1.3. Molecular therapy for LSDs

Several therapeutic approaches have been developed and clinically applied to LSDs [90], including bone marrow transplantation (BMT), enzyme replacement therapy (ERT), gene therapy (GT), and substrate reduction therapy (SRT). BMT, ERT, and *ex vivo* GT utilize hematopoietic cells transduced with the cDNA of human lysosomal enzymes, which is based on the findings that normal lysosomal enzymes secreted from the donor cells or exogenously administered can be endocytosed via glycan receptors. These receptors include mannose receptors that recognize terminal mannose residues [91] and CI-M6PR [74], as described above, that are delivered to the lysosomes where the captured enzymes can exhibit their normal catabolic functions (cross-correction). However, BMT and *ex vivo* GT have several disadvantages, including high morbidity and mortality, as well as incomplete responses to therapy depending on the clinical phenotypes. On the other hand, the intravenous ERT utilizes recombinant human lysosomal enzymes produced by mammalian cell lines (Chinese hamster ovary (CHO) and human HT1080) stably expressing their cDNA and has been found to be the most effective treatment for several LSDs involving visceral symptoms, including type 1 Gaucher disease [92], mucopolysaccharidosis (MPS) type I [93], type II [94], and type VI [95], Fabry [96], and Pompe diseases [97]. However, the intravenous ERT also has several disadvantages including long-term therapy, production of neutralizing antibodies [98], high cost, and little effectiveness to LSDs involving central nervous system (CNS) symptoms due to the blood-brain barrier (BBB). Clinical trials of the intrathecal ERT are being carried out for treating MPS type I [99], II, and IIIB.

GT has advantages such as a long-lasting treatment with a single administration utilizing recombinant viral gene transfer vectors, [100-103] including retrovirus, adenovirus, herpes simplex virus, adeno-associated virus (AAV), and lentiviruses, albeit with its own attendant concerns, such as low levels and persistence of expression, as well as insertional mutagenesis resulting in neoplasia.

Alternatively, SRT based on prevention of the biosynthesis of natural substrates by utilizing synthetic substrate analogs, has been clinically applied [90,104,105], even though its utility is limited by side effects, continuous administration, and high cost.

In contrast, no definitive treatment is clinically available for LSDs involving glycoprotein catabolism, even though preclinical experiments with animal models have been performed. Heterologous BMT in a ferine α-mannosidosis model caused by a 4-bp deletion in the feline *MAN2B1* gene showed significant therapeutic effects on the CNS symptoms, in which case the therapy began when mild clinical signs were present [106]. Brain-directed GT using the AAV vector for 8-week-old cats with α-mannosidosis also showed remarkable restoration of brain α-mannosidase activity, improvement in myelination abnormalities, reduction of substrates in the neurons, neurological signs, and prolonged life span [107]. A canine α-fucosidosis model caused by a 14-bp deletion in the canine *FUCA1* gene has also been treated with heterologous BMT, the administration of which at an early age demonstrated efficacy for CNS symptoms [108].

Moreover, a murine galactosialidosis model (*Ctsa-/-*) was treated with cell-type specific *ex vivo* GT [109,110] by using donor bone marrow-derived cells that were transduced with murine-based retroviral vectors, containing human CTSA cDNA under the control of the promoter of murine monocyte/macrophage-specific colony-stimulating factor-1 receptor. Transgenic macrophages infiltrated and resided in all organs, and correction due to the secreted CTSA was observed not only in hematopoietic tissues but also in nonhematopoietic organs, including the CNS. Systemic GT for *Ctsa-/-* mice was also performed using a liver-tropic recombinant AAV-2/8 vector [111]. Despite the restricted expression of CTSA in the liver, dose-dependent and widespread correction of the disease phenotype in other systemic organs, serum, and urine, was observed, suggesting the protein-mediated mechanism of cross-correction.

Several approaches used to develop ERT for sialidosis and galactosialidosis have been challenged. The murine sialidosis model was treated with a short-term, high-dose ERT using baculovirus-derived recombinant *Neu1* [112]. The terminal mannosylated Neu1 taken up by resident macrophages in visceral organs restored the Neu1 activity and reduced the accumulation of sialyl substrates in lysosomes; however, mice developed a severe immune response towards the exogenous Neu1 as a side effect [112]. Recently, Itoh *et al* succeeded in producing a transgenic silkworm strain that overexpresses mature human CTSA in the middle silk glands (unpublished data). Purified mature CTSA carrying the human-like, high-mannose-type oligosaccharides lacking insect-specific carbohydrate moiety was taken up by murine monocytic cell lines via MR to be delivered to lysosomes. The conjugate between CTSA and a cell-penetrating peptide was also efficiently incorporated into the fibroblasts derived from galactosialidosis patients to be delivered to lysosomes and thereafter reduced the accumulation of sialyloligosaccharides in the cells. The novel recombinant human CTSA could be applied as a low-antigenic enzyme to intrathecal ERT for treating galactosialidosis patients exhibiting neurological symptoms.

6. Conclusions

Carbohydrates are very important molecules not only as energy sources but also for a wide variety of cellular functions, ranging from cell-cell interaction to immunity (1). Examples of glycosylation disorders described above clearly demonstrate that addition of carbohydrates to proteins is crucial for maintaining normal cellular physiology and that glycosylation disorders affect various cellular activities. The sugar chains, although not the direct gene products, contain essential information for the proper cellular function. The information, encoded by carbohydrate structures, is regarded as the sugar codes and is deciphered by a collection of carbohydrate-recognizing molecules, such as selectins and galectins [113,114]. In other words, glycosylation disorders can be considered as failures in interpreting the sugar codes. Due to their structural similarity and heterogeneity, carbohydrates are the most difficult molecules to study with the methods commonly used for nucleic acids and proteins. While the structure-function relationship of carbohydrates have remained unclear for a long time, the recent progress in separation, mass spectrometry, and genome-wide association studies of carbohydrates has been bringing information more rapidly than ever[115,116]. We expect that rapidly increasing knowledge of glycan structures and functions will help not only understand the importance of glycosylation in biology and diseases but also, in the near future, exploit the way to treat glycosylation-related diseases.

Acknowledgements

We appreciate Ms. Mayuko Oe for her assistance with this review preparation. This work was in part supported by Grants-in-Aid for Scientific Research on Innovative Areas No. 24110516 (to Y.N.) from the Ministry of Education, Culture, Sports, Science, and Technology (MEXT), Japan.

Author details

Yoshiaki Nakayama[1], Naosuke Nakamura[1], Daisuke Tsuji[2], Koji Itoh[2] and Akira Kurosaka[1]

1 Laboratory of Neuroglycobiology, Department of Molecular Biosciences, Faculty of Life Sciences, Kyoto Sangyo University, Kyoto, Japan

2 Department of Medicinal Biotechnology, Institute for Medicinal Research, Graduate School of Pharmaceutical Sciences, The University of Tokushima, Tokushima, Japan

References

[1] Moremen KW, Tiemeyer M, Nairn AV. Vertebrate protein glycosylation: diversity, synthesis and function. Nature Reviews. Molecular Cell Biology 2012:13(7) 448-462

[2] Rana NA, Haltiwanger RS. Fringe benefits: functional and structural impacts of O-glycosylation on the extracellular domain of Notch receptors. Current Opinion in Structural Biology 2011:21(5) 583-589

[3] Muntoni F, Torelli S, Wells DJ, Brown SC. Muscular dystrophies due to glycosylation defects: diagnosis and therapeutic strategies. Current Opinion in Neurology 2011:24(5) 437-442

[4] Jaeken J, Vanderschueren-Lodeweyckx M, Casaer P, Snoeck L, Corbeel L, Eggermont E, R E. Familial psychomotor retardation with markedly fluctuating serum prolactin, FSH and GH levels, partial TBG-deficiency, increased serum arylsulphatase A and increased CSF protein: a new syndrome? Pediatric Research 1980:14 179

[5] Van Schaftingen E, Jaeken J. Phosphomannomutase deficiency is a cause of carbohydrate-deficient glycoprotein syndrome type I. FEBS Letters 1995:377(3) 318-320

[6] Jaeken J, Matthijs G, Saudubray JM, Dionisi-Vici C, Bertini E, de Lonlay P, Henri H, Carchon H, Schollen E, E VS. Phosphomannomutase deficiency is a cause of carbohydrate-deficient glycoprotein syndrome type I. FEBS Letters 1998:377(3) 318-320

[7] Niehues R, Hasilik M, Alton G, Korner C, Schiebe-Sukumar M, Koch HG, Zimmer KP, Wu R, Harms E, Reiter K, von Figura K, Freeze HH, Harms HK, Marquardt T.

Carbohydrate-deficient glycoprotein syndrome type Ib. Phosphomannose isomerase deficiency and mannose therapy. Journal of Clinical Investigation 1998:101(7) 1414-1420

[8] Jaeken J, Schachter H, Carchon H, De Cock P, Coddeville B, Spik G. Carbohydrate deficient glycoprotein syndrome type II: a deficiency in Golgi localised N-acetylglucosaminyltransferase II. Archives of Disease in Childhood 1994:71(2) 123-127

[9] Hansske B, Thiel C, Lubke T, Hasilik M, Honing S, Peters V, Heidemann PH, Hoffmann GF, Berger EG, von Figura K, Korner C. Deficiency of UDP-galactose: N-acetylglucosamine b1,4-galactosyltransferase I causes the congenital disorder of glycosylation type IId. Journal of Clinical Investigation 2002:109(6) 725-733

[10] Martinez-Duncker I, Dupre T, Piller V, Piller F, Candelier JJ, Trichet C, Tchernia G, Oriol R, Mollicone R. Genetic complementation reveals a novel human congenital disorder of glycosylation of type II, due to inactivation of the Golgi CMP-sialic acid transporter. Blood 2005:105(7) 2671-2676

[11] Mueller OT, Wasmuth J J, Murray JC, Lozzio CB, Lovrien EW, TB. S. Chromosomal assignment of N-acetylglucosaminylphosphotransferase, the lysosomal hydrolase targeting enzyme deficient in mucolipidosis II and III. Cytogenetics and Cell Genetics 1987:46 664

[12] Ervasti JM, Ohlendieck K, Kahl SD, Gaver MG, Campbell KP. Deficiency of a glycoprotein component of the dystrophin complex in dystrophic muscle. Nature 1990:345(6273) 315-319

[13] Winder SJ. The complexities of dystroglycan. Trends in Biochemical Sciences 2001:26(2) 118-124

[14] Ibraghimov-Beskrovnaya O, Ervasti JM, Leveille CJ, Slaughter CA, Sernett SW, Campbell KP. Primary structure of dystrophin-associated glycoproteins linking dystrophin to the extracellular matrix. Nature 1992:355(6362) 696-702

[15] Hoffman EP, Brown RH, Jr., Kunkel LM. Dystrophin: the protein product of the Duchenne muscular dystrophy locus. Cell 1987:51(6) 919-928

[16] Jacobs PA, Hunt PA, Mayer M, Bart RD. Duchenne muscular dystrophy (DMD) in a female with an X/autosome translocation: further evidence that the DMD locus is at Xp21. American Journal of Human Genetics 1981:33(4) 513-518

[17] Blake DJ, Weir A, Newey SE, Davies KE. Function and genetics of dystrophin and dystrophin-related proteins in muscle. Physiological Reviews 2002:82(2) 291-329

[18] Michele DE, Barresi R, Kanagawa M, Saito F, Cohn RD, Satz JS, Dollar J, Nishino I, Kelley RI, Somer H, Straub V, Mathews KD, Moore SA, Campbell KP. Post-translational disruption of dystroglycan-ligand interactions in congenital muscular dystrophies. Nature 2002:418(6896) 417-422

[19] Holzfeind PJ, Grewal PK, Reitsamer HA, Kechvar J, Lassmann H, Hoeger H, Hewitt JE, Bittner RE. Skeletal, cardiac and tongue muscle pathology, defective retinal trans-

mission, and neuronal migration defects in the Large(myd) mouse defines a natural model for glycosylation-deficient muscle-eye- brain disorders. Human Molecular Genetics 2002:11(21) 2673-2687

[20] Nairn AV, Aoki K, Dela Rosa M, Porterfield M, Lim JM, Kulik M, Pierce JM, Wells L, Dalton S, Tiemeyer M, Moremen KW. Regulation of glycan structures in murine embryonic stem cells: combined transcript profiling of glycan-related genes and glycan structural analysis. Journal of Biological Chemistry 2012:in press.

[21] Godfrey C, Clement E, Mein R, Brockington M, Smith J, Talim B, Straub V, Robb S, Quinlivan R, Feng L, Jimenez-Mallebrera C, Mercuri E, Manzur AY, Kinali M, Torelli S, Brown SC, Sewry CA, Bushby K, Topaloglu H, North K, Abbs S, Muntoni F. Refining genotype phenotype correlations in muscular dystrophies with defective glycosylation of dystroglycan. Brain 2007:130(Pt 10) 2725-2735

[22] Godfrey C, Foley AR, Clement E, Muntoni F. Dystroglycanopathies: coming into focus. Current Opinion in Genetics and Development 2011:21(3) 278-285

[23] Manya H, Chiba A, Yoshida A, Wang X, Chiba Y, Jigami Y, Margolis RU, Endo T. Demonstration of mammalian protein O-mannosyltransferase activity: coexpression of POMT1 and POMT2 required for enzymatic activity. Proceedings of the National Academy of Sciences USA 2004:101(2) 500-505

[24] Yoshida A, Kobayashi K, Manya H, Taniguchi K, Kano H, Mizuno M, Inazu T, Mitsuhashi H, Takahashi S, Takeuchi M, Herrmann R, Straub V, Talim B, Voit T, Topaloglu H, Toda T, Endo T. Muscular dystrophy and neuronal migration disorder caused by mutations in a glycosyltransferase, POMGnT1. Developmental Cell 2001:1(5) 717-724

[25] Beltran-Valero de Bernabe D, Currier S, Steinbrecher A, Celli J, van Beusekom E, van der Zwaag B, Kayserili H, Merlini L, Chitayat D, Dobyns WB, Cormand B, Lehesjoki AE, Cruces J, Voit T, Walsh CA, van Bokhoven H, Brunner HG. Mutations in the O-mannosyltransferase gene POMT1 give rise to the severe neuronal migration disorder Walker-Warburg syndrome. American Journal of Human Genetics 2002:71(5) 1033-1043

[26] Chiba A, Matsumura K, Yamada H, Inazu T, Shimizu T, Kusunoki S, Kanazawa I, Kobata A, Endo T. Structures of sialylated O-linked oligosaccharides of bovine peripheral nerve a-dystroglycan. The role of a novel O-mannosyl-type oligosaccharide in the binding of a-dystroglycan with laminin. Journal of Biological Chemistry 1997:272(4) 2156-2162

[27] Yoshida-Moriguchi T, Yu L, Stalnaker SH, Davis S, Kunz S, Madson M, Oldstone MB, Schachter H, Wells L, Campbell KP. O-mannosyl phosphorylation of a-dystroglycan is required for laminin binding. Science 2010:327(5961) 88-92

[28] Kobayashi K, Nakahori Y, Miyake M, Matsumura K, Kondo-Iida E, Nomura Y, Segawa M, Yoshioka M, Saito K, Osawa M, Hamano K, Sakakihara Y, Nonaka I, Naka-

gome Y, Kanazawa I, Nakamura Y, Tokunaga K, Toda T. An ancient retrotransposal insertion causes Fukuyama-type congenital muscular dystrophy. Nature 1998:394(6691) 388-392

[29] Brockington M, Blake DJ, Prandini P, Brown SC, Torelli S, Benson MA, Ponting CP, Estournet B, Romero NB, Mercuri E, Voit T, Sewry CA, Guicheney P, Muntoni F. Mutations in the fukutin-related protein gene (FKRP) cause a form of congenital muscular dystrophy with secondary laminin a2 deficiency and abnormal glycosylation of a-dystroglycan. American Journal of Human Genetics 2001:69(6) 1198-1209

[30] Brockington M, Yuva Y, Prandini P, Brown SC, Torelli S, Benson MA, Herrmann R, Anderson LV, Bashir R, Burgunder JM, Fallet S, Romero N, Fardeau M, Straub V, Storey G, Pollitt C, Richard I, Sewry CA, Bushby K, Voit T, Blake DJ, Muntoni F. Mutations in the fukutin-related protein gene (FKRP) identify limb girdle muscular dystrophy 2I as a milder allelic variant of congenital muscular dystrophy MDC1C. Human Molecular Genetics 2001:10(25) 2851-2859

[31] Inamori K, Yoshida-Moriguchi T, Hara Y, Anderson ME, Yu L, Campbell KP. Dystroglycan function requires xylosyl- and glucuronyltransferase activities of LARGE. Science 2012:335(6064) 93-96

[32] Bleckmann C, Geyer H, Lieberoth A, Splittstoesser F, Liu Y, Feizi T, Schachner M, Kleene R, Reinhold V, Geyer R. O-glycosylation pattern of CD24 from mouse brain. Biological Chemistry 2009:390(7) 627-645

[33] Martinez T, Pace D, Brady L, Gerhart M, Balland A. Characterization of a novel modification on IgG2 light chain. Evidence for the presence of O-linked mannosylation. Journal of Chromatography A 2007:1156(1-2) 183-187

[34] Kruse J, Keilhauer G, Faissner A, Timpl R, Schachner M. The J1 glycoprotein--a novel nervous system cell adhesion molecule of the L2/HNK-1 family. Nature 1985:316(6024) 146-148

[35] Yahiro K, Wada A, Yamasaki E, Nakayama M, Nishi Y, Hisatsune J, Morinaga N, Sap J, Noda M, Moss J, Hirayama T. Essential domain of receptor tyrosine phosphatase b (RPTPb) for interaction with Helicobacter pylori vacuolating cytotoxin. Journal of Biological Chemistry 2004:279(49) 51013-51021

[36] Pacharra S, Hanisch FG, Breloy I. Neurofascin 186 Is O-Mannosylated within and outside of the mucin domain. Journal of Proteome Research 2012:11(8) 3955-3964

[37] Hara Y, Balci-Hayta B, Yoshida-Moriguchi T, Kanagawa M, Beltran-Valero de Bernabe D, Gundesli H, Willer T, Satz JS, Crawford RW, Burden SJ, Kunz S, Oldstone MB, Accardi A, Talim B, Muntoni F, Topaloglu H, Dincer P, Campbell KP. A dystroglycan mutation associated with limb-girdle muscular dystrophy. New England Journal of Medicine 2011:364(10) 939-946

[38] Mercuri E, Messina S, Bruno C, Mora M, Pegoraro E, Comi GP, D'Amico A, Aiello C, Biancheri R, Berardinelli A, Boffi P, Cassandrini D, Laverda A, Moggio M, Morandi

L, Moroni I, Pane M, Pezzani R, Pichiecchio A, Pini A, Minetti C, Mongini T, Mottarelli E, Ricci E, Ruggieri A, Saredi S, Scuderi C, Tessa A, Toscano A, Tortorella G, Trevisan CP, Uggetti C, Vasco G, Santorelli FM, Bertini E. Congenital muscular dystrophies with defective glycosylation of dystroglycan: a population study. Neurology 2009:72(21) 1802-1809

[39] Lefeber DJ, Schonberger J, Morava E, Guillard M, Huyben KM, Verrijp K, Grafakou O, Evangeliou A, Preijers FW, Manta P, Yildiz J, Grunewald S, Spilioti M, van den Elzen C, Klein D, Hess D, Ashida H, Hofsteenge J, Maeda Y, van den Heuvel L, Lammens M, Lehle L, Wevers RA. Deficiency of Dol-P-Man synthase subunit DPM3 bridges the congenital disorders of glycosylation with the dystroglycanopathies. American Journal of Human Genetics 2009:85(1) 76-86

[40] Roscioli T, Kamsteeg EJ, Buysse K, Maystadt I, van Reeuwijk J, van den Elzen C, van Beusekom E, Riemersma M, Pfundt R, Vissers LE, Schraders M, Altunoglu U, Buckley MF, Brunner HG, Grisart B, Zhou H, Veltman JA, Gilissen C, Mancini GM, Delree P, Willemsen MA, Ramadza DP, Chitayat D, Bennett C, Sheridan E, Peeters EA, Tan-Sindhunata GM, de Die-Smulders CE, Devriendt K, Kayserili H, El-Hashash OA, Stemple DL, Lefeber DJ, Lin YY, van Bokhoven H. Mutations in ISPD cause Walker-Warburg syndrome and defective glycosylation of a-dystroglycan. Nature Genetics 2012:44(5) 581-585

[41] Willer T, Lee H, Lommel M, Yoshida-Moriguchi T, de Bernabe DB, Venzke D, Cirak S, Schachter H, Vajsar J, Voit T, Muntoni F, Loder AS, Dobyns WB, Winder TL, Strahl S, Mathews KD, Nelson SF, Moore SA, Campbell KP. ISPD loss-of-function mutations disrupt dystroglycan O-mannosylation and cause Walker-Warburg syndrome. Nature Genetics 2012:44(5) 575-580

[42] Manzini MC, Tambunan DE, Hill RS, Yu TW, Maynard TM, Heinzen EL, Shianna KV, Stevens CR, Partlow JN, Barry BJ, Rodriguez J, Gupta VA, Al-Qudah AK, Eyaid WM, Friedman JM, Salih MA, Clark R, Moroni I, Mora M, Beggs AH, Gabriel SB, CA. W. Exome sequencing and functional validation in zebrafish identify GTDC2 mutations as a cause of Walker-Warburg Syndrome. American Journal of Human Genetics 2012:91(3) 541-547

[43] Gill DJ, Chia J, Senewiratne J, Bard F. Regulation of O-glycosylation through Golgi-to-ER relocation of initiation enzymes. Journal of Cell Biology 2010:189(5) 843-858

[44] Topaz O, Shurman DL, Bergman R, Indelman M, Ratajczak P, Mizrachi M, Khamaysi Z, Behar D, Petronius D, Friedman V, Zelikovic I, Raimer S, Metzker A, Richard G, Sprecher E. Mutations in GALNT3, encoding a protein involved in O-linked glycosylation, cause familial tumoral calcinosis. Nature Genetics 2004:36(6) 579-581

[45] Kato K, Jeanneau C, Tarp MA, Benet-Pages A, Lorenz-Depiereux B, Bennett EP, Mandel U, Strom TM, Clausen H. Polypeptide GalNAc-transferase T3 and familial tumoral calcinosis. Secretion of fibroblast growth factor 23 requires O-glycosylation. Journal of Biological Chemistry 2006:281(27) 18370-18377

[46] ADHR_Consortium. Autosomal dominant hypophosphataemic rickets is associated with mutations in FGF23. Nature Genetics 2000:26(3) 345-348

[47] White KE, Carn G, Lorenz-Depiereux B, Benet-Pages A, Strom TM, Econs MJ. Autosomal-dominant hypophosphatemic rickets (ADHR) mutations stabilize FGF-23. Kidney International 2001:60(6) 2079-2086

[48] Kathiresan S, Melander O, Guiducci C, Surti A, Burtt NP, Rieder MJ, Cooper GM, Roos C, Voight BF, Havulinna AS, Wahlstrand B, Hedner T, Corella D, Tai ES, Ordovas JM, Berglund G, Vartiainen E, Jousilahti P, Hedblad B, Taskinen MR, Newton-Cheh C, Salomaa V, Peltonen L, Groop L, Altshuler DM, Orho-Melander M. Six new loci associated with blood low-density lipoprotein cholesterol, high-density lipoprotein cholesterol or triglycerides in humans. Nature Genetics 2008:40(2) 189-197

[49] Willer CJ, Sanna S, Jackson AU, Scuteri A, Bonnycastle LL, Clarke R, Heath SC, Timpson NJ, Najjar SS, Stringham HM, Strait J, Duren WL, Maschio A, Busonero F, Mulas A, Albai G, Swift AJ, Morken MA, Narisu N, Bennett D, Parish S, Shen H, Galan P, Meneton P, Hercberg S, Zelenika D, Chen WM, Li Y, Scott LJ, Scheet PA, Sundvall J, Watanabe RM, Nagaraja R, Ebrahim S, Lawlor DA, Ben-Shlomo Y, Davey-Smith G, Shuldiner AR, Collins R, Bergman RN, Uda M, Tuomilehto J, Cao A, Collins FS, Lakatta E, Lathrop GM, Boehnke M, Schlessinger D, Mohlke KL, Abecasis GR. Newly identified loci that influence lipid concentrations and risk of coronary artery disease. Nature Genetics 2008:40(2) 161-169

[50] Teslovich TM, Musunuru K, Smith AV, Edmondson AC, Stylianou IM, Koseki M, Pirruccello JP, Ripatti S, Chasman DI, Willer CJ, Johansen CT, Fouchier SW, Isaacs A, Peloso GM, Barbalic M, Ricketts SL, Bis JC, Aulchenko YS, Thorleifsson G, Feitosa MF, Chambers J, Orho-Melander M, Melander O, Johnson T, Li X, Guo X, Li M, Shin Cho Y, Jin Go M, Jin Kim Y, Lee JY, Park T, Kim K, Sim X, Twee-Hee Ong R, Croteau-Chonka DC, Lange LA, Smith JD, Song K, Hua Zhao J, Yuan X, Luan J, Lamina C, Ziegler A, Zhang W, Zee RY, Wright AF, Witteman JC, Wilson JF, Willemsen G, Wichmann HE, Whitfield JB, Waterworth DM, Wareham NJ, Waeber G, Vollenweider P, Voight BF, Vitart V, Uitterlinden AG, Uda M, Tuomilehto J, Thompson JR, Tanaka T, Surakka I, Stringham HM, Spector TD, Soranzo N, Smit JH, Sinisalo J, Silander K, Sijbrands EJ, Scuteri A, Scott J, Schlessinger D, Sanna S, Salomaa V, Saharinen J, Sabatti C, Ruokonen A, Rudan I, Rose LM, Roberts R, Rieder M, Psaty BM, Pramstaller PP, Pichler I, Perola M, Penninx BW, Pedersen NL, Pattaro C, Parker AN, Pare G, Oostra BA, O'Donnell CJ, Nieminen MS, Nickerson DA, Montgomery GW, Meitinger T, McPherson R, McCarthy MI, McArdle W, Masson D, Martin NG, Marroni F, Mangino M, Magnusson PK, Lucas G, Luben R, Loos RJ, Lokki ML, Lettre G, Langenberg C, Launer LJ, Lakatta EG, Laaksonen R, Kyvik KO, Kronenberg F, Konig IR, Khaw KT, Kaprio J, Kaplan LM, Johansson A, Jarvelin MR, Janssens AC, Ingelsson E, Igl W, Kees Hovingh G, Hottenga JJ, Hofman A, Hicks AA, Hengstenberg C, Heid IM, Hayward C, Havulinna AS, Hastie ND, Harris TB, Haritunians T, Hall AS, Gyllensten U, Guiducci C, Groop LC, Gonzalez E, Gieger C, Freimer NB, Ferrucci L, Erdmann J, Elliott P, Ejebe KG, Doring A, Dominiczak AF, Demissie S, Deloukas P,

de Geus EJ, de Faire U, Crawford G, Collins FS, Chen YD, Caulfield MJ, Campbell H, Burtt NP, Bonnycastle LL, Boomsma DI, Boekholdt SM, Bergman RN, Barroso I, Bandinelli S, Ballantyne CM, Assimes TL, Quertermous T, Altshuler D, Seielstad M, Wong TY, Tai ES, Feranil AB, Kuzawa CW, Adair LS, Taylor HA, Jr., Borecki IB, Gabriel SB, Wilson JG, Holm H, Thorsteinsdottir U, Gudnason V, Krauss RM, Mohlke KL, Ordovas JM, Munroe PB, Kooner JS, Tall AR, Hegele RA, Kastelein JJ, Schadt EE, Rotter JI, Boerwinkle E, Strachan DP, Mooser V, Stefansson K, Reilly MP, Samani NJ, Schunkert H, Cupples LA, Sandhu MS, Ridker PM, Rader DJ, van Duijn CM, Peltonen L, Abecasis GR, Boehnke M, Kathiresan S. Biological, clinical and population relevance of 95 loci for blood lipids. Nature 2010:466(7307) 707-713

[51] Holleboom AG, Karlsson H, Lin RS, Beres TM, Sierts JA, Herman DS, Stroes ES, Aerts JM, Kastelein JJ, Motazacker MM, Dallinga-Thie GM, Levels JH, Zwinderman AH, Seidman JG, Seidman CE, Ljunggren S, Lefeber DJ, Morava E, Wevers RA, Fritz TA, Tabak LA, Lindahl M, Hovingh GK, Kuivenhoven JA. Heterozygosity for a loss-of-function mutation in GALNT2 improves plasma triglyceride clearance in man. Cell Metabolism 2011:14(6) 811-818

[52] Merla G, Ucla C, Guipponi M, Reymond A. Identification of additional transcripts in the Williams-Beuren syndrome critical region. Human Genetics 2002:110(5) 429-438

[53] Nakamura N, Toba S, Hirai M, Morishita S, Mikami T, Konishi M, Itoh N, Kurosaka A. Cloning and expression of a brain-specific putative UDP-GalNAc: polypeptide N-acetylgalactosaminyltransferase gene. Biological and Pharmaceutical Bulletin 2005:28(3) 429-433

[54] Vonholdt BM, Pollinger JP, Lohmueller KE, Han E, Parker HG, Quignon P, Degenhardt JD, Boyko AR, Earl DA, Auton A, Reynolds A, Bryc K, Brisbin A, Knowles JC, Mosher DS, Spady TC, Elkahloun A, Geffen E, Pilot M, Jedrzejewski W, Greco C, Randi E, Bannasch D, Wilton A, Shearman J, Musiani M, Cargill M, Jones PG, Qian Z, Huang W, Ding ZL, Zhang YP, Bustamante CD, Ostrander EA, Novembre J, Wayne RK. Genome-wide SNP and haplotype analyses reveal a rich history underlying dog domestication. Nature 2010:464(7290) 898-902

[55] Li X, Wang J, Li W, Xu Y, Shao D, Xie Y, Xie W, Kubota T, Narimatsu H, Zhang Y. Characterization of ppGalNAc-T18, a member of the vertebrate-specific Y subfamily of UDP-N-acetyl-a-D-galactosamine: polypeptide N-acetylgalactosaminyltransferases. Glycobiology 2012:22(5) 602-615

[56] Nakayama Y, Nakamura N, Oki S, Wakabayashi M, Ishihama Y, Miyake A, Itoh N, Kurosaka A. A Putative polypeptide N-acetylgalactosaminyltransferase/Williams-Beuren Syndrome chromosome region 17 (WBSCR17) regulates lamellipodium formation and macropinocytosis. Journal of Biological Chemistry 2012:287(38) 32222-32235

[57] Phelan CM, Tsai YY, Goode EL, Vierkant RA, Fridley BL, Beesley J, Chen XQ, Webb PM, Chanock S, Cramer DW, Moysich K, Edwards RP, Chang-Claude J, Garcia-Clo-

sas M, Yang H, Wang-Gohrke S, Hein R, Green AC, Lissowska J, Carney ME, Lurie G, Wilkens LR, Ness RB, Pearce CL, Wu AH, Van Den Berg DJ, Stram DO, Terry KL, Whiteman DC, Whittemore AS, DiCioccio RA, McGuire V, Doherty JA, Rossing MA, Anton-Culver H, Ziogas A, Hogdall C, Hogdall E, Kruger Kjaer S, Blaakaer J, Quaye L, Ramus SJ, Jacobs I, Song H, Pharoah PD, Iversen ES, Marks JR, Pike MC, Gayther SA, Cunningham JM, Goodman MT, Schildkraut JM, Chenevix-Trench G, Berchuck A, Sellers TA. Polymorphism in the GALNT1 gene and epithelial ovarian cancer in non-Hispanic white women: the Ovarian Cancer Association Consortium. Cancer Epidemiology, Biomarkers and Prevention 2010:19(2) 600-604

[58] O'Halloran AM, Patterson CC, Horan P, Maree A, Curtin R, Stanton A, McKeown PP, Shields DC. Genetic polymorphisms in platelet-related proteins and coronary artery disease: investigation of candidate genes, including N-acetylgalactosaminyltransferase 4 (GALNT4) and sulphotransferase 1A1/2 (SULT1A1/2). Journal of Thrombosis and Thrombolysis 2009:27(2) 175-184

[59] Fakhro KA, Choi M, Ware SM, Belmont JW, Towbin JA, Lifton RP, Khokha MK, Brueckner M. Rare copy number variations in congenital heart disease patients identify unique genes in left-right patterning. Proceedings of the National Academy of Sciences USA 2011:108(7) 2915-2920

[60] Guda K, Moinova H, He J, Jamison O, Ravi L, Natale L, Lutterbaugh J, Lawrence E, Lewis S, Willson JK, Lowe JB, Wiesner GL, Parmigiani G, Barnholtz-Sloan J, Dawson DW, Velculescu VE, Kinzler KW, Papadopoulos N, Vogelstein B, Willis J, Gerken TA, Markowitz SD. Inactivating germ-line and somatic mutations in polypeptide N-acetylgalactosaminyltransferase 12 in human colon cancers. Proceedings of the National Academy of Sciences USA 2009:106(31) 12921-12925

[61] Desai AA, Zhou T, Ahmad H, Zhang W, Mu W, Trevino S, Wade MS, Raghavachari N, Kato GJ, Peters-Lawrence MH, Thiruvoipati T, Turner K, Artz N, Huang Y, Patel AR, Yuan JX, Gordeuk VR, Lang RM, Garcia JG, Machado RF. A novel molecular signature for elevated tricuspid regurgitation velocity in sickle cell disease. American Journal of Respiratory and Critical Care Medicine 2012:186(4) 359-368

[62] Wagner KW, Punnoose EA, Januario T, Lawrence DA, Pitti RM, Lancaster K, Lee D, von Goetz M, Yee SF, Totpal K, Huw L, Katta V, Cavet G, Hymowitz SG, Amler L, Ashkenazi A. Death-receptor O-glycosylation controls tumor-cell sensitivity to the proapoptotic ligand Apo2L/TRAIL. Nature Medicine 2007:13(9) 1070-1077

[63] Abuli A, Fernandez-Rozadilla C, Alonso-Espinaco V, Munoz J, Gonzalo V, Bessa X, Gonzalez D, Clofent J, Cubiella J, Morillas JD, Rigau J, Latorre M, Fernandez-Banares F, Pena E, Riestra S, Paya A, Jover R, Xicola RM, Llor X, Carvajal-Carmona L, Villanueva CM, Moreno V, Pique JM, Carracedo A, Castells A, Andreu M, Ruiz-Ponte C, Castellvi-Bel S. Case-control study for colorectal cancer genetic susceptibility in EPICOLON: previously identified variants and mucins. BMC Cancer 2011:11 339

[64] Vainchenker W, Vinci G, Testa U, Henri A, Tabilio A, Fache MP, Rochant H, Cartron JP. Presence of the Tn antigen on hematopoietic progenitors from patients with the Tn syndrome. Journal of Clinical Investigation 1985:75(2) 541-546

[65] Ju T, Cummings RD. Protein glycosylation: chaperone mutation in Tn syndrome. Nature 2005:437(7063) 1252

[66] Scriver C. Lysosomal Disorders. The online metabolic and molecular bases of inherited diseases. http://www.ommbid.com.Part 16 Chapters 134-154

[67] von Figura K, Hasilik A. Lysosomal enzymes and their receptors. Annual Review of Biochemistry 1986:55 167-193

[68] Mindell JA. Lysosomal acidification mechanisms. Annual Review of Physiology 2012:74 69-86

[69] Pshezhetsky AV, Hinek A. Where catabolism meets signalling: neuraminidase 1 as a modulator of cell receptors. Glycoconjugate Journal 2011:28(7) 441-452

[70] d'Azzo A. Galactosialidosis. In, Scriver, CR.; Beaudet, AL.; Sly, WS.; Valle, D. (eds.): The Metabolic & Moecular Bases of Inherited Disease. Vol.III (8th ed.) 2001 McGrow-Hill.

[71] Mahuran DJ. The GM2 activator protein, its roles as a co-factor in GM2 hydrolysis and as a general glycolipid transport protein. Biochimica et Biophysica Acta 1998:1393(1) 1-18

[72] Kishimoto Y, Hiraiwa M, O'Brien JS. Saposins: structure, function, distribution, and molecular genetics. Journal of Lipid Research 1992:33(9) 1255-1267

[73] Sardiello M, Palmieri M, di Ronza A, Medina DL, Valenza M, Gennarino VA, Di Malta C, Donaudy F, Embrione V, Polishchuk RS, Banfi S, Parenti G, Cattaneo E, Ballabio A. A gene network regulating lysosomal biogenesis and function. Science 2009:325(5939) 473-477

[74] Kornfeld S. Structure and function of the mannose 6-phosphate/insulinlike growth factor II receptors. Annual Review of Biochemistry 1992:61 307-330

[75] Galjart NJ, Gillemans N, Harris A, van der Horst GT, Verheijen FW, Galjaard H, d'Azzo A. Expression of cDNA encoding the human "protective protein" associated with lysosomal b-galactosidase and neuraminidase: homology to yeast proteases. Cell 1988:54(6) 755-764

[76] Itoh K, Takiyama N, Kase R, Kondoh K, Sano A, Oshima A, Sakuraba H, Suzuki Y. Purification and characterization of human lysosomal protective protein expressed in stably transformed Chinese hamster ovary cells. Journal of Biological Chemistry 1993:268(2) 1180-1186

[77] Jackman HL, Tan FL, Tamei H, Beurling-Harbury C, Li XY, Skidgel RA, Erdos EG. A peptidase in human platelets that deamidates tachykinins. Probable identity with the

lysosomal "protective protein". Journal of Biological Chemistry 1990:265(19) 11265-11272

[78] Itoh K, Kase R, Shimmoto M, Satake A, Sakuraba H, Suzuki Y. Protective protein as an endogenous endothelin degradation enzyme in human tissues. Journal of Biological Chemistry 1995:270(2) 515-518

[79] Itoh K, Oyanagi K, Takahashi H, Sato T, Hashizume Y, Shimmoto M, Sakuraba H. Endothelin-1 in the brain of patients with galactosialidosis: its abnormal increase and distribution pattern. Annals of Neurology 2000:47(1) 122-126

[80] Pshezhetsky AV, Hinek A. Serine carboxypeptidases in regulation of vasoconstriction and elastogenesis. Trends in Cardiovascular Medicine 2009:19(1) 11-17

[81] Neufeld EF, Fratantoni JC. Inborn errors of mucopolysaccharide metabolism. Science 1970:169(3941) 141-146

[82] Thomas G.H. Disorders of Glysoprotein Degradation: α-Mannosidosis, α-Mannosidosis, Fucosidosis, and Sialidosis, The Online Metabolic and Molecular Bases of Inherited Diseases. Part 16: Chapter 140.

[83] Michalski JC, Klein A. Glycoprotein lysosomal storage disorders: a- and b-mannosidosis, fucosidosis and a-N-acetylgalactosaminidase deficiency. Biochimica et Biophysica Acta 1999:1455(2-3) 69-84

[84] Malm D, Nilssen O. a-Mannosidosis. Orphanet Journal of Rare Diseases 2008:3 21

[85] Shimmoto M, Fukuhara Y, Itoh K, Oshima A, Sakuraba H, Suzuki Y. Protective protein gene mutations in galactosialidosis. Journal of Clinical Investigation 1993:91(6) 2393-2398

[86] Pshezhetsky AV, Richard C, Michaud L, Igdoura S, Wang S, Elsliger MA, Qu J, Leclerc D, Gravel R, Dallaire L, Potier M. Cloning, expression and chromosomal mapping of human lysosomal sialidase and characterization of mutations in sialidosis. Nature Genetics 1997:15(3) 316-320

[87] Bonten E, van der Spoel A, Fornerod M, Grosveld G, d'Azzo A. Characterization of human lysosomal neuraminidase defines the molecular basis of the metabolic storage disorder sialidosis. Genes and Development 1996:10(24) 3156-3169

[88] Takano T. Galactosialidosis: clinicaland molecular analysis of 19 Japanese patients. Brain Dysfunction 1991; 4: 271-280.

[89] Itoh K, Naganawa Y, Matsuzawa F, Aikawa S, Doi H, Sasagasako N, Yamada T, Kira J, Kobayashi T, Pshezhetsky AV, Sakuraba H. Novel missense mutations in the human lysosomal sialidase gene in sialidosis patients and prediction of structural alterations of mutant enzymes. Journal of Human Genetics 2002:47(1) 29-37

[90] Beck M. New therapeutic options for lysosomal storage disorders: enzyme replacement, small molecules and gene therapy. Human Genetics 2007:121(1) 1-22

[91] Achord DT, Brot FE, Bell CE, Sly WS. Human b-glucuronidase: in vivo clearance and in vitro uptake by a glycoprotein recognition system on reticuloendothelial cells. Cell 1978:15(1) 269-278

[92] Barton NW, Brady RO, Dambrosia JM, Di Bisceglie AM, Doppelt SH, Hill SC, Mankin HJ, Murray GJ, Parker RI, Argoff CE, et al. Replacement therapy for inherited enzyme deficiency--macrophage-targeted glucocerebrosidase for Gaucher's disease. New England Journal of Medicine 1991:324(21) 1464-1470

[93] Kakkis ED, Muenzer J, Tiller GE, Waber L, Belmont J, Passage M, Izykowski B, Phillips J, Doroshow R, Walot I, Hoft R, Neufeld EF. Enzyme-replacement therapy in mucopolysaccharidosis I. New England Journal of Medicine 2001:344(3) 182-188

[94] Amalfitano A, Bengur AR, Morse RP, Majure JM, Case LE, Veerling DL, Mackey J, Kishnani P, Smith W, McVie-Wylie A, Sullivan JA, Hoganson GE, Phillips JA, 3rd, Schaefer GB, Charrow J, Ware RE, Bossen EH, Chen YT. Recombinant human acid a-glucosidase enzyme therapy for infantile glycogen storage disease type II: results of a phase I/II clinical trial. Genetics in Medicine 2001:3(2) 132-138

[95] Harmatz P, Whitley CB, Waber L, Pais R, Steiner R, Plecko B, Kaplan P, Simon J, Butensky E, Hopwood JJ. Enzyme replacement therapy in mucopolysaccharidosis VI (Maroteaux-Lamy syndrome). Journal of Pediatrics 2004:144(5) 574-580

[96] Eng CM, Guffon N, Wilcox WR, Germain DP, Lee P, Waldek S, Caplan L, Linthorst GE, Desnick RJ. Safety and efficacy of recombinant human a-galactosidase A - replacement therapy in Fabry's disease. New England Journal of Medicine 2001:345(1) 9-16

[97] Winkel LP, Van den Hout JM, Kamphoven JH, Disseldorp JA, Remmerswaal M, Arts WF, Loonen MC, Vulto AG, Van Doorn PA, De Jong G, Hop W, Smit GP, Shapira SK, Boer MA, van Diggelen OP, Reuser AJ, Van der Ploeg AT. Enzyme replacement therapy in late-onset Pompe's disease: a three-year follow-up. Annals of Neurology 2004:55(4) 495-502

[98] Wang J, Lozier J, Johnson G, Kirshner S, Verthelyi D, Pariser A, Shores E, Rosenberg A. Neutralizing antibodies to therapeutic enzymes: considerations for testing, prevention and treatment. Nature Biotechnology 2008:26(8) 901-908

[99] Dickson PI, Chen AH. Intrathecal enzyme replacement therapy for mucopolysaccharidosis I: translating success in animal models to patients. Current Pharmaceutical Biotechnology 2011:12(6) 946-955

[100] Sands MS, Davidson BL. Gene therapy for lysosomal storage diseases. Molecular Therapy 2006:13(5) 839-849

[101] Haskins M. Gene therapy for lysosomal storage diseases (LSDs) in large animal models. ILAR Journal 2009:50(2) 112-121

[102] Schiffmann R. Therapeutic approaches for neuronopathic lysosomal storage disorders. Journal of Inherited Metabolic Disease 2010:33(4) 373-379

[103] Sands MS, Haskins ME. CNS-directed gene therapy for lysosomal storage diseases. Acta Paediatrica. Supplement 2008:97(457) 22-27

[104] Platt FM, Jeyakumar M. Substrate reduction therapy. Acta Paediatrica. Supplement 2008:97(457) 88-93

[105] Pastores GM. Miglustat: substrate reduction therapy for lysosomal storage disorders associated with primary central nervous system involvement. Recent Pat CNS Drug Discov 2006:1(1) 77-82

[106] Walkley SU, Thrall MA, Dobrenis K, Huang M, March PA, Siegel DA, Wurzelmann S. Bone marrow transplantation corrects the enzyme defect in neurons of the central nervous system in a lysosomal storage disease. Proceedings of the National Academy of Sciences USA 1994:91(8) 2970-2974

[107] Vite CH, McGowan JC, Niogi SN, Passini MA, Drobatz KJ, Haskins ME, Wolfe JH. Effective gene therapy for an inherited CNS disease in a large animal model. Annals of Neurology 2005:57(3) 355-364

[108] Taylor RM, Farrow BR, Stewart GJ, Healy PJ. Enzyme replacement in nervous tissue after allogeneic bone-marrow transplantation for fucosidosis in dogs. Lancet 1986:2(8510) 772-774

[109] Hahn CN, del Pilar Martin M, Zhou XY, Mann LW, d'Azzo A. Correction of murine galactosialidosis by bone marrow-derived macrophages overexpressing human protective protein/cathepsin A under control of the colony-stimulating factor-1 receptor promoter. Proceedings of the National Academy of Sciences USA 1998:95(25) 14880-14885

[110] Leimig T, Mann L, Martin Mdel P, Bonten E, Persons D, Knowles J, Allay JA, Cunningham J, Nienhuis AW, Smeyne R, d'Azzo A. Functional amelioration of murine galactosialidosis by genetically modified bone marrow hematopoietic progenitor cells. Blood 2002:99(9) 3169-3178

[111] Hu H, Gomero E, Bonten E, Gray JT, Allay J, Wu Y, Wu J, Calabrese C, Nienhuis A, d'Azzo A. Preclinical dose-finding study with a liver-tropic, recombinant AAV-2/8 vector in the mouse model of galactosialidosis. Molecular Therapy 2012:20(2) 267-274

[112] Wang D, Bonten EJ, Yogalingam G, Mann L, d'Azzo A. Short-term, high dose enzyme replacement therapy in sialidosis mice. Molecular Genetics and Metabolism 2005:85(3) 181-189

[113] Sperandio M, Gleissner CA, Ley K. Glycosylation in immune cell trafficking. Immunological Reviews 2009:230(1) 97-113

[114] Boscher C, Dennis JW, Nabi IR. Glycosylation, galectins and cellular signaling. Current Opinion in Cell Biology 2011:23(4) 383-392

[115] Antonopoulos A, North SJ, Haslam SM, Dell A. Glycosylation of mouse and human immune cells: insights emerging from N-glycomics analyses. Biochemical Society Transactions 2011:39(5) 1334-1340

[116] Zoldos V, Novokmet M, Beceheli I, Lauc G. Genomics and epigenomics of the human glycome. Glycoconjugate Journal 2012:in press.

Chapter 11

Genetics and Obesity

Maria Puiu, Adela Chirita Emandi and
Smaranda Arghirescu

Additional information is available at the end of the chapter

1. Introduction

Obesity, in both children and adults, has reached epidemic proportions in multiple countries worldwide, with serious health problems and imposing a substantial economic burden on societies [1–4]. The increase in obesity prevalence among children is particularly alarming because obesity-related complications, including obesity-associated sleep apnea,[5] non-alcoholic fatty liver disease [6], and type 2 diabetes,[7] are increasingly diagnosed in pediatric patients. Excess weight in children may increase the likelihood of heart disease in adulthood as a result of the early establishment of risk factors [8]. Pediatric obesity has been shown to have a tremendous impact on later health [8], even independent of adult weight [9]. Additionally, childhood obesity is linked with important psychosocial consequences and poor general quality of life [10].

In order to create the best management programs and determine novel therapeutic targets, it becomes essential to understand the factors causing today's rising epidemic of childhood obesity.

Obesity develops as a result of dietary and lifestyle factors, but studies also suggest a genetic influence on obesity [11]. Obesity is highly influenced by genetics; available data suggest that 40% to 77% of the observed variance in human body weight can be accounted for, by inherited factors [12–14]. Obesity, also just as clearly has environmental causes; our genetic endowments have changed minimally during the last 40 years, yet the prevalence of childhood obesity has tripled in US [15] and significantly increased worldwide [16], an observation that can only be explained by changes in external factors affecting children's energetic balance.

This chapter provides an overview of the current knowledge on genetic factors implicated in the obesity epidemic.

Methodology

This review chapter has been developed using an evidence-based approach. Data from clinical and observational studies, review articles and twin studies were all considered when shaping this review. Literature searches for topics relating to genetic obesity were carried out in PubMed and EMBASE between 10 June and 10 August 2012, using Medical Subject Heading Terms and relevant keywords. To ensure relevance to the modern day clinical setting, literature searches were limited to articles published since 1 January 2000. Older, historically significant, articles identified by the authors were also included. Only articles from the peer-reviewed literature were included in the literature search. Articles in a non-English language were not included. Abstracts from industry-sponsored meetings were not included.

2. Hypothesis for etiology of the obesity epidemic

Currently, there are quite a few theories that intend to explain the etiology of human obesity: the thrifty gene hypothesis, the fetal programming hypothesis, the predation release hypothesis, the sedentary lifestyle hypothesis, the ethnic shift hypothesis, the increased reproductive fitness hypothesis, the assortative mating hypothesis, and the complex hypothesis [17]. However, an acceptable consensus in the field is still lacking, probably due to the fact that the development of obesity comes from highly complex interactions. The vast majority of genetic factors are presumed to affect body weight enough to cause obesity, only when specific environmental conditions pertain.

The thrifty gene hypothesis was proposed by Neel in 1962 [18] and suggests we evolved genes for efficient food collection and fat deposition, in order to survive periods of famine. Now, that food is continuously available, these genes are disadvantageous because they make us obese in preparation for a famine that never comes. In respect to this hypothesis, natural selection favored individuals carrying thrifty alleles that promote the storage of fat and energy. Polynesians likely experienced long periods of cold stress and starvation during their settlement of the Pacific and today have high rates of obesity and type 2 diabetes, possibly due to past positive selection for thrifty alleles [19].

A growing body of empirical evidence suggests the concept of *fetal programming* of health and disease risk. The origins of obesity and metabolic dysfunction can be traced back to the intrauterine period of life, at which time the developing fetus is influenced by suboptimal conditions during critical periods of cellular proliferation, differentiation, and maturation by producing structural and functional changes in cells, tissues and organ systems. These changes, in turn, may have long-term consequences to increase the individual's risk for developing obesity and metabolic dysfunction [20–23]. The major nutrition-related pathways discussed in the current literature relate to the effects of maternal nutritional insults on maternal-placental-fetal glucose/insulin physiology and their downstream effects on the developing brain and peripheral systems in the fetal compartment. Also, the potential role of intrauterine stress and stress biology is brought up for discussion in developmental programming of health and disease susceptibility [23]. In the early 1990s, Hales and Barker et al. [24], published a paper in Diabetologia postulating that not only type 2 diabetes, but also the key components of the metabolic syndrome, seemed to have at least parts of their origin in early life. Authors proved, in an unselected population sample (407 men) from Hertfordshire, UK, a direct link between low weight at birth and increased risks of developing type 2 diabetes, hypertension, elevated triglycerides and insulin resistance later in life. Thus, showing the role of fetal programming in itself and equally as important, the notion that fetal programming could represent a significant player in the origin of type 2 diabetes, the metabolic syndrome and cardiovascular disease. However, the extent to which the global diabetes epidemic may be driven by a mismatch between being born with a low birth weight and the fast propagation of overnutrition and physical inactivity, seen over recent years in developing countries, needs to be further determined [25].

The *predation release hypothesis*, also called the "drifty gene" hypothesis, is opposing the thrifty gene hypothesis, because famines are relatively infrequent modern phenomena that involve insufficient mortality for thrifty genes to propagate. Speakman suggests that early hominids would have been subjected to stabilizing selection for body fatness, with obesity selected against the risk of predation. Around two million years ago predation was removed as a significant factor by the development of social behavior, weapons, and fire. The absence of predation led to a change in the population distribution of body fatness due to random mutations and drift. This novel hypothesis involves random drift, rather than directed selection, thus, explaining why, even in Western society, most people are not obese [26,27].

The *sedentary lifestyle* together with excessive energy intake is the most popular etiologic hypothesis for the worldwide increasing prevalence of overweight and obesity [28–30].

The *ethnic shift hypothesis*, claims the mounting obesity rates are due to disproportionate prevalence in the fastest growing ethnicities (namely Hispanic Americans) [31,32].

The *increased reproductive fitness hypothesis* is also debated as a possible cause for obesity epidemic. Reproductive fitness can be defined as the capacity to pass on one's DNA. It is postulated that body mass index-associated reproductive fitness (natural selection) increases obesity prevalence, due to the fact that BMI has a genetic component and because individuals genetically predisposed toward higher BMIs, reproduce at a higher rate, than do individuals genetically predisposed toward lower BMIs [33–35].

The *assortative mating hypothesis* proposed by Hebebrand et al. [36] emphasizes the fact that the current obesity epidemic has a genetic component mediated by increased rates of assortative mating for body fatness. Theoretically, the genetic consequences of assortative mating for complex traits, such as obesity, are expected to become more significant as the correlation between genotype and phenotype (penetrance) increases, even if rates of assortative mating remain constant across generations [37,38]. Spouse concordance for obesity was associated with a 20-fold higher obesity risk for biologic offspring compared with children of concordantly non-obese parents [37].

The *complex hypothesis* focuses on the shared nature of common alleles in related common disorders, including obesity. This model, the common variants/multiple disease hypothesis, emphasizes that many disease genes may not be disease specific. Common deleterious alleles, found at a relatively high frequency in the population may play a cumulative role in related clinical phenotypes in the context of different genetic backgrounds and under different environmental conditions [39].

Genes can favor fat accumulation in a given environment by increased desire to overeat; the tendency to be sedentary; a diminished ability to utilize dietary fats as fuel; an enlarged, easily stimulated capacity to store body fat. The variation in how people respond to the same environmental conditions is an additional indication that genes play an important role in the development of obesity [40]. This is also consistent with the notion that obesity results from genetic variation interacting with shifting environmental conditions. The influence of genes ranges from polygenic genetic predisposition with impact on appetite, metabolism, and the deposition of fat, to rare monogenic disorders where obesity is the primary feature. Arduous efforts have been made by the scientific society to better understand the physiological basis of obesity. Crucial to this research is the inquiry of how does our body control ingestion, digestion, absorption, and metabolism and how nutrients are distributed among various tissues, organs, and systems [41]. Simultaneously, there is a growing interest regarding the role of genetics in further explaining feeding regulatory systems [14].

3. Genetic research methods used for identification of obesity susceptibility genes

The genetic contribution to common obesity has been established initially through family, twin, and adoption studies. Twin studies have shown a relatively high heritability ranging from 40%-77% [12–14]. However, the search for obesity susceptibility genes has been an arduous task. Gene identification for the last 15 years has been based on two broad genetic epidemiological approaches (candidate gene and genome-wide linkage methods). Recently, genome-wide association studies have brought great information on obesity related genes.

Candidate gene methods

The candidacy of a gene for obesity is based on the following resources: animal models using gene knockout and transgenic approaches; cellular model systems showing their role in metabolic pathways involved in glucose metabolism; linkage and positional cloning studies using extreme cases. This approach emphasizes on an association between a variant or mutation within or near the candidate gene and a trait of interest (such as obesity). Candidate gene approach needs to be on a large scale and well powered, in order to detect the expected small effects of genetic variants involved in common traits and disease [42].

The latest update of the Human Obesity Gene Map reported 127 candidate genes for obesity-related traits. Results of large-scale studies suggest that obesity is strongly associated with genetic variants in the melanocortin-4 receptor (MC4R) gene, leptin gene, adrenergic $\beta 3$ receptor (ADRB3) gene, prohormone convertase 1 (PCSK1) gene, brain-derived neurotrophic factor (BDNF) gene, and endocannabinoid receptor 1 (CNR1) gene [43,44].

Genome-wide linkage studies

Genome-wide linkage studies, through surveying the whole genome, aim to identify new, unanticipated genetic variants associated with a disease or trait of interest. Genome-wide linkage studies rely on the relatedness of study participants and test whether certain chromosomal regions cosegregate with a disease or trait across generations [42]. The latest Human Obesity Gene Map update reported 253 loci from 61 genome-wide linkage scans, of which 15 loci have been replicated in at least three studies [45]. Yet, none of these replicated loci could be narrowed down sufficiently to pinpoint the genes or variants that underline the linkage signal.

Genome-wide association studies

Genome-wide association studies are used in genetics research to look for associations between many (typically hundreds of thousands) of specific genetic variations (most commonly, single nucleotide polymorphisms -SNP) and particular diseases or traits. Similar to genome-wide linkage, the genome-wide association approach sweeps the entire genome, unrestricted by prior assumptions. Genome-wide association studies screen the whole genome at higher resolution levels than genome-wide linkage studies and are capable to narrow down the associated locus more accurately. The genome-wide association approach has effectively replaced genome-wide linkage approach for common disease [42].

Recent success of genome-wide association studies has drawn a lot of attention. High-density multistage genome-wide association analyses have so far discovered ~30 loci consistently associated with BMI and obesity-related traits. The strongest signal remains the association with variants within FTO (the fat-mass and obesity-related gene). Other signals near BDNF, SH2B1, and NEGR1 (all implicated in aspects of neuronal function),further support the idea that obesity is a disorder of hypothalamic function [42].

4. The influential role of genes in obesity

The strongest risk factor for childhood and adolescent obesity is parental obesity [46]. The risk becomes especially elevated if both parents are obese [47]. However, obesity inheritance does not usually follow classic Mendelian patterns. A combination of gene mutations, deletions and single nucleotide polymorphisms are all known to contribute to obesity. Most cases are polygenic, the result of multiple genes interacting with a shifting environment. Each "obesity gene" only makes a small contribution to phenotype, but collectively, inherited genetic variations play a major role in determining body mass and how the body maintains a balance between physical activity and nutrition. While obesity is most commonly associated with polygenic inheritance, there are other instances in which the cause is monogenic or syndromic. Monogenic obesity typically is caused by a single gene mutation with severe obesity as the main symptom. Syndromic obesity, on the other hand, has many characteristics, of which obesity is one symptom [48].

A. Monogenic obesity, that is the obesity associated with a single gene mutation. In these cases single gene variants are sufficient by themselves to cause obesity in food abundant societies. Patients with monogenic obesity usually show extremely severe phenotypes characterized by early childhood obesity onset, often associated with additional behavioral, developmental or endocrine disorders, like hyperphagia and hypogonadism. Significant developmental delays, however, are not commonly seen.

B. Syndromic obesity includes some disorders with Mendelian inheritance, in which patients are clinically obese and are additionally characterized by mental retardation, dysmorfic features, and organ-specific developmental abnormalities.

C. Polygenic obesity, the very common kind of obesity, which concerns the great majority of obese children, arises when an individual's genetic make-up is susceptible to an environment that promotes energy consumption over energy expenditure [49].

A. Monogenic obesity

A "monogene" is by textbook definition, a gene with a strong effect on the phenotype (Mendelian traits or Mendelian - single gene conditions), giving rise to a one-on-one relationship between genotype and phenotype. A "major gene" is defined as a gene harboring, a variant which is associated with a high lifetime risk for a disease. Modifier genes and environmental factors additionally play a role in the etiology of the respective diseases [50].

The genetic causes of monogenic obesity tend to be related to the leptin-melanocortin pathway. This pathway is critical for energy balance and food intake; a disruption in this pathway will lead to severe obesity. Energy homeostasis involves the integration of afferent signals from fat (leptin) and pancreatic beta cells (insulin) and meal-related afferent signals from the gut. These inputs are integrated within the brain and regulate food intake, energy expenditure, energy partitioning and neuroendocrine status. Table 1. summarizes the peptides proposed to affect appetite regulation (adapted from Burrage and McCandless 2007) [51].

Leptin is an adipocyte-derived hormone that is secreted proportionally to body fat content, it crosses the blood–brain barrier, and stimulates a subset of neurons in the hypothalamus to produce peptides that reduce feeding and promote increased energy expenditure (leptin–melanocortin pathway). Additionally, leptin inhibits hypothalamic neurons that produce peptides promoting feeding and decreased energy expenditure.

Attention has focused on identifying the molecular events that lie downstream of the leptin receptor in hypothalamic target neurons. In particular, neurons within the hypothalamus act as primary sensors of alterations in energy stores to control appetite and energy homeostasis. Pro-opiomelanocortin (POMC) neurons produce the *anorectic* peptide a-MSH (a-melanocyte stimulating hormone) together with CART (cocaine and amphetamine-related transcript), whilst a separate group expresses the *orexigens:* neuropeptide Y (NPY) and agouti-related protein (AGRP). AGRP is a hypothalamic neuropeptide that is a potent melanocortin-3 receptor (MC3R) and melanocortin-4 receptor (MC4R) antagonist. Activation of the NPY/AGRP neurons increases food intake and decreases energy expenditure, whereas activation of the POMC neurons decreases food intake and increases energy expenditure [52].

Compounds Mainly Acting to Increase Energy Intake (Orexic)	
Central Nervous System	*Peripheral*
Neuropeptide Y	Ghrelin
Melanin-concentrating hormone (MCH)	
Orexins/hypocretins	
Agouti-related peptide (AGRP)	
Galanin	
Endogenous opioids	
Endocannabinoids	
Compounds Mainly Acting to Reduce Energy Intake (Anorexic)	
Central Nervous System	*Peripheral*
Cocaine- and amphetamine- related transcript (CART)	Leptin
Melanocortins (POMC)	Peptide YY
Corticotropin-releasing factor (CRF)	Cholecystokinin (CCK)
Insulin	Insulin
Serotonin	Amylin
Glucagon-like peptides	Glucagon-like peptides
Neurotensin	Bombesin

Table 1. Peptides proposed to affect appetite regulation. adapted from Burrage and McCandless, 2007

The cumulative prevalence of monogenic obesity among children with severe obesity is about 5% [44]. Several monogenic disorders resulting from disruption of the leptin–melanocortin pathway have been identified. In these disorders, severe obesity of early onset is itself the predominant presenting feature, although often accompanied by characteristic patterns of neuroendocrine dysfunction. Mutations in the melanocortin-4 receptor gene (*MC4R*) and the leptin receptor gene (*LEPR*) have been reported in about 2.5 % and 1.5 % of children with severe obesity. An additional 0.5 % of cases can be attributed to a chromosome 16p11.2 deletion where a gene known as *SH2B1* is deleted [48].

Congenital leptin deficiency

In 1997 two severely obese cousins were reported from a highly consanguineous family of Pakistani origin [53]. Despite their severe obesity, both children had undetectable levels of serum leptin and a mutation in the gene encoding leptin. Leptin deficiency is associated with hyperphagia and increased energy intake. Other phenotypic features include hypogonadotropic hypogonadism, elevated plasma insulin, T-cell abnormalities, and advanced bone age [54].

The role of leptin in some monogenic forms of obesity was further supported by the striking effect of leptin replacement in an extremely obese child with congenital leptin deficiency. In a 9-year-old boy with congenital leptin deficiency, daily subcutaneous injection of recombinant human leptin for a year, led to a complete reversal of obesity, with sustained fat-mass loss. Moreover, partial leptin deficiency in 13 Pakistani subjects, due to a heterozygous frame shift mutation in the leptin gene, was found to be associated with increased body fat [55,56]. However, only a handful of families with extreme forms of obesity in early infancy have mutations in these genes [57].

Mutation in the leptin receptor

Shortly after leptin deficiency was discovered, a similar phenotype, but with elevated plasma leptin levels, was identified [58]. The cause was a homozygous mutation in the leptin receptor. A later study suggested that approximately 3% of severe morbid obesity in a population including both non-consanguineous and consanguineous families could be explained by mutations in the leptin receptor [59].

Melanocortin-4 receptor deficiency (MC4R)

Mutations in another component of the leptin–melanocortin pathway melanocortin-4 receptor have also been associated with obesity. MC4R deficiency represents the most common monogenic obesity disorder that has been identified so far. It is present in about 5-6% of obese individuals from different ethnic groups, with a higher prevalence in cases with increased severity and earlier age of onset [60,61]. Affected subjects exhibit hyperphagia, but this is not as severe as that seen in leptin deficiency, although it often starts in the first year of life. Alongside the increase in fat mass, MC4R-deficient subjects also have an increase in lean mass, that is not seen in leptin deficiency and a marked increase in bone mineral density. The accelerated linear growth is apparently not related to a dysfunction of the GH axis and may be a consequence of the disproportionate early hyperinsulinaemia. Interestingly, both heterozygous and homozygous mutations in MC4R have been implicated in obesity, but extreme obesity is incompletely penetrant in heterozygous patients. In other words, some individuals with a single copy of the mutation are obese, whereas others are not obese [51].

Currently, there is no specific therapy for MC4R deficiency, however, it is highly likely that these subjects would respond well to pharmacotherapy that overcame the reduction in the hypothalamic melanocortinergic tone that exists in these patients [12].

Pro-opiomelanocortin (POMC) deficiency

Small numbers of patients have been described with mutations in the gene encoding pro-opiomelanocortin, which is involved in the leptin-melanocortin pathway [62,63]. In neonatal life, these patients present with adrenal crisis due to ACTH deficiency (POMC is a precursor of ACTH in the pituitary), also, the children have pale skin and red hair due to the lack of MSH action at melanocortin-1 receptors in the skin and hair follicles. POMC deficiency results in hyperphagia and early-onset obesity due to loss of melanocortin signaling at the melanocortin-4 receptor (MC4R) [12].

Prohormone convertase-1 (PC1) deficiency

Jackson et al described a woman with severe early-onset obesity, hypogonadotropic hypogonadism, postprandial hypoglycaemia, hypocortisolemia, and evidence of impaired processing of POMC and proinsulin who was a compound heterozygote for prohormone convertase-1 mutations [63].

Although great hope was invested in the studies of patients with early-onset severe obesity, they have revealed the identity of very few genes associated with obesity. Interestingly, the few gene mutations associated with morbid obesity appear to influence body weight primarily by altering appetite. Some of the molecules may also impact activity, but this has not yet been shown to be a significant contributor to obesity. A significant limitation of the strategy of focusing on morbid obesity is that mutations or genetic variants in these genes may not be associated with more common forms of the condition [51].

B. Syndromic obesity

Syndromic obesity is represented by at least 20 rare syndromes (shown in Table 2), that are caused by discrete genetic defects or chromosomal abnormalities, both autosomal and X-linked, that are characterized by obesity. Most of these obesity syndromes associate mental retardation.

It was expected that the syndromic forms of obesity could help unravel novel genes relevant for idiopathic obesity. However, although the genes for several of the syndromic forms have been detected, the relevance of these genes for general obesity is still unclear [45,57].

1	Achondroplasia
2	Alström Syndrome
3	Bannayan-Riley-Ruvalcaba Syndrome
4	Beckwith-Wiedemann Syndrome
5	Biedl Bardet Syndrome
6	Borjeson-Forssman-Lehmann Syndrome
7	Carpenter syndrome
8	CDG 1a
9	Cohen Syndrome
10	Fragile X Syndrome
11	Mehmo Syndrome
12	Meningomyelocoele
13	Prader Willi Syndrome
14	Psdeuohypoparathyroidism 1a
15	Simpson-Golabi-Behmel Syndrome
16	Smith-Magenis Syndrome
17	Sotos Syndrome
18	Wilson-Turner Syndrome
19	Ulnar-Mammary Schinzel Syndrome
20	Weaver Syndrome

Table 2. Syndromes characterized by obesity.

Prader–Willi syndrome

Prader–Willi syndrome (PWS) is the most frequent of these syndromes (1 in 25,000 births). It is an autosomal-dominant disorder, characterized by obesity, hyperphagia, muscular hypotonia, mental retardation, short stature and hypogonadotropic hypogonadism. It is usually caused by a paternally inherited deletion at the chromosomal region 15q11.2–q12, and less frequently by maternal uniparental disomy (Orphanet). The cause of hyperphagia in PWS is not proven, although PWS phenotypes are consistent with a combined hypothalamic impairment, causing several endocrine abnormalities. Also, it was suggested that the elevated production of the stomach secreted peptide ghrelin seen in PWS might increase appetite by interacting with the POMC/CART and NPY hypothalamic neurons [57].

Single Minded Homologue 1 (SIM-1)

The loss of the single minded homologue 1 (SIM1) gene has also been associated with hyperphagia in syndromic obesity. This gene encodes a transcription factor that has a pivotal role in neurogenesis. In humans, deletion or disruption of the SIM1 region results in either a "Prader–Willi-like" phenotype or a form of early-onset obesity, associated with excessive food intake [64].

WAGR Syndrome

The WAGR syndrome (Wilms tumor, aniridia, genitourinary anomalies and mental retardation syndrome and obesity) is caused by heterozygous contiguous gene deletions that involve at least two genes, *WT1* and *PAX6*, which are present in the 11p13 region. Although persons with the WAGR syndrome typically have low-normal birth weight, marked obesity subsequently develops in a substantial subgroup [65].

Pseudohypoparathyroidism type 1A (PHP1A)

PHP1A syndrome is due to a maternally transmitted mutation in GNAS1, which encodes the α-subunit of the Gs protein. Food-intake abnormalities in patients with this syndrome might be due to the expression of the resulting variant Gs protein in the hypothalamic circuitry that controls energy balance, which involves many G-protein coupled receptors [66].

Bardet–Biedl syndrome (BBS)

Bardet–Biedl syndrome is characterized by six main features: Rod-Cone Dystrophy (the most frequent phenotype), polydactyly, learning disabilities, hypogonadism in males, renal abnormalities and obesity. In BBS patients, obesity has early onset, usually arising within the first few years of life. However, one study of post-pubertal BBS patients found that only 52% were clinically obese; therefore, this syndrome can present with a heterogeneous phenotype [67].

Albright's hereditary osteodystrophy

Albright's hereditary osteodystrophy describes a constellation of physical features, including short adult stature, obesity, brachydactyly, and ectopic ossifications. It is an autosomal dominant disorder due to germline mutations in GNAS1, which encodes for a-subunit of the stimulatory G protein (Gsa) [68].

Fragile X syndrome

Fragile X syndrome is characterized by moderate to severe mental retardation, macroorchidism, large ears, macrocephaly, prominent jaw (mandibular prognathism), high-pitched jocular speech and obesity. Fragile X syndrome is an X-linked, single gene disorder caused by dysfunction in the transcription of the *FMR1* gene that codes for fragile X mental retardation protein (FMRP) [69].

Borjeson–Forssman–Lehmann syndrome

Borjeson, Forssman and Lehmann described a syndrome characterized by moderate to severe mental retardation, epilepsy, hypogonadism, and obesity with marked gynecomastia [70]. Mutations in a novel, widely expressed zinc-finger gene plant homeodomain (PHD)-like finger (PHF6) have been identified in affected families, although the functional properties of this protein remain unclear [71].

Alstrom syndrome

Alstrom syndrome is a homogeneous autosomal recessive disorder that is characterized by childhood obesity associated with hyperinsulinaemia, chronic hyperglycemia and neurosensory deficits. Subsets of affected individuals present with additional features such as dilated cardiomyopathy, hepatic dysfunction, hypothyroidism, male hypogonadism, short stature and mild to moderate developmental delay. Symptoms first appear in infancy and progressive development of multi-organ pathology leads to a reduced life expectancy. Variability in age of onset and severity of clinical symptoms, even within families, is likely due to genetic background. Mutations in a single gene, ALMS1, have been found to be responsible for all cases of Alstrom syndrome [72].

C. Complex polygenic obesity

Complex polygenic obesity represents the end result of behavioral, environmental, and genetic factors that may influence individual responses to diet and physical activity. Changes in our environment over the last decades, in particular the unlimited supply of cheap, highly palatable, energy-dense foods; plus a sedentary lifestyle, the so called "obesogenic" environment together with a genetic susceptibility are the culprits for today's obesity epidemic [73].

Compared with obesity syndromes or single-gene obesity, the recent rapid increase in prevalence of childhood obesity suggests that environmental factors most likely have a larger impact on body weight in common obesity patients, although individual responses to these environmental factors are influenced by genetic factors -"susceptibility genes".

Some traits can be due to simultaneous presence of DNA variation in multiple genes. Any of a group of alleles, at distinct gene loci that collectively control the inheritance of a quantitative phenotype or modify the expression of a qualitative character, are termed "polygenic" variants. It is generally assumed that for quantitative traits, each allele has a small effect, but the allelic effects can be additive or non-additive. Potentially, many such polygenic variants play a role in body weight regulation. It is estimated that the total number of genes with a small effect most likely exceeds 100 [50].

SNP	Chr	Position	Nearest gene	Sample size in original publication	Frequency of the risk allele	Effect on BMI in the original publication
rs2815752	1	72,524,461	NEGR1	32,387	62% (A)	+0.10 kg/m2 per A allele[b]
rs2568958	1	72,537,704	NEGR1	25,344	58% (A)	+0.43 kg/m2 for AA genotype[c]
rs10913469	1	176,180,142	SEC16B,RASAL2	25,344	20% (C)	+0.50 kg/m2 for CC genotype[c]
rs6548238	2	624,905	TMEM18	32,387	84% (C)	+0.26 kg/m2 per C allele[b]
rs7561317	2	634,953	TMEM18	25,344	84% (G)	+0.70 kg/m2 for GG genotype[c]
rs7566605	2	118,552,495	INSIG2	9,881	37% (C)	+1.00 kg/m2 for CC genotype
rs7647305	3	187,316,984	SFRS10, ETV5, DGKG	25,344	77% (C)	+0.54 kg/m2 for CC genotype[c]
rs10938397	4	45,023,455	GNPDA2	32,387	48% (G)	+0.19 kg/m2 per G allele[b]
rs4712652	6	22,186,593	PRL	2,796	41% (A)	+0.031 kg/m2 per A allele in children[d]
rs10508503	10	16,339,956	PTER	2,796	8.5% (C)	+0.144 kg/m2 per C allele in children[d]
rs6265 (V66M)	11	27,636,492	BDNF	25,344	85% (G)	+0.67 kg/m2 for GG genotype[c]
rs10838738	11	47,619,625	MTCH2	32,387	34% (G)	+0.07 kg/m2 per G allele[b]
rs7138803	12	48,533,735	BCDIN3D, FAIM2	25,344	37% (A)	+0.54 kg/m2 for AA genotype[c]
rs7498665	16	28,790,742	SH2B1	32,387	41% (G)	+0.15 kg/m2 per G allele[b]
rs7498665	16	28,790,742	SH2B1, ATP2A1	25,344	44% (G)	+0.45 kg/m2 for GG genotype[c]
rs8050136	16	52,373,776	FTO	25,344	41% (A)	+1.07 kg/m2 for AA genotype[c]
rs9939609	16	52,378,028	FTO	38,759	40% (A)	+0.40 kg/m2 per A allele
rs9939609	16	52,378,028	FTO	32,387	41% (A)	+0.33 kg/m2 per A allele[b]
rs1421085	16	52,358,455	FTO	2,796	40% (C)	+0.112 kg/m2 per C allele[d]
rs1424233	16	78,240,251	MAF	2,796	43% (A)	+0.091 kg/m2 per A allele in children[d]
rs1805081	18	19,394,429	NPC1	2,796	44% (A)	-0.087 kg/m2 per A allele in children[d]
rs17782313	18	56,002,077	MC4R	16,876	24% (C)	+0.22 kg/m2 per C allele
rs17782313	18	56,002,077	MC4R	32,387	22% (C)	+0.22 kg/m2 per C allele[b]
rs17782313	18	56,002,077	MC4R	2,796	17,5% (C)	+0.097 kg/m2 per C alleled
rs12970134	18	56,035,730	MC4R	25,344	30% (A)	+0.36 kg/m2 for AA genotypec
rs52820871 (I251L)	18	56,189,806	MC4R	16,797	0.75% (251L)	-0.35 SD of their BMI Z-score/ 251L allele
rs2229616 (V103I)	18	56,190,256	MC4R	7,713	2% (103I)	-0.48 kg/m2 per 103I allele
rs29941	19	39,001,372	CHST8,KCTD15	25,344	70% (C)	+0.46 kg/m2 for CC genotype[c]
rs11084753	19	39,013,977	KCTD15	32,387	67% (G)	+0.06 kg/m2 per G allele[b]

Table 3. [a] Either in the GWAS or the initial sample [b] Reported in the population-based cohorts EPIC, FINRISK97, BPPP and METSIM (N = 18,812) [c] Reported for the Islandic sample (N = 25,344) [d] Reported for children from the Northern Finland Birth Cohort (N = 5,291)NEGR1: neuronal growth factor regulator 1; SEC16B; cerevisiae, homolog of, B; RASAL2: RAS protein activator like 2; TMEM18: transmembrane protein 18, INSIG2: insulin induced gene 2, SFRS10: splicing factor, arginine/serine-rich, 10; ETV5:etsvariant 5; DGKG diacylglycerol kinase, gamma, 90kD, GNPDA2: glucosamine-6-phosphate deaminase 2; PRL: prolactin; PTER: phosphotriesterase related; BDNF: brain derived neurotrophic factor; MTCH2: mitochondrial carrier homolog 2 (C. elegans); BCDIN3D: BCDIN3 domain containing; FAIM2: Fas apoptotic inhibitory molecule 2; SH2B1: SH2B adaptor protein 1; ATP2A1: ATPase, Ca++ transporting, cardiac muscle, fast twitch 1; FTO: fat mass and obesity associated; MAF: v-maf musculoaponeurotic fibrosarcoma oncogene homolog (avian); NPC1: Niemann-Pick disease, type C1; MC4R: melanocortin 4 receptor; CHST8: carbohydrate (N-acetylgalactosamine 4-0) sulfotransferase 8; KCTD15: potassium channel tetramerisation domain containing 15Genetic variants with a polygenic effect on body weight in humans [50]

A large number of candidate gene association studies, of variable power, have been searched in obesity and related phenotypes. By far the most strongly replicated candidate gene from these analyses is melanocortin 4 receptor, but other replicated associations include those with adipokine and adipokine receptor genes. Further confirming the central role of behavioral stimuli in obesity, alleles of genes encoding dopamine, serotonin, and cannabinoid receptors (DRD2, HTR2C, and CBI) [74–76] are also reported to be associated with feeding behavior and related traits.

Genome-wide association studies have led to the identification of new candidate genes in obesity, most notably the "fat mass and obesity associated" gene (FTO). Rodent studies indicate that FTO mRNA is highly expressed in brain areas important for regulation of energy- and reward driven consumption. Food deprivation alters FTO expression in the hypothalamus in rats and mice. The contribution of the FTO variant is fairly modest, with adult homozygotes for the risk allele having only a 2- to 3-kg increase in weight [77], but the obesity high-risk allele is common in Caucasian populations and its effects begin early in life. Higher fat mass is observable from the age of 2 weeks, and carriage of the allele is associated with higher BMI and reduced satiety in children [11,50].

Other loci detected in genome wide association studies were identified in large study groups and via meta-analyses. Genome wide association studies (GWAS) reported novel obesity genes with small effects on human body weight. A total of more than 150,000 individuals was analyzed. Hinney et al. made a comprehensive review of these new loci in their paper published in 2010 in European Child Adolescent Psychiatry, see Table 3-adapted from Hinney et al [50].

Alternatively, the missing heritability may be accounted for by other genetic factors like genomic copy number variation and epigenetic modifications.

5. Epigenetics

Some people have a different response of to environmental conditions and this may be the result of genetic variation alone, but there is increasing recognition that genetic expression related to disease risk may be modified by the environment during development. The "epigenetic changes" include methylation and alterations to histone proteins that alter the likelihood that specific genes are transcribed. Epigenetic changes usually occur during prenatal development or the early postnatal period. Maternal nutrition is a major factor leading to epigenetic changes. Thus, the levels of vitamins consumed in pregnancy, such as folate, methionine, and vitamin B12, which affect methylation become very important [78]. Undernutrition during prenatal development has been suggested to lead to postnatal consumption of a fatty diet. On the other hand, overnutrition of the mother is just as influential. The most convincingly shown factor is glycemic status during pregnancy. Hyperglycemia clearly affects infants' birth weight but, beyond its effects on body weight, may increase the risk for subsequent development of insulin resistance and obesity. Nutritional signals reaching the developing hypothalamus during pregnancy may influence the sensitivity of these neurons to respond to similar signals postnatally. Infant nutrition in the neonatal period may also potentially affect future risk for obesity and its complications [79].

6. Assessment of the obese child

In order to establish the diagnosis of overweight or obese in a child, the clinician must evaluate the BMI and compare it to the standardized reference chart, appropriate for the age and sex of the child. According to World Health Organization the definition of overweight and obesity in children is established at the following cut-offs [80]:

Overweight: >+1Standard Deviations (equivalent to BMI 25 kg/m^2 at 19 years)

Obesity: >+2 Standard Deviations (equivalent to BMI 30 kg/m^2 at 19 years).

The cumulative prevalence of monogenic obesity among children with severe obesity is about 5%. There are a lot of genes implicated in obesity and too many obese patients in the world to perform molecular study for everyone. Most genetic and hormonal causes of obesity are rare. The decision to test for these abnormalities should depend upon the presence of particular phenotypes and clinical features suggesting the possibility of a diagnosable disorder [table 4). The presence of severe obesity in a young child (<5 yr old) associated to extreme hyperphagia, severe insulin resistance disproportionate for the degree of obesity and a positive family history of early-onset obesity may support a genetic analysis.

History	Suggested Diagnosis
Early onset (!!! 5 years of age)	genetic disorders
Visual impairment and deafness	genetic disorders
Primary hypogonadotropic hypogonadism or hypogenitalism	genetic disorders
Family history: consanguineous relationships, other children affected	genetic disorders
Hyperphagia-often denied, ask specific questions such as waking at night to eat, demanding food very soon after a meal	if severe, suggests a genetic cause for obesity
Mood disturbance and central obesity	Cushing's syndrome
Frequent infections and fatigue	ACTH deficiency due to POMC mutations
Dry skin, constipation, intolerance to cold, or fatigue	hypothyroidism
Developmental delay	behavioral disorders
Short duration of obesity	endocrine or central cause
Onset and tempo of pubertal development	endocrine disorders
Damage to the CNS (e.g. infection, trauma, hemorrhage, radiation therapy, seizures)	hypothalamic obesity, pituitary GH deficiency or pituitary hypothyroidism

History	Suggested Diagnosis
Morning headaches, vomiting, visual disturbances, excessive urination or drinking	tumor or mass in the hypothalamus
Treatment with certain drugs or medications known to promote weight gain	obesity related to drugs
Examination	**Suggested Diagnosis**
Dysmorphic features or skeletal dysplasia	genetic disorders
Red hair (if not familial)	mutations in POMC in white Caucasians
Tall stature (on the upper centiles)	common obesity, but also MC4R deficiency
Selective fat deposition (60%)	leptin and leptin receptor deficiency
Short stature or a reduced rate of linear growth	GH deficiency, hypothyroidism, cortisol excess, pseudohypoparathyroidism, or a genetic syndrome such as Prader–Willi
Central body fat distribution with purple striae	Cushing's syndrome
Diminished growth rate and pubertal development	growth hormone deficiency, hypothyroidism, cortisol excess, and genetic syndromes
Accelerated growth rate and pubertal development	precocious puberty and some girls with PCOS
Acanthosis nigricans	insulin resistance
Investigations when clinically indicated	
- Fasting and 2-hour glucose and insulin levels - Proinsulin if PC-1 deficiency considered - Fasting lipid panel - Thyroid function tests - Serum leptin - Karyotype, DNA for molecular diagnosis - Bone age, Growth hormone (GH) secretion and function tests, when indicated - Assessment of reproductive hormones, when indicated - Serum calcium, phosphorus, and parathyroid hormone levels to evaluate for suspected pseudohypoparathyroidism - MRI scan of the brain with focus on the hypothalamus and pituitary - ACTH, adrenocorticotropic hormone; - POMC, pro-opiomelanocortin; MAOI, monoamine oxidase inhibitor; MC4R, melanocortin-4 receptor; PC-1, prohormone convertase-1.	

Table 4. Assessment of the obese child.

7. Conclusions

Obesity is caused by complex interactions between environment, behavior and genetic predisposition. The increased heath risk that obesity brings is well established by now. There is growing evidence that genetic predisposition presents a cornerstone role in the development of obesity. Nevertheless, despite the enormous success of genetic studies, there are still important gaps in knowledge. Obesity-specific gene expression pattern may help in understanding the pathogenic mechanisms of obesity and its associated metabolic diseases. Recent advances in identifying genetic risk factors for obesity have contributed to understanding disease pathology, which, in term, may lead to development of new therapeutic strategies, including personalized medicine. In the everyday practice of a clinician, when facing a patient with obesity, it is important to identify particular phenotypes and clinical features that can help to recognize the children who need genetic screening.

Author details

Maria Puiu[1*], Adela Chirita Emandi[2] and Smaranda Arghirescu[2]

*Address all correspondence to: maria_puiu@umft.ro

1 University of Medicine and Pharmacy "Victor Babes" Timisoara - Genetics Department; Emergency Hospital for Children "Louis Turcanu" Timisoara - Genetics Department, Romania

2 University of Medicine and Pharmacy "Victor Babes" Timisoara - Pediatrics Department; Emergency Hospital for Children "Louis Turcanu" Timisoara - Pediatrics Department, Romania

References

[1] De Onis, M., & Blössner, M. (2000). Prevalence and trends of overweight among preschool children in developing countries. *Am. J. Clin. Nutr. Oct*, 72(4), 1032-9.

[2] Jackson-Leach, R., & Lobstein, T. (2006). Estimated burden of paediatric obesity and co-morbidities in Europe. Part 1. The increase in the prevalence of child obesity in Europe is itself increasing. *Int J Pediatr Obes*, 1(1), 26-32.

[3] John, J., Wenig, C. M., & Wolfenstetter, S. B. (2010). Recent economic findings on childhood obesity: cost-of-illness and cost-effectiveness of interventions. *Curr Opin Clin Nutr Metab Care.*, 13(3), 305-13.

[4] Wang, Y., & Lobstein, T. (2006). Worldwide trends in childhood overweight and obesity. *Int J Pediatr Obes*, 1(1), 11-25.

[5] Muzumdar, H., & Rao, M. (2006). Pulmonary dysfunction and sleep apnea in morbid obesity. *Pediatr Endocrinol Rev.*, 3(4), 579-83.

[6] Ogden, C. L., Yanovski, S. Z., Carroll, M. D., & Flegal, K. M. (2007). The epidemiology of obesity. *Gastroenterology.*, 132(6), 2087-102.

[7] Dabelea, D., Bell, R. A., D'Agostino, R. B., Jr Imperatore, G., Johansen, J. M., Linder, B., et al. (2007). Incidence of diabetes in youth in the United States. *JAMA.*, 297(24), 2716-24.

[8] Baker, J. L., Olsen, L. W., & Sorensen, T. I. A. (2007). Childhood body-mass index and the risk of coronary heart disease in adulthood. *N. Engl. J. Med.*, 357(23), 329-37.

[9] Maffeis, C., & Tatò, L. (2001). Long-term effects of childhood obesity on morbidity and mortality. *Horm. Res*, 55(1), 42-5.

[10] Swallen, K. C., Reither, E. N., Haas, S. A., & Meier, A. M. (2005). Overweight, obesity, and health-related quality of life among adolescents: the National Longitudinal Study of Adolescent Health. *Pediatrics.*, 115(2), 340-7.

[11] Blakemore, A. I. F., & Froguel, P. (2008). Is Obesity Our Genetic Legacy? *J Clin Endocrinol Metab.*, 11(93, 1), S51-56.

[12] Farooqi, I. S. (2005). Genetic and hereditary aspects of childhood obesity. *Best Pract. Res. Clin. Endocrinol. Metab.*, 19(3), 359-74.

[13] O'Rahilly, S., & Farooqi, I. S. (2008). Human obesity as a heritable disorder of the central control of energy balance. *Int J Obes (Lond).*, 32(7), 55-61.

[14] Llewellyn, C. H., van Jaarsveld, C. H. M., Boniface, D., Carnell, S., & Wardle, J. (2008). Eating rate is a heritable phenotype related to weight in children. *Am. J. Clin. Nutr.*, 88(6), 1560-6.

[15] Ogden, C. L., Carroll, M. D., & Flegal, K. M. (2008). High body mass index for age among US children and adolescents, 2003-2006. *JAMA.*, 299(20), 2401-5.

[16] de Onis, M., Blössner, M., Borghi, E., Frongillo, E. A., & Morris, R. (2004). Estimates of Global Prevalence of Childhood Underweight in 1990 and 2015. *JAMA: The Journal of the American Medical Association.*, 291(21), 2600-2606.

[17] Marti, A., Goyenechea, E., & Martínez, J. A. (2010). Nutrigenetics: A Tool to Provide Personalized Nutritional Therapy to the Obese. *In: Simopoulos AP, Milner JA, editors. World Review of Nutrition and Dietetics. Basel: KARGER.*

[18] Neel, J. V. (1962). Diabetes mellitus: a "thrifty" genotype rendered detrimental by "progress"? *Am. J. Hum. Genet.*, 14, 353-62.

[19] Myles, S., Lea, R. A., Ohashi, J., Chambers, G. K., Weiss, J. G., Hardouin, E., et al. (2011). Testing the thrifty gene hypothesis: the Gly482Ser variant in PPARGC1A is associated with BMI in Tongans. *BMC Med Genet.*, 18(12), 10.

[20] Gluckman, P. D., & Hanson, M. A. (2004). Living with the past: evolution, development, and patterns of disease. *Science.*, 305(5691), 1733-6.

[21] Holness, M. J., Langdown, M. L., & Sugden, M. C. (2000). Early-life programming of susceptibility to dysregulation of glucose metabolism and the development of Type 2 diabetes mellitus. *Biochem. J.*, 349 Pt 3, 657-65.

[22] Mc Millen, I. C., & Robinson, J. S. (2005). Developmental origins of the metabolic syndrome: prediction, plasticity, and programming. *Physiol. Rev.*, 85(2), 571-633.

[23] Entringer, S., Buss, C., Swanson, J. M., Cooper, D. M., Wing, D. A., Waffarn, F., et al. (2012). Fetal Programming of Body Composition, Obesity, and Metabolic Function: The Role of Intrauterine Stress and Stress Biology. *J Nutr Metab.*

[24] Barker, D. J., Hales, C. N., Fall, C. H., Osmond, C., Phipps, K., & Clark, P. M. (1993). Type 2 (non-insulin-dependent) diabetes mellitus, hypertension and hyperlipidaemia (syndrome X): relation to reduced fetal growth. *Diabetologia.*, 36(1), 62-7.

[25] Vaag, A. A., Grunnet, L. G., Arora, G. P., & Brons, C. (2012). The thrifty phenotype hypothesis revisited. *Diabetologia.*, 55(8), 2085-8.

[26] Speakman, J. R. (2007). A nonadaptive scenario explaining the genetic predisposition to obesity: the "predation release" hypothesis. *Cell Metab.*, 6(1), 5-12.

[27] Speakman, J. R. (2008). Thrifty genes for obesity, an attractive but flawed idea, and an alternative perspective: the "drifty gene" hypothesis. *Int J Obes (Lond).*, 32(11), 1611-7.

[28] Altenburg, T. M., Singh, A. S., van Mechelen, W., Brug, J., & Chinapaw, M. J. (2012). Direction of the association between body fatness and self-reported screen time in Dutch adolescents. *Int J Behav Nutr Phys Act.*, 24(9), 4.

[29] Rennie, K. L., Johnson, L., & Jebb, S. A. (2005). Behavioural determinants of obesity. *Best Pract. Res. Clin. Endocrinol. Metab.*, 19(3), 343-58.

[30] Pate, R. R., O'Neill, J. R., & Lobelo, F. (2008). The evolving definition of "sedentary. ". *Exerc Sport Sci Rev.*, 36(4), 173-8.

[31] Walley, A. J., Asher, J. E., & Froguel, P. (2009). The genetic contribution to non-syndromic human obesity. Nat. Rev. Genet. Jul; , 10(7), 431-42.

[32] Talbert, M. (2009). Positional Cloning of Adiposity Genes in Ethnic Minorities of the Insulin Resistance Atherosclerosis Family Study.

[33] Keith, S. W., Redden, D. T., Katzmarzyk, P. T., Boggiano, M. M., Hanlon, E. C., Benca, R. M., et al. (2006). Putative contributors to the secular increase in obesity: exploring the roads less traveled. *International Journal of Obesity.*, 30(11), 1585-94.

[34] Weng, H. H., Bastian, L. A., Taylor, D. H., Moser, B. K., & Ostbye, T. (2004). Number of Children Associated with Obesity in Middle-Aged Women and Men: Results from the Health and Retirement Study. *Journal of Women's Health.*, 13(1), 85-91.

[35] Frisch, R. E. (1987). Body fat, menarche, fitness and fertility. *Hum. Reprod.*, 2(6), 521-33.

[36] Hebebrand, J., Wulftange, H., Goerg, T., Ziegler, A., Hinney, A., Barth, N., et al. (2000). Epidemic obesity: are genetic factors involved via increased rates of assortative mating? *International Journal of Obesity.*, 24(3), 345-53.

[37] Jacobson, P., Torgerson, J. S., Sjöström, L., & Bouchard, C. (2007). Spouse Resemblance in Body Mass Index: Effects on Adult Obesity Prevalence in the Offspring Generation. *Am. J. Epidemiol.*, 165(1), 101-8.

[38] Allison, D., Neale, M., Kezis, M., Alfonso, V., Heshka, S., & Heymsfield, S. (1996). Assortative mating for relative weight: Genetic implications. *Behavior Genetics*, 26(2), 103-11.

[39] Becker, K. G. (2004). The common variants/multiple disease hypothesis of common complex genetic disorders. *Medical Hypotheses.*, 62(2), 309-17.

[40] Via, S., & Hawthorne, D. J. (2005). Back to the future: genetic correlations, adaptation and speciation. *Genetica*, 123(1-2), 147-156.

[41] Garaulet, M., & Madrid, J. A. (2010). Chronobiological aspects of nutrition, metabolic syndrome and obesity. *Adv. Drug Deliv. Rev.*, 62(9-10), 967-978.

[42] Cheung, W. W., & Mao, P. (2012). Recent Advances in Obesity: Genetics and Beyond. *ISRN Endocrinol.*

[43] Bochukova, E. G., Huang, N., Keogh, J., Henning, E., Purmann, C., Blaszczyk, K., et al. (2010). Large, rare chromosomal deletions associated with severe early-onset obesity. *Nature*, 463(7281), 666-70.

[44] Perrone, L., Marzuillo, P., Grandone, A., & del Giudice, E. M. Chromosome 16p11.2 deletions: another piece in the genetic puzzle of childhood obesity. *Ital J Pediatr.*, 36, 43.

[45] Rankinen, T., Zuberi, A., Chagnon, Y. C., Weisnagel, S. J., Argyropoulos, G., Walts, B., et al. (2006). The human obesity gene map: the 2005 update. *Obesity (Silver Spring).*, 14(4), 529-644.

[46] Reilly, J. J., Armstrong, J., Dorosty, A. R., Emmett, P. M., Ness, A., Rogers, I., et al. (2005). Early life risk factors for obesity in childhood: cohort study. *BMJ.*, 330(7504), 1357.

[47] Magnusson, P. K. E., & Rasmussen, F. (2002). Familial resemblance of body mass index and familial risk of high and low body mass index. A study of young men in Sweden. *Int. J. Obes. Relat. Metab. Disord.*, 26(9), 1225-31.

[48] Stein, Q. P., Mroch, A. R., De Berg, K. L., & Flanagan, J. D. (2011). The influential role of genes in obesity. *S D Med.* [12-5], 12-5.

[49] Chirita, Emandi. A., Puiu, M., & Micle, I. (2011). Obesity in rare diseases and genetic factors in the "frequent" childhood obesity. *Romanian Journal Of Rare Diseases.*, 1, 22-8.

[50] Hinney, A., Vogel, C. I. G., & Hebebrand, J. (2010). From monogenic to polygenic obesity: recent advances. *Eur Child Adolesc Psychiatry.*, 19(3), 297-310.

[51] Burrage, L. C., & Mc Candless, S. E. (2007). Genetics of childhood obesity. *US Pediatrics Review.*, 1, 60-3.

[52] Schwartz, M. W., Woods, S. C., Porte, D., Jr Seeley, R. J., & Baskin, D. G. (2000). Central nervous system control of food intake. *Nature*, 404(6778), 661-71.

[53] Montague, C. T., Farooqi, I. S., Whitehead, J. P., Soos, Rau. H., Wareham, N. J., et al. (1997). Congenital leptin deficiency is associated with severe early-onset obesity in humans. *Nature*, 387(6636), 903-8.

[54] Farooqi, I. s., & O'Rahilly, S. (2004). Monogenic Human Obesity Syndromes. *Recent Prog Horm Res.*, 59(1), 409-24.

[55] Farooqi, I. S., Jebb, S. A., Langmack, G., Lawrence, E., Cheetham, C. H., Prentice, A. M., et al. (1999). Effects of recombinant leptin therapy in a child with congenital leptin deficiency. *N. Engl. J. Med.*, 341(12), 879-84.

[56] Farooqi, I. S., Keogh, J. M., Kamath, S., Jones, S., Gibson, W. T., Trussell, R., et al. (2001). Partial leptin deficiency and human adiposity. *Nature*, 414(6859), 34-5.

[57] Bell, C. G., Walley, A. J., & Froguel, P. (2005). The genetics of human obesity. *Nat Rev Genet.*, 6(3), 221-34.

[58] Clement, N. D., Duckworth, A. D., Baker, A. D. L., & Porter, D. E. (2012). Skeletal growth patterns in hereditary multiple exostoses: a natural history. *J Pediatr Orthop B.*, 21(2), 150-4.

[59] Farooqi, I. S., Wangensteen, T., Collins, S., Kimber, W., Matarese, G., Keogh, J. M., et al. (2007). Clinical and molecular genetic spectrum of congenital deficiency of the leptin receptor. *N. Engl. J. Med.*, 356(3), 237-47.

[60] Lubrano-Berthelier, C., Durand, E., Dubern, B., Shapiro, A., Dazin, P., Weill, J., et al. (2003). Intracellular retention is a common characteristic of childhood obesity-associated MC4R mutations. *Hum. Mol. Genet.*, 12(2), 145-53.

[61] Farooqi, I. S., Keogh, J. M., Yeo, G. S. H., Lank, E. J., Cheetham, T., & O'Rahilly, S. (2003). Clinical spectrum of obesity and mutations in the melanocortin 4 receptor gene. *N. Engl. J. Med.*, 348(12), 1085-95.

[62] Krude, H., Biebermann, H., Luck, W., Horn, R., Brabant, G., & Grüters, A. (1998). Severe early-onset obesity, adrenal insufficiency and red hair pigmentation caused by POMC mutations in humans. *Nat. Genet.*, 19(2), 155-7.

[63] Jackson, R. S., Creemers, J. W., Ohagi, S., Raffin-Sanson, M. L., Sanders, L., Montague, C. T., et al. (1997). Obesity and impaired prohormone processing associated with mutations in the human prohormone convertase 1 gene. *Nat. Genet.*, 16(3), 303-6.

[64] Faivre, L., Cormier-Daire, V., Lapierre, J. M., Colleaux, L., Jacquemont, S., Geneviéve, D., et al. (2002). Deletion of the SIM1 gene (6q16.2) in a patient with a Prader-Willi-like phenotype. *J. Med. Genet.*, 39(8), 594-6.

[65] Fischbach, B. V., Trout, K. L., Lewis, J., Luis, CA, & Sika, M. (2005). WAGR syndrome: a clinical review of 54 cases. *Pediatrics*, 116(4), 984-8.

[66] Spiegel, A. M., & Weinstein, L. S. (2004). Inherited diseases involving g proteins and g protein-coupled receptors. *Annu. Rev. Med.*, 55, 27-39.

[67] Mutch, D. M., & Clément, K. (2006). Unraveling the Genetics of Human Obesity. *PLoS Genet.*, 2(12).

[68] Weinstein, L. S., Yu, S., Warner, D. R., & Liu, J. (2001). Endocrine Manifestations of Stimulatory G Protein α-Subunit Mutations and the Role of Genomic Imprinting. *Endocrine Reviews.*, 22(5), 675-705.

[69] Verkerk, A. J., Pieretti, M., Sutcliffe, J. S., Fu, Y. H., Kuhl, D. P., Pizzuti, A., et al. (1991). Identification of a gene (FMR-1) containing a CGG repeat coincident with a breakpoint cluster region exhibiting length variation in fragile X syndrome. *Cell*, 65(5), 905-14.

[70] Borjeson, M., Forssman, H., & Lehmann, O. (1962). An X-linked, recessively inherited syndrome characterized by grave mental deficiency, epilepsy, and endocrine disorder. *Acta Med Scand.*, 171, 13-21.

[71] Berland, S., Alme, K., Brendehaug, A., Houge, G., & Hovland, R. (2011). PHF6 Deletions May Cause Borjeson-Forssman-Lehmann Syndrome in Females. *Mol Syndromol.*, 1(6), 294-300.

[72] Marshall, J. D., Maffei, P., Collin, G. B., & Naggert, J. K. (2011). Alström Syndrome: Genetics and Clinical Overview. *Curr Genomics*, 12(3), 225-35.

[73] Barsh, G. S., Farooqi, I. S., & O'Rahilly, S. (2000). Genetics of body-weight regulation. *Nature*, 404(6778), 644-51.

[74] Zhao, J., Bradfield, J. P., Li, M., Wang, K., Zhang, H., Kim, CE, et al. (2009). The role of obesity-associated loci identified in genome wide association studies in the determination of pediatric BMI. *Obesity (Silver Spring).*, 17(12), 2254-7.

[75] Benzinou, M., Chèvre-C, J., Ward, K. J., Lecoeur, C., Dina, C., Lobbens, S., et al. (2008). Endocannabinoid receptor 1 gene variations increase risk for obesity and modulate body mass index in European populations. *Hum. Mol. Genet.*, 17(13), 1916-21.

[76] Russo, P., Strazzullo, P., Cappuccio, F. P., Tregouet, D. A., Lauria, F., Loguercio, M., et al. (2007). Genetic variations at the endocannabinoid type 1 receptor gene (CNR1) are associated with obesity phenotypes in men. *J. Clin. Endocrinol. Metab.*, 92(6), 2382-6.

[77] Frayling, T. M., Timpson, N. J., Weedon, M. N., Zeggini, E., Freathy, R. M., Lindgren, C. M., et al. (2007). A common variant in the FTO gene is associated with body mass index and predisposes to childhood and adult obesity. *Science.*, 316(5826), 889-94.

[78] Waterland, R. A. (2005). Does nutrition during infancy and early childhood contribute to later obesity via metabolic imprinting of epigenetic gene regulatory mechanisms? Nestle Nutr Workshop Ser Pediatr Program discussion 171-174., 56, 157-171.

[79] Crocker, M. K., & Yanovski, J. A. (2011). Pediatric obesity: etiology and treatment. Pediatr. Clin. North Am. xi., 58(5), 1217-1240.

[80] De Onis, M., Onyango, A. W., Borghi, E., Siyam, A., Nishida, C., & Siekmann, J. (2007). Development of a WHO growth reference for school-aged children and adolescents. *Bull. World Health Organ.*, 85(9), 660-7.

Chapter 12

Bone Marrow Microenvironment Defects in Fanconi Anemia

Wen Xing, Mingjiang Xu and Feng-Chun Yang

Additional information is available at the end of the chapter

1. Introduction

In 1927, the Swiss pediatrician Guido Fanconi first reported a family with aplastic anemia and physical anomalies known as FA now, as reviewed by Lobitz et al (Lobitz and Velleuer 2006). FA is a chromosomal fragility disorder characterized by cytopenia, progressive bone marrow failure (BMF) under production, variable developmental anomalies and a strong propensity for cancer. The prevalence of FA is 1 to 5 per million, and heterozygous carrier frequency is about 1 in 300. Clinically, FA patients develop heterogeneous manifestations. 80% of FA patients develop progressive BMF with a mean age of death occurring at 19 years (D'Andrea, Dahl et al. 2002; Bagby and Alter 2006;Giri, Batista et al. 2007). The other 20% of patients usually die of malignancies resulting from the acquisition of myeloid cell leukemia particularly acute myelogenous leukemia and myelodysplastic syndrome. In addition, FA Patients are susceptible to solid tumors, including gynecologic squamous cell carcinoma, head and neck squamous cell carcinoma, esophageal carcinoma, liver tumors, brain tumors, skin tumors, and renal tumors(Kutler, Singh et al. 2003).

To date, at least 15 distinct *FANC* genes, including *FANCA, FANCB, FANCC, FANCD1/ BRCA2, FANCD2/BRCA1, FANCE, FANCF, FANCG/XRCC9, FANCI, FANCJ/BRIP1, FANCL, FANCM/HEF, FANCN/PALB2, FANCO/ RAD51c* and *FANCP/SLX4*, are found in FA patients, and *FANCA, FANCC, FANCG* and *FANCD2* are the most frequentin clinic (Moldovan and D'Andrea 2009; Vaz, Hanenberg et al. 2010; Kim, Lach et al. 2011; Stoepker, Hain et al. 2011). Except for *FANCB* which is on the X chromosome (Meetei, Levitus et al. 2004), all these *FANC* genes are located on autosomes.

FA pathway is inactive in normal cells but turned on during the S phase of cell cycle or in the presence of DNA damage proteins, and it also plays a pivotal role in DNA repair pathway in cellular defense against DNA interstrandcrosslinkers(Moldovan and D'Andrea 2009;

Kee and D'Andrea 2010). Following the activation, eight of 15 *FANC* gene productions, including FANCA, B, C, E, F, G, L and M proteins assemble into a nuclear E3 ubiquitin ligase complex. This complex is known as FA core complex and one of the main functions of this core complex is to monoubiquitinate and to activate the proteins of FANCD2 and FANCI, which co-localizes with BRCA1 and BRCA2, at the sites of DNA repair(D'Andrea 2010). The monoubiquitinated FANCD2/FANCI is then translocated to chromatin and interacts with other downstream FA proteins FANCD1, J, N and O to form a nuclear DNA-repair complex (D'Andrea 2010). FA patients display spontaneous chromosomal breakage and chromosomal abnormalities (Schroeder, Anschutz et al. 1964; Sasaki 1975). In addition, these DNA instability can be significantly enhanced by DNA cross-linking agents, such as mitomycin C (MMC) (Schroeder, Anschutz et al. 1964; Sasaki 1975).

2. *FANC* genes regulate HSC/HPC functions

Because of the earlier bone marrow failure and the predisposition to malignancy, especially the high risk of developing acute myeloid leukemia(AML), FA has been clinically categorized as a hematopoietic disease due to hematopoietic dysfunction. The defective hematopoietic functions are known related to an excess of genetic instability. FA bone marrow cells have clonal evolution, which predispose patients to the development of malignancies. Vinciguerra et al reported an increased number of ultrafine DNA bridges and binucleated cells in both bone marrow stromal cells from FA patients and in primary murine FA pathway-deficient hematopoietic stem/progenitor cells (HSCs/HPCs)(Vinciguerra, Godinho et al. 2010). Using primary and immortalized cell cultures as well as *ex vivo* materials from patients, multiple studies showed oxidant hypersensitivity of these FA cells as reviewed by Du et al. (Du, Adam et al. 2008).

3. Murine models of FA

To our best knowledge, 9 of 15 *Fanc* genes have been inactivated in mice, resulting in *Fanca, Fancc, Fancg, Fancd1, Fancd2, Fancl, Fancm, Fancn*and *Fancp* knockout mice.

Cheng et al first created *Fanca*$^{-/-}$ mice by deletion of *Fanca* exons 4-7(Cheng, van de Vrugt et al. 2000). The *Fanca*$^{-/-}$ mice developed a significant thrombocytopenia, while no other severe hematological abnormalities were observed. Using the same murine model, Rio and colleagues reported that megakaryocyte progenitors, but not granulocyte-macrophage progenitors from the bone marrow of the *Fanca*$^{-/-}$ mice have impaired proliferation *in vitro*(Rio, Segovia et al. 2002). In addition, embryonic fibroblasts (MEFs) derived from these knocknout mice are hypersensitive to the crosslinker MMC and both male and female mice showed reduced fertility due to hypogonadism(Cheng, van de Vrugt et al. 2000; Rio, Segovia et al. 2002). Different from FA patients, these knockout mice do not spontaneously develop congenital anomalies(Cheng, van de Vrugt et al. 2000; Rio, Segovia et al. 2002). Later, Wong and colleagues established another *Fanca*$^{-/-}$ murine model by deletion of exons 1-6 of *Fanca*gene (Wong, Alon et al. 2003). The homozygous germline-line deletion of the functionally exons 1-6 of *Fanca*leads to multiple developmental deficits, including growth retardation, microphthalmia, craniofacial malformations, as well as hypogonadism, resembling those observed in FA patients (Wong, Alon et al. 2003).

Two different *Fancc*$^{-/-}$ murine models were generated by deletion of *Fancc* exon 9 or exon 8 (Chen, Tomkins et al. 1996; Whitney, Royle et al. 1996). Similar to *Fanca*$^{-/-}$ mice, these mice do not spontaneously develop peripheral hematological abnormalities. However the bone marrow HSCs/HPCs of these mice display impaired functions *in vitro*, such as abnormal colony forming capacity, hypersensitive to interferon-γ. Furthermore, these *Fancc*$^{-/-}$ mice also have impaired fertility and increased incidence of a congenital microphthalmia without skeletal abnormalities, replicating some of the features of the FA patients(Chen, Tomkins et al. 1996; Whitney, Royle et al. 1996).

Fancg$^{-/-}$ micewere generated by deletion of *Fancg* exons 2-9 (Yang, Kuang et al. 2001; Koomen, Cheng et al. 2002). Similar to *Fanca*$^{-/-}$ and *Fancc*$^{-/-}$ mice, *Fancg*$^{-/-}$ mice do not develop spontaneously hematological abnormalities and congenital anomalies either, although MEFs of*Fancg*$^{-/-}$ mice are hypersensitive to MMC (Yang, Kuang et al. 2001; Koomen, Cheng et al. 2002).

BRCA2 has a close functional relationship with the classical FA pathway. Genetic deletion of *Fancd1/Brca2* in mice results in embryonic lethality (Sharan, Morimatsu et al. 1997). Using mice with hypomorphic mutations in *Brca2* (*Brca2*$^{\Delta 27/\Delta 27}$), Navarro et al reported thatbone marrow cells of *Brca2*$^{\Delta 27/\Delta 27}$mice display spontaneous chromosomal aberrations and are more hypersensitive to MMC (Navarro, Meza et al. 2006), consistent with FANCD1/BRCA2 as downstream of FA core complex in FA pathway and plays a critical role in DNA repair process. Different from *Fanca*$^{-/-}$ mice, *Fancd1*$^{-/-}$ mice are hypersensitive to ionizing radiation and do not have defect in fertility (Navarro, Meza et al. 2006).

Fancd2 undergoes monoubiquitylation by the complex and is targeted into nuclear foci and co-localizes with Brca1. *Fancd2*$^{-/-}$ mice were generated by targeted deletion of *Fancd2* exons 26 and 27 (Houghtaling, Timmers et al. 2003).*Fancd2* mutant mice display cellular sensitivity to DNA interstrand cross-links and germ cell loss, which is similar to human FA patients and other FA mouse models. Interestingly, different from other mice carrying disruptions of proximal FA genes, these *Fancd2* mutant mice exhibited phenotypes including microphthalmia, perinatal lethality, and epithelial cancers. There is similarity between*Fancd2* mutant mice and*Brca2/Fancd1*hypomorphic mutation mice, implying a common function for both proteins in the same pathway.

Although *Fancg*$^{-/-}$, *Fancc*$^{-/-}$, and *Fancd2*$^{-/-}$ mice do not develop spontaneous hematopoietic malignancies seen in FA patients, HSCs/HPCs from *Fancg*$^{-/-}$, *Fancc*$^{-/-}$, and *Fancd2*$^{-/-}$ mice have defective engraftment and reconstitution of the short and long term hematopoiesis in a competitive transplantation assay (Haneline, Gobbett et al. 1999; Parmar, Kim et al. 2010; Barroca, Mouthon et al. 2012). The defective homing and reconstitution may associated with an impaired cell migration and adhesion of *Fancg*$^{-/-}$ hematopoietic cells as reported by Barroca et al(Zhang, Shang et al. 2008; Barroca, Mouthon et al. 2012). In addition, the mobilization of HSCs/HPCs in *Fanca*$^{-/-}$ mice in response to G-CSF was defective in the absence of bone marrow failure (Milsom, Lee et al. 2009).

Fancl, also known as *Pog*(proliferation of germ cells), belongs to the multisubunit FA complex.*Fancl*$^{-/-}$ mice were generated by deletion of *Pog* gene exons 4-14 (Agoulnik, Lu et al. 2002). *Fancl*$^{-/-}$ mice have defects in fertility, growth retardation, although no obvious hematological abnormalities (Agoulnik, Lu et al. 2002). *Fancm*$^{-/-}$ mice were generated by deletion of *Fancm* exon 2 (Bakker, van de Vrugt et al. 2009). Similar to other FA mouse models, *Fancm*$^{-/-}$ mice do not spontaneously develop hematological abnormalities and congenital anomalies, whereas, *Fancm*$^{-/-}$ mice showed increased cancer incidence.

Fancn/Palb2 $^{-/-}$micewere generated by insertion of a gene trap construct located between exon 1 and exon 2 of the *Palb2* gene (Rantakari, Nikkila et al. 2010;Bouwman, Drost et al. 2011). Homozygous deletion of *Palb2* leads to embryonic lethality which die at E9.5 at the latest (Rantakari, Nikkila et al. 2010; Bouwman, Drost et al. 2011)

As described above, differing from FA patients who often spontaneously develop bone marrow failure in their lives, most of the models have relatively normal hematological function. It is possible that FA proteins have divergent functions which are independent of FANCD2/FANCI monoubiquitination in hematopoietic cells. To test if deletion of multiple *Fanc*genes would result in a more aggressive hematopoietic phenotype, Pulliam-Leath and colleagues generated*Fancc*$^{-/-}$;*Fancg*$^{-/-}$(*DKO*)miceby genetically intercrossing *Fancc*$^{+/-}$mice with*Fancg*$^{+/-}$ mice(Pulliam-Leath, Ciccone et al. 2010).Combined inactivation of *Fancc* and *Fancg* leads to a defective hematopoietic stem cell function, supporting the hypothesis that besidestheir common role in FANCD2/FANCI monoubiquitination, FANCC and FANCG function in divergent molecular pathways of relevance to hematopoiesis. This *DKO* model best recapitulates the spontaneous clinical hematopoietic phenotypes of human FA, including hematopoietic malignancies and bone marrow aplasia.

4. Bone marrow microenvironmental abnormalities in hematopoietic diseases

Hematopoiesis is a dynamic and highly regulated process,which relies on the ordered self-renewal and differentiation of HSCs/HPCs within the bone marrow (BM) (Kotton, Ma et al. 2001; Krause 2002; Zhang, Niu et al. 2003; Li and Li 2006; Yin and Li 2006). This process involves intrinsic and extrinsic cues including both cellular and humoral regulatory signals generated by the HSC microenvironment, also known as "niche". The concept of hematopoietic niche has been proposed in the 1970s (Schofield 1978). Studies have shown that the cellular composition of this "niche" contains heterogeneous populations, including endothelial cells, osteoblasts, adipocytes (Calvi, Adams et al. 2003; Zhang, Niu et al. 2003; Arai, Hirao et al. 2005; Sacchetti, Funari et al. 2007), and mesenchymal stem/progenitor cells (MSPCs) (Badillo and Flake 2006),a common progenitor for many of these cells composing the HSC niche. The regulatory signals of the BM microenvironment represent a demarcated anatomical compartment that provides stimulatory signals to HSCs via the following mechanisms: (1) cell/cell direct interactions, (2) secreting soluble factors, and (3) extracellular matrix. These cellular and humoral regulatory signals dictate HSC cell fate, such as self-renewal, proliferation, differentiation, and apoptosis.

The osteoblastic niche and the vacular niche are well described by independent groups (Heissig, Hattori et al. 2002; Calvi, Adams et al. 2003; Zhang, Niu et al. 2003;Avecilla, Hattori et al. 2004).Studies have shown that BM microenvironment is critical for the physiologic as well as pathologic development of hematopoiesis through the following mechanisms: cell/cell interactions, soluble factors and extracellular matrix(Koh, Choi et al. 2005; Williams and Cancelas 2006). There is increasing evidence suggesting a role of the hematopoietic microenvironment in initiating hematopoietic disorders, such as myeloproliferative disorders (MPD).

Recently, using a murine model in which Dicer1 was specifically deleted in osteoprogenitors, Raaijmakers et al demonstrated that bone marrow microenvironment plays a causative role in the development of myelodysplasia and secondary leukaemia(Raaijmakers, Mukherjee et al. 2010). The vascular microvessel density is increased in the bone marrow of many hematopoietic disorders including AML, acute lymphoblastic leukemia (ALL), myelosyndromes (MDS) and myeloproliferative neoplasms (MPN). The adipocytes are also found to be accumulated in BMF (Li, Chen et al. 2009). Although the mechanism for the accumulation of adipocytes in bone marrow is still largely unknown, the accumulated adipocytes may act as negative regulators in the hematopoietic microenvironment (Naveiras, Nardi et al. 2009).

5. Dysregulated bone marrow microenvironment in FA patients and FA murine models

Besides the hematopoietic defects, mesenchymal tissue-derived congenital malformations are also prevalent in FA patients, such as the renal/limb abnormalities and short stature. Despite these clinical observations suggesting multiple mesenchymal defects, little attention has been directed to the association between the pathological HSC functions and the microenvironment in FA.

Using a murine model with targeted disruption of the *Fancg* gene (*Fancg*$^{-/-}$), Li and colleagues first reported that *Fancg*$^{-/-}$ MSPCs have decreased clonogenic growth, diminished proliferating capability and increased apoptosis and senescence (Li, Chen et al. 2009). *Fancg*$^{-/-}$ MSPCs have impaired function in supporting the proliferation, recruitment, adhesion and homing of HSPCs *in vitro* and *in vivo*. Importantly, some cellular defects such as survival and proliferation of murine MSPCs can be restored by introduction of human*Fancg*cDNA(Li, Chen et al. 2009).

Consistently, study by Zhang et al showed that MSPCs derived from the bone marrow of *Fancd2*$^{-/-}$ mice showed less support for progenitor growth than that from wild type mice in a CAFC assay (Zhang, Marquez-Loza et al. 2010).

Using the MSPCs derived from patients with *FANCA* mutation, Lecourt et al showed that human FA MSPCs also have poor proliferation and increased senescence, while no defective hematopoietic supportive activity was observed *in vitro*(Lecourt, Vanneaux et al. 2010), suggesting a species-specific effect between human and murine system.

6. Current treatments for FA

The long-term curative therapy for the BMF of FA patients is HSC transplantation, ideally from an HLA-matched sibling(Gluckman, Broxmeyer et al. 1989; Davies, Khan et al. 1996; Guardiola, Pasquini et al. 2000; Kutler, Singh et al. 2003; Mathew 2006) Allogeneic BM transplantation (BMT) or cord blood (CB) transplantation is available to up-to 30% of FA patients. However, allogeneic BMT or CB transplantation is frequently associated with an increased risk of secondary cancers, particularly squamous cell carcinoma of the head and neck(Kutler, Auerbach et al. 2003; Rosenberg, Socie et al. 2005). Since the conditioning regimens such as irradiation clearly heightens the risk of transformation of the ongoing genetic susceptibility of non-hematopoietic tissue. This complication is even more severe in high-risk FA patients, transplanted with non-matched donors and those develop chronic graft-versus-host disease. Therefore, even with successful allogeneic transplantation for BMF, the risk of secondary malignancies results in a high mortality over 10-15 years. Gene therapy using autologous HSCs is a second theoretical modality to correct defects in the HSC compartment. Transplantation of genetically corrected autologous HSCs without genotoxic conditioning regiments could provide a therapeutic strategy that avoids the increased risks of secondary cancer(Si, Ciccone et al. 2006). However, a significant obstacle for this therapy is the limited number of HSCs that can be harvested from mobilized blood or BM. In addition, in preliminary phase 1 clinical trials in FANCC and FANCA patients using retroviral mediated gene transfer, despite an efficient gene transfer of the mobilized progenitors (40-80%), and no long-term engraftment of retroviral marked stem cells was achieved(Liu, Kim et al. 1999; Williams, Croop et al. 2005; Kelly, Radtke et al. 2007). Although inefficient gene transfer of repopulating HSCs can not be excluded, inefficient engraftment and homing of exogenous genetically modified cells could also be contributory, particularly given the low numbers of HSC targets that are available for gene transfer/transplantation(Gothot, Pyatt et al. 1998; Glimm, Oh et al. 2000; Orschell-Traycoff, Hiatt et al. 2000). Since mesenchymalstem/progenitor cells were excluded in these studies, it is possible that the lack of an appropriate microenvironment could have impaired the ability of transduced cells to home and proliferate *in vivo*.

7. Biology of MSPCs and their potential clinical application in transplantation therapy for FA patients

Friedenstein and colleagues first reported a rare, plastic-adherent and fibroblast-like subpopulation expanded from the culture of bone marrow in 1970s (Friedenstein, Chailakhjan et al. 1970), this type of stromal cells, now commonly known as MSCs/MSPCs, has captivated more and more investigators, especially in the past two decades. As a group cells with heterogeneity, three criteria have been proposed to define human MSPCs, including plastic-adherence, surface expression of CD105, CD73 and CD90, and the absence of CD45, CD34, CD14 or CD11b, CD79a, CD19, CD14 or CD11b and HLA-DR, and trilineage differentiation to osteoblasts, adipocytes and chondrocytes *in vitro*(Dominici, Le Blanc et al. 2006).

It is well known that MSPCs lack expression of MHC class II and most of the classical co-stimulatory molecules such as CD80, CD86, or CD40 (Pittenger, Mackay et al. 1999; Tse, Pendleton et al. 2003). This phenotypic characteristic endows MSPCs with nonimmunogenicity, and therefore transplantation of MSPCs into allogeneic host could be implemented without using immunosuppressive agents. MSPCs are known promote the reconstitution of hematopoiesis. We have recently provided evidence for the first time that *Fancg-/-* MSPCs exhibited profoundly diminished supportive activity for normal HSCs, and intratibial injection of WT or genetically corrected FA MSPCs enhanced donor HSC reconstitution (Li, Chen et al. 2009). This data suggests that normal MSPCs transplantation may have a potential clinical application in FA patients.

8. Future directions

FA is an inherited disease caused by germ-line mutations in *FANC* genes. Investigators are now paying more attentions on the emerging role of the *Fanc* gene inactivation-caused defective bone marrow microenvironment in the pathogenesis of FA. Co-transplantation of HSCs and MSPCs is hypothesized as a potentially more effective option than HSC transplantation alone for treating the hematopoietic abnormalities in FA. Therefore, much more effort is warranted to understand the mechanisms of the utility of MSPCs to treat FA patients. These efforts should include: 1) unveiling the cellular fates of the co-injected MSPCs *in vivo*, such as at what degree these MSPCs are able to reconstitute the marrow microenvironment and how long a significant degree of MSPC engraftment could persist; 2) clarifying whether an immune suppression activity mediated by the injected MSPCs contributes to the enhanced HSC engraftment by co-transplantation of MSPCs; and 3) elucidating at what extend the co-injected MSPCs could normalize the altered marrow microenvironment cytokine/growth factors profiling in FA patients.

Author details

Wen Xing[1*], Mingjiang Xu[2*] and Feng-Chun Yang[2*]

1 State Key Laboratory of Experimental Hematology, Institute of Hematology and Blood Disease Hospital, Chinese Academy of Medical Sciences and Peking Union Medical College, China

2 Herman B Wells Center for Pediatric Research, Indiana University School of Medicine; Indianapolis, Indiana, USA

References

[1] Agoulnik, A. I., Lu, B., et al. (2002). A novel gene, Pog, is necessary for primordial germ cell proliferation in the mouse and underlies the germ cell deficient mutation, gcd.". *Hum Mol Genet*, 11(24), 3047-3053.

[2] Arai, F., Hirao, A., et al. (2005). Regulation of hematopoiesis and its interaction with stem cell niches.". *Int J Hematol*, 82(5), 371-376.

[3] Auerbach, A. D., Buchwald, M., et al. (2002). Fanconianemia. In: Vogelstein B, Kinzler KW, eds.", *The Genetic Bases of Human Cancer 2nd Edition*, (New YorK: McGraw-Hill, Inc.):, 289-306.

[4] Avecilla, S. T., Hattori, K., et al. (2004). Chemokine-mediated interaction of hematopoietic progenitors with the bone marrow vascular niche is required for thrombopoiesis.". *Nat Med*, 10(1), 64-71.

[5] Badillo, A. T., & Flake, A. W. (2006). The regulatory role of stromal microenvironments in fetal hematopoietic ontogeny.". *Stem Cell Rev*, 2(3), 241-246.

[6] Bagby, G. C., & Alter, B. P. (2006). Fanconianemia.". *SeminHematol*, 43, 147-156.

[7] Agoulnik, A. I., Lu, B., et al. (2002). A novel gene, Pog, is necessary for primordial germ cell proliferation in the mouse and underlies the germ cell deficient mutation, gcd.". *Hum Mol Genet*, 11(24), 3047-3053.

[8] Arai, F., Hirao, A., et al. (2005). Regulation of hematopoiesis and its interaction with stem cell niches.". *Int J Hematol*, 82(5), 371-376.

[9] Auerbach, A. D., Buchwald, M., et al. (2002). Fanconianemia. In: Vogelstein B, Kinzler KW, eds.", *The Genetic Bases of Human Cancer 2nd Edition*, (New YorK: McGraw-Hill, Inc.):, 289-306.

[10] Avecilla, S. T., Hattori, K., et al. (2004). Chemokine-mediated interaction of hematopoietic progenitors with the bone marrow vascular niche is required for thrombopoiesis.". *Nat Med*, 10(1), 64-71.

[11] Badillo, A. T., & Flake, A. W. (2006). The regulatory role of stromal microenvironments in fetal hematopoietic ontogeny.". *Stem Cell Rev*, 2(3), 241-246.

[12] Bagby, G. C., & Alter, B. P. (2006). Fanconianemia.". *SeminHematol*, 43, 147-156.

[13] Bagby, G. C., Jr , , Segal, G. M., et al. (1993). Constitutive and induced expression of hematopoietic growth factor genes by fibroblasts from children with Fanconianemia.". *ExpHematol*, 21(11), 1419-1426.

[14] Bakker, S. T., van de Vrugt, H. J., et al. (2009). Fancm-deficient mice reveal unique features of Fanconianemia complementation group M.". *Hum Mol Genet*, 18(18), 3484-3495.

[15] Barroca, V., Mouthon, M. A., et al. (2012). Impaired functionality and homing of Fancg-deficient hematopoietic stem cells.". *Hum Mol Genet*, 21(1), 121-135.

[16] Bouwman, P., Drost, R., et al. (2011). Loss of 53 partially rescues embryonic development of Palb2 knockout mice but does not foster haploinsufficiency of Palb2 in tumour suppression.". *J Pathol*, 224(1), 10-21.

[17] Calvi, L. M., Adams, G. B., et al. (2003). Osteoblastic cells regulate the haematopoietic stem cell niche.". *Nature*, 425(6960), 841-846.

[18] Chen, M., Tomkins, D. J., et al. (1996). Inactivation of Fac in mice produces inducible chromosomal instability and reduced fertility reminiscent of Fanconi anaemia.". *Nat Genet*, 12(4), 448-451.

[19] Cheng, N. C., van de Vrugt, H. J., et al. (2000). Mice with a targeted disruption of the Fanconianemia homolog Fanca.". *Hum Mol Genet*, 9(12), 1805-1811.

[20] D'Andrea, A. D. (2010). Susceptibility pathways in Fanconi'sanemia and breast cancer.". *N Engl J Med*, 362(20), 1909-1919.

[21] D'Andrea, A. D., Dahl, N., et al. (2002). Marrow failure.". *Hematology Am SocHematolEduc Program:*, 58-72.

[22] Davies, S. M., Khan, S., et al. (1996). Unrelated donor bone marrow transplantation for Fanconianemia.". *Bone Marrow Transplant*, 17(1), 43-47.

[23] Dominici, M., Le Blanc, K., et al. (2006). Minimal criteria for defining multipotentmesenchymal stromal cells. The International Society for Cellular Therapy position statement.". *Cytotherapy*, 8(4), 315-317.

[24] Du, W., Adam, Z., et al. (2008). Oxidative stress in Fanconianemiahematopoiesis and disease progression.". *Antioxid Redox Signal*, 10(11), 1909-1921.

[25] Friedenstein, A. J., Chailakhjan, R. K., et al. (1970). The development of fibroblast colonies in monolayer cultures of guinea-pig bone marrow and spleen cells.". *Cell Tissue Kinet*, 3(4), 393-403.

[26] Giri, N., Batista, D. L., et al. (2007). Endocrine Abnormalities in Patients with FanconiAnemia.". *J ClinEndocrinolMetab*, 92(7), 2624-2631.

[27] Glimm, H., Oh, I. H., et al. (2000). Human hematopoietic stem cells stimulated to proliferate in vitro lose engraftment potential during their S/G(2)/M transit and do not reenter G(0).". *Blood*, 96(13), 4185-4193.

[28] Gluckman, E., Broxmeyer, H. A., et al. (1989). Hematopoietic reconstitution in a patient with Fanconi'sanemia by means of umbilical-cord blood from an HLA-identical sibling.". *N Engl J Med*, 321(17), 1174-1178.

[29] Gothot, A., Pyatt, R., et al. (1998). Assessment of proliferative and colony-forming capacity after successive in vitro divisions of single human CD34+ cells initially isolated in G0.". *ExpHematol*, 26(7), 562-570.

[30] Guardiola, P., Pasquini, R., et al. (2000). Outcome of 69 allogeneic stem cell transplantations for Fanconianemia using HLA-matched unrelated donors: a study on behalf of the European Group for Blood and Marrow Transplantation.". *Blood*, 95(2), 422-429.

[31] Haneline, L. S., Gobbett, T. A., et al. (1999). Loss of FancC function results in decreased hematopoietic stem cell repopulating ability.". *Blood*, 94(1), 1-8.

[32] Heissig, B., Hattori, K., et al. (2002). Recruitment of stem and progenitor cells from the bone marrow niche requires MMP-9 mediated release of kit-ligand.". *Cell*, 109(5), 625-637.

[33] Houghtaling, S., Timmers, C., et al. (2003). Epithelial cancer in Fanconianemia complementation group D2 (Fancd2) knockout mice.". *Genes Dev*, 17(16), 2021-2035.

[34] Kee, Y., & D'Andrea, A. D. (2010). Expanded roles of the Fanconianemia pathway in preserving genomic stability.". *Genes Dev*, 24(16), 1680-1694.

[35] Kelly, P. F., Radtke, S., et al. (2007). Stem cell collection and gene transfer in Fanconianemia.". *MolTher*, 15(1), 211-219.

[36] Kim, Y., Lach, F. P., et al. (2011). Mutations of the SLX4 gene in Fanconianemia.". *Nat Genet*, 43(2), 142-146.

[37] Koh, S. H., Choi, H. S., et al. (2005). Co-culture of human CD34+ cells with mesenchymal stem cells increases the survival of CD34+ cells against the 5-aza-deoxycytidine- or trichostatin A-induced cell death.". *BiochemBiophys Res Commun*, 329(3), 1039-1045.

[38] Kook, H. (2005). Fanconianemia: current management.". *Hematology 10 Suppl*, 1, 108-110.

[39] Koomen, M., Cheng, N. C., et al. (2002). Reduced fertility and hypersensitivity to mitomycin C characterize Fancg/Xrcc9 null mice.". *Hum Mol Genet*, 11(3), 273-281.

[40] Kopen, G. C., Prockop, D. J., et al. (1999). Marrow stromal cells migrate throughout forebrain and cerebellum, and they differentiate into astrocytes after injection into neonatal mouse brains.". *ProcNatlAcadSci U S A*, 96(19), 10711-10716.

[41] Kotton, D. N., et, B. Y., & al, . (2001). Bone marrow-derived cells as progenitors of lung alveolar epithelium.". *Development*, 128(24), 5181-5188.

[42] Krause, D. S. (2002). Plasticity of marrow-derived stem cells.". *Gene Ther*, 9(11), 754-758.

[43] Kutler, D. I., Auerbach, A. D., et al. (2003). High incidence of head and neck squamous cell carcinoma in patients with Fanconianemia.". *Arch Otolaryngol Head Neck Surg*, 129(1), 106-112.

[44] Kutler, D. I., Singh, B., et al. (2003). A 20-year perspective on the International FanconiAnemia Registry (IFAR).". *Blood*, 101(4), 1249-1256.

[45] Lecourt, S., Vanneaux, V., et al. (2010). Bone marrow microenvironment in fanconianemia: a prospective functional study in a cohort of fanconianemia patients.". *Stem Cells Dev*, 19(2), 203-208.

[46] Li, Y., Chen, S., et al. (2009). Mesenchymal stem/progenitor cells promote the reconstitution of exogenous hematopoietic stem cells in Fancg-/- mice in vivo.". *Blood*, 113(10), 2342-2351.

[47] Li, Z., & Li, L. (2006). Understanding hematopoietic stem-cell microenvironments.". *Trends BiochemSci*, 31(10), 589-595.

[48] Liu, J. M., Kim, S., et al. (1999). Engraftment of hematopoietic progenitor cells transduced with the Fanconianemia group C gene (FANCC).". *Hum Gene Ther*, 10(14), 2337-2346.

[49] Lobitz, S., & Velleuer, E. (2006). Guido Fanconi (1892-1979): a jack of all trades.". *Nat Rev Cancer*, 6(11), 893-898.

[50] Mathew, C. G. (2006). Fanconi anaemia genes and susceptibility to cancer.". *Oncogene*, 25(43), 5875-5884.

[51] Meetei, A. R., Levitus, M., et al. (2004). X-linked inheritance of Fanconianemia complementation group B.". *Nat Genet*, 36(11), 1219-1224.

[52] Milsom, M. D., Lee, A. W., et al. (2009). Fanca-/- hematopoietic stem cells demonstrate a mobilization defect which can be overcome by administration of the Rac inhibitor NSC23766.". *Haematologica*, 94(7), 1011-1015.

[53] Moldovan, G. L., & D'Andrea, A. D. (2009). How the fanconianemia pathway guards the genome.". *Annu Rev Genet*, 43, 223-249.

[54] Munoz-Elias, G., Marcus, A. J., et al. (2004). Adult bone marrow stromal cells in the embryonic brain: engraftment, migration, differentiation, and long-term survival.". *J Neurosci*, 24(19), 4585-4595.

[55] Navarro, S., Meza, N. W., et al. (2006). Hematopoietic dysfunction in a mouse model for Fanconianemia group D1.". *MolTher*, 14(4), 525-535.

[56] Naveiras, O., Nardi, V., et al. (2009). Bone-marrow adipocytes as negative regulators of the haematopoietic microenvironment.". *Nature*, 460(7252), 259-263.

[57] Orschell-Traycoff, C. M., Hiatt, K., et al. (2000). Homing and engraftment potential of Sca-1(+)lin(-) cells fractionated on the basis of adhesion molecule expression and position in cell cycle.". *Blood*, 96(4), 1380-1387.

[58] Parmar, K., Kim, J., et al. (2010). Hematopoietic stem cell defects in mice with deficiency of Fancd2 or Usp1.". *Stem Cells*, 28(7), 1186-1195.

[59] Pittenger, M. F., Mackay, A. M., et al. (1999). Multilineage potential of adult human mesenchymal stem cells.". *Science*, 284(5411), 143-147.

[60] Pulliam-Leath, A. C., Ciccone, S. L., et al. (2010). Genetic disruption of both Fancc and Fancg in mice recapitulates the hematopoietic manifestations of Fanconianemia.". *Blood*, 116(16), 2915-2920.

[61] Raaijmakers, M. H., Mukherjee, S., et al. (2010). Bone progenitor dysfunction induces myelodysplasia and secondary leukaemia.". *Nature*, 464(7290), 852-857.

[62] Rantakari, P., Nikkila, J., et al. (2010). Inactivation of Palb2 gene leads to mesoderm differentiation defect and early embryonic lethality in mice.". *Hum Mol Genet*, 19(15), 3021-3029.

[63] Rio, P., Segovia, J. C., et al. (2002). In vitro phenotypic correction of hematopoietic progenitors from Fanconianemia group A knockout mice.". *Blood*, 100(6), 2032-2039.

[64] Rosenberg, P. S., Socie, G., et al. (2005). Risk of head and neck squamous cell cancer and death in patients with Fanconianemia who did and did not receive transplants.". *Blood*, 105(1), 67-73.

[65] Sacchetti, B., Funari, A., et al. (2007). Self-renewing osteoprogenitors in bone marrow sinusoids can organize a hematopoietic microenvironment.". *Cell*, 131(2), 324-336.

[66] Sasaki, M. S. (1975). Is Fanconi's anaemia defective in a process essential to the repair of DNA cross links?". *Nature*, 257(5526), 501-503.

[67] Schofield, R. (1978). The relationship between the spleen colony-forming cell and the haemopoietic stem cell.". *Blood Cells*, 4(1-2), 7-25.

[68] Schroeder, T. M., Anschutz, F., et al. (1964). Spontaneous chromosome aberrations in familial panmyelopathy.". *Humangenetik*, 1(2), 194-196.

[69] Sharan, S. K., Morimatsu, M., et al. (1997). Embryonic lethality and radiation hypersensitivity mediated by Rad51 in mice lacking Brca2.". *Nature*, 386(6627), 804-810.

[70] Si, Y., Ciccone, S., et al. (2006). Continuous in vivo infusion of interferon-gamma (IFN-gamma) enhances engraftment of syngeneic wild-type cells in Fanca-/- and Fancg-/- mice.". *Blood*, 108(13), 4283-4287.

[71] Stoepker, C., Hain, K., et al. (2011). SLX4, a coordinator of structure-specific endonucleases, is mutated in a new Fanconianemia subtype.". *Nat Genet*, 43(2), 138-141.

[72] Tse, W. T., Pendleton, J. D., et al. (2003). Suppression of allogeneic T-cell proliferation by human marrow stromal cells: implications in transplantation.". *Transplantation*, 75(3), 389-397.

[73] Vaz, F., Hanenberg, H., et al. (2010). Mutation of the RAD51C gene in a Fanconianemia-like disorder.". *Nat Genet*, 42(5), 406-409.

[74] Vinciguerra, P., Godinho, S. A., et al. (2010). Cytokinesis failure occurs in Fanconia-nemia pathway-deficient murine and human bone marrow hematopoietic cells.". *J Clin Invest*, 120(11), 3834-3842.

[75] Whitney, M. A., Royle, G., et al. (1996). Germ cell defects and hematopoietic hyper-sensitivity to gamma-interferon in mice with a targeted disruption of the Fanconiane-mia C gene.". *Blood*, 88(1), 49-58.

[76] Williams, D. A., & Cancelas, J. A. (2006). Leukaemia: niche retreats for stem cells.". *Nature*, 444(7121), 827-828.

[77] Williams, D. A., Croop, J., et al. (2005). Gene therapy in the treatment of Fanconiane-mia, a progressive bone marrow failure syndrome.". *CurrOpinMolTher*, 7(5), 461-466.

[78] Wong, J. C., Alon, N., et al. (2003). Targeted disruption of exons 1 to 6 of the Fanco-niAnemia group A gene leads to growth retardation, strain-specific microphthalmia, meiotic defects and primordial germ cell hypoplasia.". *Hum Mol Genet*, 12(16), 2063-2076.

[79] Yang, Y., Kuang, Y., et al. (2001). Targeted disruption of the murine Fanconianemia gene, Fancg/Xrcc9.". *Blood*, 98(12), 3435-3440.

[80] Yin, T., & Li, L. (2006). The stem cell niches in bone.". *J Clin Invest*, 116(5), 1195-1201.

[81] Zhang, J., Niu, C., et al. (2003). Identification of the haematopoietic stem cell niche and control of the niche size.". *Nature*, 425(6960), 836-841.

[82] Zhang, Q. S., Marquez-Loza, L., et al. (2010). Fancd2-/- mice have hematopoietic de-fects that can be partially corrected by resveratrol.". *Blood*, 116(24), 5140-5148.

[83] Zhang, X., Shang, X., et al. (2008). Defective homing is associated with altered Cdc42 activity in cells from patients with Fanconianemia group A.". *Blood*, 112(5), 1683-1686.

Chapter 13

Role of the Genetic Factors in the Development of Myopia

Malgorzata Mrugacz

Additional information is available at the end of the chapter

1. Introduction

Myopia, also known as nearsightedness, is the most common eye disorder worldwide. In myopic peoples, the image of distant objects falls in front of the retina, either as the eye is too long (axial myopia), the cornea is too convex or the index of refraction of the lens is too high (refractive myopia). The light enteringthe eye is not focused correctly and distant objects look blurred [1]. The myopic eye is generally vulnerable and persons with ≤-6.0 diopters (D) are more liable to a wide range of ocular pathologies. The development of high-grade myopia involves anterior-posterior enlargement of the eye, scleral thinning, changes in the diameter of scleral collagen fibrils, and frequent detachment of the retina resulting from stress related with axial elongation [2].

2. Epidemiology

The prevalence of myopia often varies with age, country, sex, race, ethnicity, occupation and environment [3]. In general, myopia firstly occurs in school-age children, and typically progresses until about the age of 21, because the eye continues to grow during childhood. However, myopia may also develop in adults due to visual stress or health conditions such as diabetes [4].

Myopia affects 25% people over age 40 in the Western Europe and the United States, making this condition the most common eye disorder in the West and constituting a significant public health and economic problem [5,6]. The cost of optical correction to provide clear distinct vision is considerable. Moreover, the development of high-grade myopia (≤-6.0 diopters [D]) [7] is a significant risk factor for other ocular diseases, includingperipheral retinal and choroidal degenerations, glaucoma, retinal detachment, premature cataracts, and finally blindness [8-10]. Consequently, great efforts have been undertaken to identify and understand the mechanisms underlying the development and progression of myopia. The estimated prevalence of high grade myopia is ~2.5 to 9.6% in the elderly world population [7,8]. However, its highest prevalence rates are in Asians, in whom almost 50 to 80% of the adult populations are myopic [10-12]. Recent population-based studies suggest that the prevalence is increasing, specifically in Asian populations. In some areas, such as China, India and Malaysia, up to 41% of the adult population is myopic to -1 diopters, up to 80% to -0.5 diopters. In some urban areas in East Asia, the prevalence of myopia amnong teenagers and young adults exceeds 70% [13]. A recent review observed that 26.6% of Western Europeans aged 40 or over have at least -1.0 diopters of myopia, and 4.5% have at least -5.0 diopters [7]. In China, myopia rate was the highest in the world: 400 milion people are myopic out of its 1.3 bilion people. The prevalence of mtopia is 77.3% in high school students in China, and is more than 80% in college students. The prevalence of myopia has been reported as high as 70%-90% in some Asian countries, 30%-40% in Europe and the Unites States, and 10%-20% in Africa. By the year 2020, it is estimated that 2.5 bilion people- 30% of the world's population- will be affected by myopia alone. Myopia is less common in the african population and associated diaspora. In American people between the age of 12 and 54, myopia has been observed to affect African Americans less than Caucasians. Asians had the highest prevalence followed by Hispanics. Caucasians had the lowest prevalence of myopia [7].

In addition, a number of studies have found that the incidence of myopia increases with level of education and many studies have shown a correlation between myopia and higher intelligence quotient (IQ), possibly due to the confunding factor of formal education [4].

3. Environmental and genetic factors in myopia

Myopia has a diverse etiology, with both environmental and genetic factors believed to be involved in the condition's development and progression. Whether myopia is due to interethnic differences in the genetic predisposition to myopia or to culture-specific environmental influences remains uncertain.

The environmental factors implicated in myopia include near work, light exposure, lack of physical activity, diet, a higher level of education, and urbanization [14-17]. For instance, population-based studies have ahown associations between myopia and higher socioeconomic status and greater levels of educational attainment [18]. High prevalences and progression rates of myopia have been reported in individuals in visually intensive occupations such as clinical microscopists, carpet weavers and visual display workers [19]. Within the context of the myopization proces, education, socioeconomic status, and occupation are generally considered to be indirect surrogates for more proximal risk factors such as near-work visual demand. Studies of the effect of reading have attempted to show a more direct relationship between myopia and near work activity. Children with myopia spent more time studying, reading, and less time playing sports than children without myopia. Studies on the effect of reading on the rate of progression of myopia have provided conflicting results. In the study of Singaporean school children, near work was not associated with worsening myopia [20]. On the other hand, myopis children in Finland who spent more time reading had faster rates of myopia progression [21]. The relationship between reading, near work activity and myopia is complex and still poorly understood. Assesment of exposure to near worki s subject to considerable measurement error and is prone to bias in retrospective studies. Effect estimates may vary depending on the unit of measurement chosen (i.e. intensity, duration, reading distance or cumulative dose), outcome definitions (myopia, refractive error, rates of progression), or the ages, ethnicities and social circumstances. The current ubiquity of technologies such as computers, cellular and smart phones, and gaming devices has added a layer of complexity to the near work question. Indeed, it could be argued that the recent increase in myopia prevalence in East Asia reported in some studies may be the result of a steady rise in the use of modern electronic devices over the past three decades. Nevertheless, a direct link between the utilization of electronic devices and myopia development has yet to be convincingly established and future studies should attempt to validate and quantify this relationship [22].

While excessive reading or near work activity increase the risk of myopia, other environmental factors (such as playing sports and time spent outdoors) have shown protective relationships. Recent studies have shown that time spent outdoors and participation in outdoor sports during childhood is associated with a decreased risk of myopia [15]. Moreover, the beneficial effect of outdoor activity appears not to be the result of a concomitant reduction in near work. There is also evidence that genetic factors may interact with outdoor activity on the risk of myopia. The inverse relationship between outdoor activity and myopia development may be limited to children with a strong familial predisposition to myopia such as children with two myopic parents compared to children with either no, or one myopic parent.

While behawior and environment play important roles in refractive development, it has been convincingly established that heritable (presumbly genetic) factors, are also important in ocular refraction. Familial aggregation studies have estimated sibling recurrence risks of common forms of refractive errors to range from 2 to 5.61 for myopia [23,24]. Moreover, children of myopic parents tend to have longer eyes and are more likely to develop myopia during childhood or adolescence. The strong familial effects for refraction phenotypes are present across populations with varying underlying distributions of refractive error. This observation is consistent with the hypothesis that environmental influences may drive regional and ethnic differences in refractive distribution, but that within-population variation is largely due to genetic factors.

However, HM is highly heritable and often appears as familial ocular disorder, where genetic predisposition seems to be a dominant factor of its development and progression [25-27]. Each type of Mendelian inheritance for familial HM has been described [28,29]. Myopia related genes include about 70 genetic loci to which primary myopias have been mapped, although the numer is constantly increasing and depends to some extent on definition. Of these, several are associated with additional abnormalities, mostly as part of developmental syndromes. These tend to result from mutations in genes encoding transcriptional activators, and most of these have been identified by sequencing candidate genes in patients with developmental syndromes [3].

To date, several genetic loci for nonsyndromic myopia (*MYP*) have been mapped, including 12 loci linked to HM: *MYP1*, chromosome Xq28, *MYP2* 18p11.31, *MYP3* 12q21-q23, *MYP4* 7q36, *MYP5* 17q21-q22, *MYP11* 4q22-q27, *MYP12* 2q37.1, *MYP13* Xq23-q25, *MYP15* 10q21.1, *MYP16* 5p15.33-p15.2 ; *MYP18* 14q22.1-q24.2, and *MYP19* 5p15.1-p13.3 [30-45]. Moreover, two recent independent genome-wide association studies involving large cohorts of refractive error patients identified loci at chromosome 15q14 and 15q25 [46,47].

Candidate gene association studies have revealed several HM susceptibility genes, including: collagen, type I, alpha 1 (*COL1A1*), transforming growth factor, beta 1 (*TGFB1*), transforming growth beta-induced factor (*TGIF*), lumican (*LUM*), hepatocyte growth factor (*HGF*), myocilin (*MYOC*), paired box 6 (*PAX6*), and uromodulin-like 1 (*UMODL1*) [48-62]. However, positive results have not been replicated, and inconsistent data have been published. Thus, the causative mutation(s) has not yet been found, suggesting genetic heterogeneity among studied populations.

A genetic association between the three single nucleotide polymorphism (SNP)s rs6214, rs10860860, and rs2946834 and familial myopia in a large, international cohort of myopia pedigrees of Caucasian origin, suggests that insulin-like growth factor 1 (*IGF-1*) may be a candidate gene for HM [63]. These three SNPs are located within the *MYP3* locus mapped to chromosomal region 12q21-q23. This locus was previously reported to be associated with autosomal dominant HM. The SNP rs6214 (reference allele G) lies in the 3′-untranslated region (UTR) of *IGF-1*, whereas the SNPs rs10860860 (reference allele A) and rs2946834 (reference allele C) are located in the noncoding sequence in close proximity to *IGF-1* [34,35].

The *IGF-1* gene encodes insulin-like growth factor (pIGF-1), which is a member of the signaling system involved in development, cellular growth, differentiation, protein translation, metabolism, apoptosis, and aging [64,65]. The association of *IGF-1* with numerous human diseases, such as diabetes, cancer, and growth failure has been reported. *IGF-1* has been also implicated in ocular diseases, including retinopathy of prematurity, age-related macular degeneration, and diabetic retinopathy [66-73]. The *IGF-1* gene polymorphisms investigations in Polish families do not suport the studies reporting association of the SNPs rs 6214, rs10860860, and rs2946834 in the *IGF-1* gene with HM and any myopia phenotypes [74]. Haplotype analysis with informative crossovers in affected individuals defined a 12.2; 10.9; and 9.5 Mb genomic regions for high-grade myopia spanned between SNP markers rs11977885/rs10950639, rs11770622/rs9719399, and rs4763417/rs10842388 on chromosomes 7p22.1–7p21.1, 7p12.3–7p11.2, and 12p12.3–12p12.1 [75]. However, the polymorphism of rs12423791in the Chinese population showed positive association with extreme myopia [76,77]. Further replication studies involving other populations are needed to investigate the possible role of *IGF-1* as a potential myopia candidate gene.

Quantitative analyses of 225 Caucasian families identified two additional potential loci at chromosome 6q13-16.1 and chromosome 5q35.1-35.2 for myopia [78].

4. Preventive measures and treatment

Treatments that are currently available for slowing the progression of myopia include spectacle lenses, contact lenses, and pharmaceutical agents such as a non-selective muscarinic antagonist (Atropine). Several large studies conducted indifferent parts of world have shown that the prevalence of myopia in children with more outdoor activity hours is lower than in children with fewer hours.

5. Conclusion

Uncorrected refractive errors such as myopia and hyperopia aren the most common causes of visual impairment worldwide. It is estimated that 2.5 bilion people will be affected by myopia within the next decade. Epidemiologica, experimental and clinical research has shown that refractive development is influenced environmental and genetic factors for myopia. Genetic linkage studies have mapped the dozen loci, while association studies have found more than 70 different genes. Many of these genes are involved in common biological pathways to known to mediate extracellular matrix composition and regulate connective tissue remodelling. Other associated genomic regions suggest novel mechanisms in the etiology of high myopia, such as mitochondrial-mediated cell death and photoreceptor-mediated visual signal transmission. The interactions between genes and environmental factors may be significant in determing individual risks of high myopia, and may help explain the pathogenetic mechanisms of myopia in human population.

Author details

Malgorzata Mrugacz*

Address all correspondence to: malgorzata.mrugacz@umb.edu.pl

Medical University of Bialystok, Poland

References

[1] Llorente L, Barbero S, Cano D, Dorronsoro C, Marcos S. Myopic versus hyperopic eyes: axial length, corneal shape and optical aberrations. J Vis. 2004;4:288-98.

[2] Burton TC. The influence of refractive error and lattice degeneration on the incidence of retinal detachment. Trans Am Ophthalmol Soc. 1989;87:143-55.

[3] Yu L, Li ZK, Gao JR, Liu JR Xu CT. Epidemiology, genetics and treatments for myopia. Int J Ophthalmol. 2011;4(6):658-669.

[4] Siegwart JT Jr, Norton TT. Perspective: how might emmetropization and genetic factors produce myopia in normal eyes? Optom Vis Sci. 2011;88(3):365-372.

[5] Pararajasegaram R. VISION 2020-the right to sight: from strategies to action. Am J Ophthalmol. 1999;128:359-60.

[6] Vitale S, Cotch MF, Sperduto R, Ellwein L. Costs of refractive correction of distance vision impairment in the United States, 1999–2002. Ophthalmology 2006;113:2163-70.

[7] Kempen JH, Mitchell P, Lee KE, Tielsch JM, Broman AT, Taylor HR, Ikram MK, Congdon NG, O'Colmain BJ. The prevalence of refractive errors among adults in the United States, Western Europe, and Australia. Arch Ophthalmo.l 2004;122:495-505.

[8] Wong TY, Foster PJ, Hee J, Ng TP, Tielsch JM, Chew SJ, Johnson GJ, Seah SK. Prevalence and risk factors for refractive errors in adult Chinese in Singapore. Invest Ophthalmol Vis Sci. 2000;41:2486-94.

[9] Hosaka A. Population studies–myopia experience in Japan. Acta Ophthalmol Suppl. 1988; 185:37-40.

[10] Chandran S. Comparative study of refractive errors in West Malaysia. Br J Ophthalmol. 1972;56:492-5.

[11] Wu HM, Seet B, Yap EP, Saw SM, Lim TH, Chia KS. Does education explain ethnic differences in myopia prevalence? A population-based study of young adult males in Singapore. Optom Vis Sc.i 2001;78:234-9.

[12] Kleinstein RN, Jones LA, Hullett S, Kwon S, Lee RJ, Friedman NE, Manny RE, Mutti DO, Yu JA, Zadnik K. Refractive error and ethnicity in children. Arch Ophthalmol. 2003; 121:1141-7.

[13] Lin LL, Shih YF, Tsai CB, Chen CJ, Lee LA, Hung PT, Hou PK. Epidemiologic study of ocular refraction among schoolchildren in Taiwan in 1995. Optom Vis Sci. 1999;76:275-81.

[14] Mutti DO, Mitchell GL, Moeschberger ML, Jones LA, Zadnik K. Parental myopia, near work, school achievement, and children's refractive error. Invest Ophthalmol Vis Sci. 2002; 43:3633-40.

[15] Jones LA, Sinnott LT, Mutti DO, Mitchell GL, Moeschberger ML, Zadnik K. Parental history of myopia, sports and outdoor activities, and future myopia. Invest Ophthalmol Vis Sci. 2007; 48:3524-32.

[16] Cordain L, Eaton SB, Brand MJ, Lindeberg S, Jensen C. An evolutionary analysis of the aetiology and pathogenesis of juvenile-onset myopia. Acta Ophthalmol Scand. 2002; 80:125-35.

[17] Czepita D, Goslawski W, Mojsa A, Muszyñska-Lachota I. Role of light emitted by incandescent or fluorescent lamps in the development of myopia and astigmatism. Med Sci Monit. 2004;10:168-71.

[18] Wong TY, Foster PJ, Johnson GJ. Education, socioeconomic status and ocular dimenssions in Chinese adults. The Tanjong Pagar Survey. Br J Ophthalmol. 2001;86:963-968.

[19] Siemensen B, Thorud LO. Adult-onset myopia and occupation. Acta ophthalmologica. 1994;2:469-471.

[20] Saw SM, Nieto FJ, Katz J. Factors related to the progression of myopia in Singaporean children. Optom Vis Sci. 2000;77:549-554.

[21] Parssinen O, Hemminki E, Klemetti A. Effect of spectacle use and accomodation on myopic progression: final results of a three-years randomised clinical trials among schoolchildren. Br J Ophthalmol. 1989;73:547-551.

[22] Wojciechowski R. Nature and nurture: the complex genetics of myopia and refractive errors. Clin Genet. 2011;79(4):301-320.

[23] Wojciechowski R, Congdon N, Bowie H. Heritability of refractive errors and familial aggregation of myopia in an elderly American population. Ivest Ophthalmol Vis Sci. 2005;46:1588-1592.

[24] Guggenheim JA, Pong-Wong R, Haley CS. Correlations in refractive errors between siblings in the Singapore Cohort Study of risk factors for myopia. Br J Ophthalmol. 2007;91:781-784.

[25] Hammond CJ, Snieder H, Gilbert CE, Spector TD. Genes and environment in refractive error: the twin eye study. Invest Ophthalmol Vis Sci. 2001; 42:1232-6.

[26] Dirani M, Chamberlain M, Shekar SN, Islam AF, Garoufalis P, Chen CY, Guymer RH, Baird PN. Heritability of refractive error and ocular biometrics: the Genes in Myopia (GEM) twin study. Invest Ophthalmol Vis Sci. 2006; 47:4756-61.

[27] Liang CL, Yen E, Su JY, Liu C, Chang TY, Park N, Wu MJ, Lee S, Flynn JT, Juo SH. Impact of family history of high myopia on level and onset of myopia. Invest Ophthalmol Vis Sci. 2004; 45:3446-52.

[28] Sorsby A, Benjamin B. Modes of inheritance of errors of refraction. J Med Genet. 1973; 10:161-4.

[29] Young TL, Metlapally R, Shay AE. Complex trait genetics of refractive error. Arch Ophthalmol. 2007;125:38-48.

[30] Schwartz M, Haim M, Skarsholm D. X-linked myopia: Bornholm eye disease–linkage to DNA markers on the distal part of Xq. Clin Genet. 1990;38:281-6.

[31] Young TL, Deeb SS, Ronan SM, Dewan AT, Alvear AB, Scavello GS, Paluru PC, Brott MS, Hayashi T, Holleschau AM, Benegas N, Schwartz M, Atwood LD, Oetting WS, Rosenberg T, Motulsky AG, King RA. X-linked high myopia associated with cone dysfunction. Arch Ophthalmol. 2004;122:897-908.

[32] Young TL, Ronan SM, Drahozal LA, Wildenberg SC, Alvear AB, Oetting WS, Atwood LD, Wilkin DJ, King RA. Evidence that a locus for familial high myopia maps to chromosome 18p. Am J Hum Genet. 1998; 63:109-19.

[33] Lam DS, Tam PO, Fan DS, Baum L, Leung YF, Pang CP. Familial high myopia linkage to chromosome 18p. Ophthalmologica 2003;217:115-8.

[34] Young TL, Ronan SM, Alvear AB, Wildenberg SC, Oetting WS, Atwood LD, Wilkin DJ, King RA. A second locus for familial high myopia maps to chromosome 12q. Am J Hum Genet. 1998; 63:1419-24.

[35] Nürnberg G, Jacobi FK, Broghammer M, Becker C, Blin N, Nürnberg P, Stephani U, Pusch CM. Refinement of the MYP3 locus on human chromosome 12 in a German family with Mendelian autosomal dominant high-grade myopia by SNP array mapping. Int J Mol Med. 2008; 21:429-38.

[36] Farbrother JE, Kirov G, Owen MJ, Pong-Wong R, Haley CS, Guggenheim JA. Linkage analysis of the genetic loci for high myopia on 18p, 12q, and 17q in 51 U.K. families. Invest Ophthalmol Vis Sci. 2004;45:2879-85.

[37] Naiglin L, Gazagne C, Dallongeville F, Thalamas C, Idder A, Rascol O, Malecaze F, Calvas P. A genome wide scan for familial high myopia suggests a novel locus on chromosome 7q36. J Med Genet. 2002;39:118-24.

[38] Paluru P, Ronan SM, Heon E, Devoto M, Wildenberg SC, Scavello G, Holleschau A, Mäkitie O, Cole WG, King RA, Young TL. New locus for autosomal dominant high myopia maps to the long arm of chromosome 17. Invest Ophthalmol Vis Sci. 2003; 44:1830-6.

[39] Zhang Q, Guo X, Xiao X, Jia X, Li S, Hejtmancik JF. A new locus for autosomal dominant high myopia maps to 4q22-q27 between D4S1578 and D4S1612. Mol Vis. 2005; 11:554-60.

[40] Paluru PC, Nallasamy S, Devoto M, Rappaport EF, Young TL. Identification of a novel locus on 2q for autosomal dominant high-grade myopia. Invest Ophthalmol Vis Sci. 2005; 46:2300-7.

[41] Zhang Q, Guo X, Xiao X, Jia X, Li S, Hejtmancik JF. Novel locus for X linked recessive high myopia maps to Xq23-q25 but outside MYP1. J Med Genet. 2006; 43:e20

[42] Nallasamy S, Paluru PC, Devoto M, Wasserman NF, Zhou J, Young TL. Genetic linkage study of high-grade myopia in a Hutterite population from South Dakota. Mol Vis. 2007; 13:229-36.

[43] Lam CY, Tam PO, Fan DS, Fan BJ, Wang DY, Lee CW, Pang CP, Lam DS. A genome-wide scan maps a novel high myopia locus to 5p15. Invest Ophthalmol Vis Sci. 2008; 49:3768-78.

[44] Yang Z, Xiao X, Li S, Zhan Q. Clinical and linkage study on a consanguineous Chinese family with autosomal recessive high myopia. Mol Vis. 2009;15:312-8.

[45] Ma JH, Shen SH, Zhang GW, Zhao DS, Xu C, Pan CM, Jiang H, Wang ZQ, Song HD. Identification of a locus for autosomal dominant high myopia on chromosome 5p13.3-p15.1 in a Chinese family. Mol Vis. 2010;16:2043-54.

[46] Solouki AM, Verhoeven VJ, van Duijn CM, Verkerk AJ, Ikram MK, Hysi PG, Despriet DD, van Koolwijk LM, Ho L, Ramdas WD, Czudowska M, Kuijpers RW, Amin N, Struchalin M, Aulchenko YS, van Rij G, Riemslag FC, Young TL, Mackey DA, Spector TD, Gorgels TG, Willemse-Assink JJ, Isaacs A, Kramer R, Swagemakers SM, Bergen AA, van Oosterhout AA, Oostra BA, Rivadeneira F, Uitterlinden AG, Hofman A, de Jong PT, Hammond CJ, Vingerling JR, Klaver CC. A genome-wide association study identifies a susceptibility locus for refractive errors and myopia at 15q14. Nat Genet. 2010;42:897-901.

[47] Hysi PG, Young TL, Mackey DA, Andrew T, Fernández-Medarde A, Solouki AM, Hewitt AW, Macgregor S, Vingerling JR, Li YJ, Ikram MK, Fai LY, Sham PC, Manyes L, Porteros A, Lopes MC, Carbonaro F, Fahy SJ, Martin NG, van Duijn CM, Spector TD, Rahi JS, Santos E, Klaver CC, Hammond CJ. A genome-wide association study for myopia and refractive error identifies a susceptibility locus at 15q25. Nat Genet. 2010;42:902-5.

[48] Inamori Y, Ota M, Inoko H, Okada E, Nishizaki R, Shiota T, Mok J, Oka A, Ohno S, Mizuki N. The COL1A1 gene and high myopia susceptibility in Japanese. Hum Genet. 2007; 122:151-7.

[49] Metlapally R, Li YJ, Tran-Viet KN, Abbott D, Czaja GR, Malecaze F, Calvas P, Mackey D, Rosenberg T, Paget S, Zayats T, Owen MJ, Guggenheim JA, Young TL. COL1A1 and COL2A1 genes and myopia susceptibility: evidence of association and suggestive linkage to the COL2A1 locus. Invest Ophthalmol Vis Sci. 2009;50:4080-6.

[50] Hayashi T, Inoko H, Nishizaki R, Ohno S, Mizuki N. Exclusion of transforming growth factor-beta1 as a candidate gene for myopia in the Japanese. Jpn J Ophthalmol. 2007;51:96-9.

[51] Zha Y, Leung KH, Lo KK, Fung WY, Ng PW, Shi MG, Yap MK, Yip SP. TGFB1 as a susceptibility gene for high myopia: a replication study with new findings. Arch Ophthalmol. 2009;127:541-8.

[52] Scavello GS, Paluru PC, Ganter WR, Young TL. Sequence variants in the transforming growth beta-induced factor (TGIF) gene are not associated with high myopia. Invest Ophthalmol Vis Sci. 2004;45:2091-7.

[53] Pertile KK, Schäche M, Islam FM, Chen CY, Dirani M, Mitchell P, Baird PN. Assessment of TGIF as a candidate gene for myopia. Invest Ophthalmol Vis Sci. 2008; 49:49-54.

[54] Wang P, Li S, Xiao X, Jia X, Jiao X, Guo X, Zhang Q. High myopia is not associated with the SNPs in the TGIF, lumican, TGFB1, and HGF genes. Invest Ophthalmol Vis Sci. 2009;50:1546-51.

[55] Lin HJ, Wan L, Tsai Y, Chen WC, Tsai SW, Tsai FJ. The association between lumican gene polymorphisms and high myopia. Eye (Lond). 2010;24:1093-101.

[56] Han W, Yap MK, Wang J, Yip SP. Family-based association analysis of hepatocyte growth factor (HGF) gene polymorphisms in high myopia. Invest Ophthalmol Vis Sci. 2006; 47:2291-9.

[57] Yanovitch T, Li YJ, Metlapally R, Abbott D, Viet KN, Young TL. Hepatocyte growth factor and myopia: genetic association analyses in a Caucasian population. Mol Vis. 2009; 15:1028-35.

[58] Tang WC, Yip SP, Lo KK, Ng PW, Choi PS, Lee SY, Yap MK. Linkage and association of myocilin (MYOC) polymorphisms with high myopia in a Chinese population. Mol Vis. 2007;13:534-44.

[59] Zayats T, Yanovitch T, Creer RC, McMahon G, Li YJ, Young TL, Guggenheim JA. Myocilin polymorphisms and high myopia in subjects of European origin. Mol Vis. 2009; 15:213-22.

[60] Hewitt AW, Kearns LS, Jamieson RV, Williamson KA, van Heyningen V, Mackey DA. PAX6 mutations may be associated with high myopia. Ophthalmic Genet. 2007;28:179-82.

[61] Ng TK, Lam CY, Lam DS, Chiang SW, Tam PO, Wang DY, Fan BJ, Yam GH, Fan DS, Pang CP. AC and AG dinucleotide repeats in the PAX6 P1 promoter are associated with high myopia. Mol Vis. 2009;15:2239-48.

[62] Nishizaki R, Ota M, Inoko H, Meguro A, Shiota T, Okada E, Mok J, Oka A, Ohno S, Mizuki N. New susceptibility locus for high myopia is linked to the uromodulin-like 1 (UMODL1) gene region on chromosome 21q22.3. Eye 2009; 23:222-9.

[63] Metlapally R, Ki CS, Li YJ, Tran-Viet KN, Abbott D, Malecaze F, Calvas P, Mackey DA, Rosenberg T, Paget S, Guggenheim JA, Young TL. Genetic association of insulin-like growth factor-1 polymorphisms with high-grade myopia in an international family cohort. Invest Ophthalmol Vis Sci. 2010;51:4476-9.

[64] Werner H, Leroith D. New concepts in regulation and function of the insulin-like growth factors: implications for understanding normal growth and neoplasia. Cell Mol Life Sci. 2000; 57:932-42.

[65] Bartke A. The somatotropic axis and aging: Mechanisms and persistent questions about practical implications. Exp Gerontol. 2009;44:372-4.

[66] Dunger DB, Ong KK, Sandhu MS. Serum insulin-like growth factor-I levels and potential risk of type 2 diabetes. Horm Res. 2003;60:131-5.

[67] Pollak M. Insulin and insulin-like growth factor signalling in neoplasia. Nat Rev Cancer. 2008;8:915-28.

[68] Netchine I, Azzi S, Houang M, Seurin D, Perin L, Ricort JM, Daubas C, Legay C, Mester J, Herich R, Godeau F, Le Bouc Y. Partial primary deficiency of insulin-like

growth factor (IGF)-I activity associated with IGF1 mutation demonstrates its critical role in growth and brain development. J Clin Endocrinol Metab. 2009;94:3913-21.

[69] Hellström A, Engström E, Hard AL, Albertsson-Wikland K, Carlsson B, Niklasson A, Löfqvist C, Svensson E, Holm S, Ewald U, Holmström G, Smith LE. Postnatal serum insulin-like growth factor I deficiency is associated with retinopathy of prematurity and other complications of premature birth. Pediatrics. 2003; 112:1016-20.

[70] Pérez-Muñuzuri A, Fernández-Lorenzo JR, Couce-Pico ML, Blanco-Teijeiro MJ, Fraga-Bermúdez JM. Serum levels of IGF1 are a useful predictor of retinopathy of prematurity. Acta Paediatr. 2010;99:519-25.

[71] Rosenthal R, Wohlleben H, Malek G, Schlichting L, Thieme H, Bowes Rickman C, Strauss O. Insulin-like growth factor-1 contributes to neovascularization in age-related macular degeneration. Biochem Biophys Res Commun. 2004;323:1203-8.

[72] Bergman PB, Moravski CJ, Edmondson SR, Russo VC, Bach LA, Wilkinson-Berka JL, Werther GA. Expression of the IGF system in normal and diabetic transgenic (mRen-2)27 rat eye. Invest Ophthalmol Vis Sci. 2005;46:2708-15.

[73] Wilkinson-Berka JL, Wraight C, Werther G. The role of growth hormone, insulin-like growth factor and somatostatin in diabetic retinopathy. Curr Med Chem. 2006;13:3307-17.

[74] Rydzanicz M, Nowak DM, Karolak JA, Frajdenberg A, Podfigurna-Musielak M, Mrugacz M, Gajecka M. IGF-1 gene polymorphisms in Polish families with high-grade myopia. Mol Vis. 2011;17:2428-2439.

[75] Rydzanicz M, Nath SK, Sun C, Podfigurna-Musielak M, Frajdenberg A, Mrugacz M, Winters D, Ratnamala U, Radhakrishna U, Bejjani BA, Gajecka M. Identification of novel suggestive loci for high-grade myopia in Polish families. Mol Vis. 2011;17:2028-39.

[76] Zhuang W, Yang P, Li Z, Sheng X, Zhao J, Li S, Yang X, Xiang W, Rong W, Liu Y, Zhang F. Association of insulin-like growth factor-1 polymorphisms with high myopia in the Chinese population. Mol Vis. 2012;18:634-644.

[77] Mak JY, Yap MK, Fung WY, Ng PW, Yip SP. Association of IGF1 gene haplotypes with high myopia in Chinese adults. Arch Ophthalmol. 2012;130(2):209-216.

[78] Abbott D, Li YJ, Guggenheim J, Metlapally R, Malecaze F, Calvas P, Rosenberg T, Paget S, Zayats T, Mackey D, Feng S, Young TL. An international collaborative family-based whole genome quantitative trait linkage scan for myopic refractive error. Mol Vis. 2012;18:720-729.

Chapter 14

Cystic Fibrosis: Does CFTR Malfunction Alter pH Regulation?

Douglas B. Luckie and Mauri E. Krouse

Additional information is available at the end of the chapter

1. Introduction

"Woe to the child kissed on the forehead who tastes salty, for it is cursed and soon must die," is a form of diagnosis for cystic fibrosis that dates back to the Middle Ages in Eastern Europe [1]. This observation was rediscovered and made relevant in 1948 during a heat wave in New York City. Paul di Sant'Agnese at Columbia University noticed that CF patients had a larger incidence of heat prostration than others, due to excessive salt loss [2]. This ultimately led to the use of the "sweat test" (measurement of sweat electrolytes) as the definitive test for diagnosing cystic fibrosis. Originally, Dorothy Andersen in 1938 created the term cystic fibrosis [4] in describing the appearance of the pancreas from certain individuals. Later she went on to show that CF was a genetic disease [5].

Cystic fibrosis is the most common lethal genetic disease in the Caucasian population. As first postulated by Paul Quinton it is now known that it is due to a lack of chloride flux, and hence salt movement, in all affected organs [3]. For instance, in the coiled tube of the sweat gland, fluid initially has roughly the same salt concentration as blood plasma (high Na+ and Cl-). This fluid passes upward toward the skin surface through the sweat duct. Ions are reabsorbed into the body through the Na+ and Cl- (CFTR) channels. Thus salt is normally reabsorbed out of the sweat and the concentration falls to about 1/5 of blood plasma. But in the disease cystic fibrosis the Cl- channels are either absent or non-functioning and the salt concentration in the sweat remains high as it reaches the skin surface, which one can taste on the forehand of a child with CF.

The gene itself was discovered through a remarkable collaboration by the lab of Francis Collins at the University of Michigan and those of Jack Riordan and Lap-Chee Tsui at the University of Toronto in 1989 [6-8]. It was expressed and found to code for a small linear chloride channel by Christine Bear and others [9].

But the question remained, how did a missing chloride channel cause CF airway lung disease? In many organs (pancreas, lungs, and reproductive organs) it was not understood how the lack of salt movement led to the blockage of the pancreas, the disappearance of the vas deferens and bacterial infection in the lung. But the link between genotype and phenotype might have been more difficult to understand perhaps because we, the CF research field, were initially focused too narrowly on just chloride.

It is easy to think only about sodium and chloride, as they are the main salt component of plasma. But the second most common anion is bicarbonate. The CFTR channel is permeable to bicarbonate [10] thus whenever it opens both chloride and bicarbonate can move through it. With bicarbonate movement you can get corresponding changes in pH which have broad effects. In CF, while the disease pathology in many organs is attributed primarily to impaired Cl- conductance [11], manifestations in some organs have been difficult to attribute solely to a defect in Cl- conductance [12]. Since CFTR is permeable to HCO3- and has also been shown to regulate other membrane proteins [13,14] its absence in CF may lead to significant changes in intracellular or extracellular fluid composition in impacted organs. It is the investigation into changes in pH and bicarbonate that are associated with the disease cystic fibrosis, which we hope to summarize in this review.

2. Context #1: Organized by organ systems

During many years of research, scientists develop a mental encyclopedia for their field. These expert mental databases often have the same knowledge flexibly organized in different manners. Much like a software database, an expert can re-conceptualize data in different contexts. In the field of cystic fibrosis, an expert researcher tends to think about findings in several context-dependent ways like: impacted organs, research groups, animal models and chronology. We will organize several sections of this review in a similar format and then conclude with a brief discussion of the latest findings.

It all began with the pancreas. The diagnosis and naming of the disease, cystic fibrosis, resulted when Dorothy Andersen saw a pattern of fibrotic cysts that formed on the pancreas of a group of patients. That organ was first in the understanding of the disease and that organ was also first in detecting abnormalities related to pH. In the 1980s the in vivo pathology that ravages the pancreas in cystic fibrosis was directly tied the CFTR malfunction altering fluid and bicarbonate secretion in the pancreatic ducts [15,16]. Lost regulation of pH is a problem caused by cystic fibrosis in that organ.

2.1. The pancreas

The pancreas is both an endocrine organ, releasing hormones such as insulin and glucagon into the blood, and an exocrine organ, releasing digestive enzymes in a bicarbonate rich fluid (pancreatic juice) into the intestines and eventually out of the body. Both of these systems often become defective in individuals with cystic fibrosis. In healthy humans the pancreas can produce 2 liters of concentrated sodium bicarbonate solution (140 mM) per day [17]. The exact mechanism for this remarkable feat is still controversial and certainly depends on the exact species under investigation (the bicarbonate concentration in mice is only 70 mM).

Simply put, the model for a healthy functioning human pancreas requires an active apical anion channel, that has some bicarbonate permeability, to be present in pancreatic duct cells, which turns out to be CFTR. The other proteins involved are a basolaterally located sodium bicarbonate cotransporter (NBC) needed to move bicarbonate into the duct cells and a Na-K pump to maintain the sodium gradient and intracellular voltage. During secretion the intracellular chloride concentration becomes so low that chloride secretion cannot be maintained and all the secretion is bicarbonate. This model was developed by many people [18] but was put to an elegant test in a paper by Whitcomb & Ermentrout [19] where they mathematically modeled the ductal secretion with predicted results that aligned exactly with those found by organ studies. The controversy in this field is simply explained as whether another protein, an apical chloride-bicarbonate exchanger, exists or is needed to produce the very high bicarbonate concentrations detected. Muallem and others [20] have shown that there is an apical membrane located chloride-bicarbonate exchanger found in mice. The activity of this exchanger appears to be coupled somehow to CFTR. But it is not certain whether this same system also is also normally active in the human pancreas.

On the other hand, the model for a poorly or non-functioning human pancreas impacted by the disease cystic fibrosis involves chloride, bicarbonate and pH. When the critical apical anion channel needed in duct cells, CFTR, is broken or missing, the system breaks down and the pancreas cannot produce the alkaline solution it normally would. Likely the lack of enough pancreatic juice to help dilute the enzymes secreted by the pancreatic acinar cells leads to pancreatic insufficiency. There is also evidence from measurements in the duodenum that support the idea that liquid secreted from the CF pancreas has a much more acidic pH [21]. The changed environment in the fluid secreted into the CF pancreatic duct leads the pancreatic enzymes to form protein plugs and block the pancreatic ducts [17]. In addition the secreted digestive enzymes, which are normally activated by acidic pH in the duodenum, may activate early and start to destroy the individual ducts. Eventually, with the help of an abnormal immune response, enough ducts are destroyed or blocked that very few enzymes reach the intestines to help digest fats and proteins, leading to the characteristic steatorrhea seen in cystic fibrosis patients. Roughly 10% of CF individual are born without a functioning pancreas. Over time this number climbs to 85% as more and more pancreatic ducts are destroyed. Those 10-15% of CF patients with pancreatic sufficiency are associated with mild CFTR mutations, or mutations that preserve some channel function.

It was work by Choi et al in 2001 [22] that brought the topic of the pancreas back to the forefront of CF research. The amazing finding was that when they compared different mutations of CFTR, they found that those channels with measureable residual bicarbonate conductance were associated with the mild form of CF in pancreatic sufficient patients and the mutations of CFTR where bicarbonate secretion was lost were always associated with the more severe version of CF, pancreatic insufficient. Later that year Jeff Wine [23] wrote a paper bringing into question some of their findings. While there may be a correlation between bicarbonate conductance and pancreatic sufficiency in cells in culture artificially expressing

CFTR, in the sweat gland under normal conditions all the patients with pancreatic insufficiency had high chloride concentration in their sweat gland secretions (the definitive test of CF is the sweat chloride level as mentioned above) and those with pancreatic sufficiency had intermediate sweat chloride levels, indicative of mild mutations that allowed for residual chloride conductance. While these sweat chloride measures supported that the chloride conductance is important in the pancreas, bicarbonate has not since left the spotlight.

The destruction of the pancreas does not stop with just damaging the exocrine function but eventually spreads to the endocrine pancreas. Cystic fibrosis related diabetes (CFRD) develops when the ducts and cells responsible for delivering insulin to the blood supply are finally destroyed and the patient develops diabetes and needs insulin. CFRD is rare at birth and develops over time. Patients with CFRD have a 6-fold higher mortality rate. It is unfortunate that the loss of an anion channel in the pancreas can lead to such devastation. Fortunately there is at least enzyme replacement therapy and insulin treatment for CF patients. This has circumvented the mortality associated with the digestive system and failure-to-thrive so that now 90% of all CF deaths are due to lung disease.

2.2. The lungs

In the 1940's cystic fibrosis transitioned from a disease of the pancreas to a disease of the airway. Many doctors were involved in clinical research at this time and it was Dr. Harry Schwachman who tried to further the idea that what was known then as "cystic fibrosis of the pancreas" was in fact a disease of many organs. At the same time Dr. Paul Di Sant'Agnese was using the newly discovered drug penicillin to treat lung infections associated with cystic fibrosis. In the 1950's Hans Ussing invented a method for investigating epithelium named the Ussing chamber. The method helped standardize experiments on epithelia and led to an increase in the scientific investigation of the organs affected in cystic fibrosis. It wasn't until the 1980s that the basic defect that leads to cystic fibrosis in the airways was found.

Initially, Drs. Knowles, Gatsy and Boucher [24] measured the difference in voltage across the nasal epithelium in 24 CF patients. They reported a much larger voltage in CF individuals and this voltage could be greatly reduced by blocking the epithelial sodium channel with amiloride. They speculated that excess sodium absorption could lead to excess salt and liquid absorption in the airway, leading to CF lung disease. Two years later they published another paper [25] "excessive active Na+ transport can account for the abnormalities" seen in CF airway. And today excessive sodium absorption is still the leading hypothesis of how CF lung disease develops.

To review what was mentioned earlier, in 1983 Paul Quinton published the seminal paper, which correctly identified the CF defect as a loss of chloride permeability [3]. He focused his studies on the sweat gland where any abnormality found could be attributed to the CF defect. It wasn't until 1989 that Collins, Riordan and Tsui discovered the gene. They called it the cystic fibrosis transmembrane conductance regulator (CFTR) because it was not yet certain as to its function. In 1991 Bear and others expressed the CFTR gene and discovered a small linear anion channel as the gene product. It is with this background that bicarbonate and pH became important in the airway.

One of the first reports of bicarbonate secretion in the airway was in the Ussing chamber. A special method of studying epithelial cells as a monolayer in which only the electrical currents moving into or out of the cells is measured. When cells are bathed in a solution that lacks chloride the other major anion in airway fluid and blood plasma, bicarbonate, takes its place. Smith and Welsh [26] reported that in airway epithelium under these special circumstances an elevation of cyclic AMP (cAMP) in the cell opened a channel, which could carry bicarbonate in normal tissue but was absent in CF tissue. The same thing happened when the calcium inside the cells was increased except a different set of anion channels were opened and bicarbonate can pass through in both normal and CF tissues. The following year Smith and Welsh [27] published a paper studying electrolyte transport in cultured airway epithelia cells. It was found that both normal and CF tissue secreted H+ in exchange for K+. They discovered an apical hydrogen-potassium ATPase that works to absorb potassium while secreting H+. It was noted that the H-K ATPase did not account for all the luminal acidification and other mechanisms of H+ secretions may be present. In normal airway cells the addition of forskolin to raise intracellular cAMP inhibited luminal acidification probably by stimulating bicarbonate secretion through the activated CFTR channel. Poulsen [28] then showed the same thing in transfected cells expressing the CFTR gene. C127 (mammary epithelia) and NIH-3T3 (fibroblasts) expressing normal wild-type CFTR could be made acidic inside under certain conditions and the acidity was reduced only in healthy cells when forskolin was added to the solution raising cAMP and opening CFTR channels. The alkalinization was not seen either in cells transfected with the mutant ΔF508 CFTR or non-transfected cells that expressed no CFTR. They went on to measure the ratio of chloride to bicarbonate permeability through the CFTR channel to be near 4:1 (3.9). Linsdell [10] then found the same result of chloride to bicarbonate permeability of 4:1 (4.0) using single channel studies. Hence 1 million bicarbonate ions could accompany the 4 million chloride ions that moved through the CFTR channel every few seconds.

A second group later repeated the experiments on airway epithelium [29]. In a different culture system both the apical culture liquid pH and the K+ concentration were measured. In unstimulated culture both the pH (or bicarbonate concentration) and the potassium concentration fell over 24 hours. Activating CFTR resulted in alkalinization of the surface liquid in normal cultures while CF tissues were unaffected and just continued becoming more acidic. They also went on to conclude the CFTR could conduct bicarbonate under normal conditions.

A seminal paper in 1992 was published that led a few of scientist to consider a different origin of CF lung disease. The paper by Englehardt et al [30] showed by antibody staining of CFTR channels was concentrated in the submucosal glands of the human bronchus. The new paradigm was that since most of the CFTR was in the glands it was likely that CF lung disease starts in the glands. Two scientists then led the investigation of airway submucosal glands, Steve Ballard at the University of South Alabama studied intact glands in pig airway and Jeffrey Wine at Stanford University initially studied a cell line model of gland cerous cells (Calu-3) and later went on to study intact human glands. Lee et al in [31] and Devor et al in [32] had previously established the fact that Calu-3 cells secrete bicarbonate and we, Krouse et al [33], went on to study acid and base secretion in Calu-3 cells. The cells secreted base (bicarbonate) via CFTR and secreted acid via an H-K ATPase. We quickly became very interested in the study of abnormal properties of the mucus secreted into the lungs from the glands. In cystic fibrosis this demonstrated that even before newly made mucus reached to the airway surface there was a mechanism to control the mucus pH that was altered dramatically in cystic fibrosis.

3. Context #2: Organized by research groups

Dorothy Andersen and her student Paul di Sant'Agnese at Columbia University led the first CF research groups. To gain an understanding of the work done to date, we now present a sample of the researchers in the United States who have helped make great strides in the understanding of how bicarbonate movement and pH changes may influence the pathophysiology of cystic fibrosis.

3.1. Michael Welsh and Jeffrey Smith, University of Iowa, Iowa City, IA

Dr. Michael J. Welsh is one of the most productive scientists in the field of cystic fibrosis and at the University of Iowa Medical Center has led one of the most respected CF research programs in the US. His work with Dr. Jeffrey J. Smith has been significant for scientists interested in examining pH abnormalities in CF. While the relevance of pH for the CF pancreas is accepted and understood, the thought that pH might also be important in the pathology of the human CF airway has only recently gained wide interest. The Welsh group takes advantage of a variety of methods in their studies but cell culture studied by electrophysiology, and in particular use of the Ussing Chamber, is a common technique they apply.

As early as 1992, in the Journal of Clinical Investigation, Smith and Welsh [26] reported that in studies with cultured canine and human epithelial cells cAMP stimulation of the CFTR channel increases bicarbonate secretion across normal, but not cystic fibrosis, airway epithelia. In this paper they posed the question, might HCO3- may play role in CF? A year later Welsh and Smith [27] reported their findings on how human epithelia cells control the quantity and composition of respiratory tract fluid. To do so they measured fluid and electrolyte transport by cultured human nasal epithelia and found that elevated cAMP stimulated fluid secretion across some epithelia, but for others the reverse, cAMP stimulated fluid absorption. They also reported "The finding that cAMP agonists inhibited luminal acidification may be explained by the recent finding that cAMP increases apical HCO3- conductance." These results provided new insights into how the intact airway epithelium may actively modify the composition of the respiratory tract fluid which drew colleagues' interest to the very thin film of liquid lining the interior of the lung, the airway surface liquid (ASL).

In 1996 Michael Welsh and Jeffrey Smith [34] published a widely read paper in the journal Cell where the reported a finding that cystic fibrosis airway epithelia fail to kill bacteria because of abnormal airway surface fluid. Their evidence pointed to an abnormally high concentration of salt, NaCl, in the ASL that inhibits the killing of bacteria. This finding was reminiscent of the high salt seen in CF sweat glands. This paper led to a very exciting time in recent CF research. Numerous labs tried to measure the salt concentration in the lung. Some found low salt in normal lung but most found the same salt concentration in the ASL of the CF lung. The alternative hypothesis put forward, of how lung diseased develops, was the model of Richard Boucher and others that the hyper absorption of the sodium leads to a depletion of the airway surface liquid, as mentioned earlier. Many people tried to find this depleted ASL in CF lungs but it has yet to found in vivo but does exist in cultures of airway cells. In 2001 Smith and Welsh returned [35] to canine and human cells to test for the presence of HCO3- transport in epithelial cells. They reported that their data suggest that cAMP and Ca2+ stimulate HCO3- secretion across airway epithelium, and suggest that HCO3- leaves the cell across the apical membrane via conductive pathways. They found the cAMP-induced secretory response was absent in cystic fibrosis (CF) airway epithelial cells, although Ca2+-stimulated secretion was intact. This result suggested that HCO3- exist at the apical membrane is through the Cl- channel that is defectively regulated in CF epithelia. These results also raise the possibility that a defect in HCO3- secretion may contribute to the pathophysiology of CF pulmonary disease.

Most recently in 2012 [36] the Welsh group reported a dramatic finding, that their data suggests in the CF pig model that reduced airway surface liquid pH impairs bacterial killing in the cystic fibrosis lung. It was found that the ASL pH is more acidic in pigs with cystic fibrosis, so in the end increasing pH in ASL restored the bactericidal activity to the ASL from the CF pigs. This finding will draw much attention in the years to come.

3.2. Robert Bridges, Rosalind Franklin University & University of Chicago, Chicago, IL

Robert Bridges joined the CF research group at the University of Alabama (UAB), Birmingham in the mid 1980s. Dr. Krouse, an author, remembers meeting Dr. Bridges at a meeting organized by the Cystic Fibrosis Foundation, where a number of researchers were discussing the purported rectifying anion channel as the CF channel. He was complaining prophetically that this small linear channel kept getting in the way of his single channel recordings. In 1992 he teamed with Bear et al [9] to show that this small linear channel was in fact the correct gene product of the CF gene (CFTR). Bob Bridges teamed with many different CF scientists at UAB. With Neil Bradbury he help explore the role of CFTR in endo- and exo- cystosis. In their Science paper from [37] they concluded, "CFTR is critical for cAMP-dependent regulation of membrane recycling in epithelial tissues, and this function of CFTR could explain in part the pleiotropic nature of cystic fibrosis." Simply put, stimulation of CFTR not only opens the channel but causes insertion of CFTR containing vesicles into the membrane and slowing removal of CFTR from the membrane. Thus increasing the number of CFTR channels in the membrane.

In the mid 90's Dr. Bridges moved to the University of Pittsburgh in Pennsylvania. There he continued working on cystic fibrosis. His work with Dan Devor resulted in two papers in 1996 [38,39] that helped formulate the idea that chloride and bicarbonate secretion is dependent on the driving force for each anion. This work culminated in another paper in 1999

[32] where they showed that Calu-3 cells secreted bicarbonate and this secretion is dependent upon the mode of stimulation. They ended their abstract with possibly the understatement of the year: "If these results with Calu-3 cells accurately reflect the transport properties of native submucosal gland serous cells, then HCO3- secretion in the human airways warrants greater attention." In early 2000 Dr Bridges teamed with Martin Hug to investigate intact submucosal glands [40]. They found that the gland cells secrete bicarbonate in response to stimulation. In order for cells to transport bicarbonate there must be a way for bicarbonate to enter the cells. In collaboration with Kriendler et al [41] they identified two sodium bicarbonate cotransporters on the basolateral side of Calu-3 cells.

Dr Bridges' other passion, like most CF scientists, is for finding a cure for cystic fibrosis. He has collaborated with a variety of people testing various compounds for CFTR corrector activity. His papers are too numerous to mention here. After moving to Rosalind Franklin University and Chicago Medical School he continued his interest in CFTR correctors. He is head of the Cystic Fibrosis Foundation Therapeutics CFTR Modulator Chemical Compound program. Each year he gives out compounds for others scientists to use and screens thousands of new possible compounds that may "cure" CF.

3.3. Shmuel Muallem, University of Texas Southwestern, Dallas, TX

Dr. Shmuel Muallem is the leader of a significant research group at the University of Texas Southwestern and now at the NIH. One thread of his work relates bicarbonate transport to the disease cystic fibrosis and has carefully examined and identified every potential element in the mechanism of bicarbonate secretion by epithelial cells. He has done work using a variety of methodologies centered on electrophysiology and patch clamp supported by molecular genetic approaches in his group's studies to determine which genes are important for bicarbonate secretion. His research group also has published considerable research on other proteins which are essential for bicarbonate secretion, focusing on bicarbonate-secreting exchanger proteins. His work has greatly contributed to understanding the molecular mechanisms that explain cellular bicarbonate secretion and it's role in the disease cystic fibrosis.

If we limit ourselves to this decade, Muallem's first papers regarding the relationship between bicarbonate transport and CF was published in 2001 [42]. It examined at the relationship between CFTR and a Na/H+ exchanger (NHE3) in pancreatic duct cells. His group found evidence to support that CFTR indirectly regulated and inhibited Na/H+ exchange activity at the apical membrane via PDZ binding domains, which inhibited NHE3 activity. In another study published in Nature [22] his research group found evidence that CFTR mutations associated with pancreatic insufficiency, the more severe version of cystic fibrosis, had no HCO3- transport. And some of them still had good Cl- conductance. From a pH perspective they found "alkaline fluids are secreted by normal tissues, whereas acidic fluids are secreted by mutant CFTR-expressing tissues, indicating the importance of this activity." This Nature paper impacted the field in its suggestion that CF is not a result of Cl- transport problems but rather it was all about CFTR's conductance of bicarbonate ions. However, this view did not exist long unchallenged as Jeff Wine published a paper establishing that the measurements of chloride conductance in these experiments did not agree with the data from the sweat gland.

Muallem's group followed a significant paper in Nature with another in 2002 in the Journal of Biological Chemistry [20], which presented evidence that CFTR, and NBC3 (sodium bicarbonate cotransporter) are part of the same HCO3-transporting complex assembled with the aid of PDZ domain-containing scaffolds, and this interaction is how CFTR regulates NBC3 activity. A few years later in 2006 [43] Muallem hypothesized that the Slc26a6 gene product (a Cl/HCO3- exchanger) regulates and primarily inhibits CFTR activity. He followed that up by adding that the SLC26 family of transporters may be part of a transporter complex with CFTR where all regulate each other. The complex could be organized in PDZ domain scaffolds (with NHE3 and NBC3) and each transporter protein has a specific role and all in the apical membrane of epithelia. When taken altogether, the bicarbonate transport chain is formed and in cystic fibrosis it does not function and leads to the disease state. Their model supports that HCO3- secretion is vital to epithelia cells and is mediated by a cotransporter pNBC1 at the basolateral membrane and exits the luminal side via the CFTR. Since 2009 his group has published several papers identifying the mechanism by which this CFTR-NHE-NBC complex is regulated by IRBIT and WNK/SPAK kinase pathways in the process of HCO3- secretion.

3.4. Alan Verkman, University of California San Francisco, San Francisco, CA

Alan Verkman's research group is a force of nature with an incredible variety of productivity. Dr. Verkman's research group works at the University of California San Francisco; and his group uses microscopy and fluorescent dyes to enable the detection of ion concentrations, pH, and even precise measurements of the volume of the smallest intracellular compartment. Their findings have greatly informed the field.

In the recent decade their work has focused on whether there are changes in Na, Cl, pH and salts in general in the pathophysiology of cystic fibrosis. They often tested controversial findings from researchers in the field and either supported or refuted their work. In the early years of this decade [44] they tested and refuted the "high salt" hypothesis of the Welsh and Smith group. They found a similar ASL tonicity and pH in cystic fibrosis (CFTR-null) mice as well as human bronchi. Their findings regarding Na and Cl levels being unchanged led them to conclude this provided "direct evidence that the ASL is approximately isotonic and not saltier in cystic fibrosis." In 2001 they also published a report that measured the ionic composition and viscosity of fluid from airway submucosal glands. Neither Na+ nor pH differed in gland fluid from CF airways versus controls but mucus viscosity was significantly elevated compared to normal airways [45]. In 2002 they reported that Cl- flux is important to support the normal acidification process that occurs in the cell's endosomes but CFTR does not really change the acidification of endosomes because other Cl- channels, ClC-5, are present, at least in mice [46]. This refuted a variety of hypotheses that endosome pH was abnormal in cystic fibrosis, which perhaps altered the characteristics of mucus produced in the airway.

In a Journal of General Physiology paper in 2003 [47] they reported findings with a novel lung preparation designed to measure ASL composition and depth in small distal airways. Distal ASL was studied with ion- or pH-sensitive dyes. The ASL pH was found to be 7.28 and not affected when CFTR was inhibited by the drug CFTRinh-172.

In 2004 they started seeing pH differences. They tested airway submucosal gland fluid by using a selective CFTR inhibitor (CFTRinh-172) in pig and human airways. Gland fluid pH was 7.1 and was reduced by 0.4 units after CFTR inhibition [48].

In 2006 they investigated whether gland fluid pH is abnormal in early CF, using nasal biopsies from pediatric subjects having minimal CF lung disease [49]. Having minimal disease is very important as Fischer and Widdecombe published a paper showing the airway surface pH changes with the longitudinal progression of different disease states. Gland fluid pH, was 6.57 in biopsies from six CF subjects, much lower than the recorded pH of 7.18 in eight non-CF biopsies. In pig trachea and human bronchi, gland fluid pH was also reduced by up to 0.45 units by CFTR inhibitors. They found evidence for CFTR-dependent bicarbonate transport by the tracheal epithelium and stated: "These results provide evidence for intrinsic hyperacidity in CF gland fluid secretions, which may contribute to CF airway pathology." Their group's recent papers have focused again on intracellular pH in the lysosomes of macrophages and epithelia from humans and mice and found no evidence it is altered in CF. "We conclude that biologically significant involvement of CFTR in organellar acidification is unlikely." [50].

3.5. Paul Quinton and Malla Reddy, University of California, La Jolla, CA

In a publication in 1983 Paul Quinton [3] was the first investigator to make the connection that cystic fibrosis might be caused by a broken Cl- channel. He also may have been the first CF researcher to have the disease. When he was 19 he diagnosed himself, "I started reading up on bronchitis and bronchiectasis out of curiosity about my own lung problems. When I noticed a footnote that referenced cystic fibrosis, the definition of the disease gave me chills because everything seemed to fit with what I was already experiencing." Paul Quinton works at the University of California-San Diego; his research with Dr. Malla Reddy has used human cells and electrophysiological techniques to explore the problems in CF.

In the recent decade their work has focused on how changes in pH and bicarbonate ion concentrations could lead in the pathophysiology of cystic fibrosis through changes in mucus. In the year 2000 Quinton and Reddy [51] reported that they found the CFTR anion channel is somewhat permeable to bicarbonate anions. At the time Quinton was unsure that this new fact was relevant to the pathogenesis of cystic fibrosis at normal physiological levels. In a 2001 paper in the Journal of the Pancreas [52], Quinton and Reddy found evidence that the presence of mutated CFTR correlated to a decrease in cell membrane permeability to bicarbonate ions. They also found that the severity of disease was related to the phenotypic ability of a mutant CFTR to express a bicarbonate conductance and different CF mutations may have differing level of bicarbonate conductance, this is very similar to the views expressed by Shmuel Muallem about the loss of bicarbonate conductance being the most important this in the pancreas. They surmised that the severity of the pathogenesis in CF might be closely related to the phenotypic ability of a mutant CFTR to express a HCO3- conductance.

Very recently, in 2010, Paul Quinton reported in the Journal of Physiology [53] that CF epithelial cells in the cervix could secrete fluid normally, but unlike wild type cells, they could not secrete bicarbonate. And furthermore that mucus released in CF epithelial was severely impaired even though stimulated fluid secretion was similar to healthy cells. They reported "Mucus release was severely inhibited in the absence of serosal HCO3-, HCO3- transport, or functional CFTR." In the same year in an American Journal of Physiology report the [54] Quinton group found that extracellular bicarbonate is necessary for mucoviscosity. They hypothesized that extracellular bicarbonate could chelate calcium from the mucins at the moment of secretion to allow the mucins to fully expand. In CF disease the mucins don't fully expand and appear as "dehydrated mucus." Lastly in a 2010 review, Quinton [55] put forward the possibility that mucus build up in cystic fibrosis patients may largely be caused by bicarbonate disruption, not by salt/fluid imbalance as traditionally explained. This now has supplemented an existing hypothesis of how lung disease develops, that is that the mucus from the submucosal glands is already defective as it emerges and adheres to the glands and airway surface providing an island for bacterial growth. In this case though, Paul Quinton has put forward a mechanism (mentioned above) whereby lack of bicarbonate leads to this sticky mucus. This will lead to many more experiments as it is tested.

3.6. Steve Ballard, University of South Alabama, Mobile, AL

Steve Ballard started his career in cystic fibrosis research working with Richard Boucher and John Gatzy at the University of North Carolina at Chapel Hill. His first paper [56 helped form the basis for one of the leading model of CF lung disease. That is that alveolar cells secrete fluid and the rest of the lung absorbs that fluid. After moving to the University of South Alabama in Mobile, Ballard and others [57] showed in distal bronchi that most of the secretion comes from submucosal glands. This helped form the basis for a second model of CF lung disease. That is that the disease pathophysiology of cystic fibrosis originates in the submucosal glands. In subsequent papers [58,59] the Ballard lab showed that bronchial secretion was due to both chloride secretion and bicarbonate secretion.

In 1997 Steve Ballard and others [60] published a paper on the visualization of bronchial submucosal glands from pigs. Dr. Krouse, an author, remembers watching their movies of submucosal glands secretion, with the gland orifice opening, mucus streaming out and cilia beating, showing that glands were an exciting dynamic part of airway fluid secretion. In the same year they discovered that "inhibition of the anion (chloride and bicarbonate) secretion response to acetylcholine leads to mucus obstruction of submucosal gland ducts that resembles the early pathological changes observed in CF." This result provided another link between cystic fibrosis and submucosal gland function. In the following paper [61] they also noted that the mucus (after inhibition of anion secretion) on the airway surface was different, having less water and altered rheology, similar to CF.

By the turn of the century the Ballard lab had established that most of the secretion in the upper airway was due to chloride and bicarbonate secretion through CFTR in the submucosal glands. That inhibition of anion secretion leads to impacted mucus within glands and defective mucus on the airway surface. In a paper by Trout et al. [62] they showed that much more of the airway is covered by defective mucus when the glands are stimulated to secrete and there was no measureable goblet cell secretion. They concluded that the source of the defective mucus on the airway surface was from the submucosal glands. They concluded, "that inhibition of anion and liquid secretion in porcine lungs disrupts the normal morphology of airway surface mucus, providing further evidence that impaired anion secretion alone could account for critical aspects of CF lung disease." In 2004 Ballard and Inglis [63] published an excellent review summarizing their findings.

3.7. Terry Machen and Horst Fischer, University of California Berkeley, Berkeley CA

Drs. Terry Machen and Horst Fischer have been collaborators at the University of California Berkeley for two decades and were perhaps the first group to put forward the idea that pH and HCO3- may be aberrant in the disease cystic fibrosis. They most frequently use the methods of electrophysiology, including transepithelial short-circuit current measurements by Ussing Chamber (sometimes with pH-stat technique), whole cell and single cell patch clamp techniques, and nasal potential difference (PD) measurements from living subjects. An early PNAS paper [28] directed the field's attention to the topic HCO3- permeability through the CFTR channel. Their study assessed intracellular pH and channel activity of mouse wild type or mutant CFTR-expressing epithelial cells. They found evidence that HCO3- could move into cells through CFTR channels and hypothesized since the electrochemical gradients of both Cl- and HCO3- are physiologically directed outward, "HCO3- secretion may be important for controlling pH of the luminal, but probably not the cytoplasmic, fluid in CFTR-containing epithelia. In CF, a decreased secretion of HCO3- may lead to decreased pH of the luminal fluid."

In a 1996 Pflugers Archives paper [64] this research group studied intracellular pH regulation using a florescent dye, BCECF, and cultured bovine epithelial cells. They again found evidence that HCO3-dependent, Na and Cl- independent, pHi recovery may be due largely to an influx of HCO3- via CFTR Cl- channels. They suggested that CFTR may mediate HCO3- secretion and contribute to regulation of pH in periciliary fluid. In the following American Journal of Physiology paper [65] they extended this line of inquiry in Ussing Chambers and using a variety of channel blockers. The found "Blocker effects were absent in human CF tracheal cells homozygous for the delta F508 mutation of CFTR (CFT1); Cl- and HCO3- currents were rescued in CFT1 cells recombinantly expressing wild-type CFTR. Thus CFTR functions as a HCO3- and Cl- conductor, and genistein and bromotetramisole maximize CFTR activity in airway epithelial cells." In 1999 in Pflugers Archives [66] they evaluated a new cell model for airway submucosal gland cells, Calu-3, and reported data elucidating the ion selectivity of the CFTR channel.

Their research group also explored another question related to pH, whether the intracellular organelles like the endosome, lysosome or golgi which acidify themselves are altered in cystic fibrosis. In a Chandy et al [67] paper they used pH-sensitive dyes targeted to the golgi apparatus and reported "Comparison of genetically matched DeltaF508 and wt-CFTR cells showed that the absence of CFTR statistically increased Golgi acidity by 0.2 pH units, though this small difference was unlikely to be physiologically important." In 2006 Fischer co-authored a review paper with Jonathan Widdicombe [68] which directed the fields attention to mechanisms that might explain pH changes in the lung's airway surface liquid, ASL, could alter the function of antimicrobial factors that mean to keep the lung sterile. They also point out: "CFTR Cl- channel conducts HCO3- and, therefore, may contribute to ASL pH. However, the acidity of the ASL indicated parallel mechanisms for H+ secretion. Recent investigations identified several H(+) transporters in the apical membrane of the airway epithelium." Thus we should not ignore the role proton channels will also play in modifying pH in the airway surface liquid. In a recent publication [69] this research group explored human nasal mucosa pH and rate of acid and base secretion using Ussing chambers and the pH-stat technique. They found the pH of nasal epithelia from CF patients was pH = 7.08 while that in normal subjects was pH = 7.34. They conclude with "Our data suggests that CF patients exhibited significantly lower base secretion by the nasal airway epithelium. It is possible that improper regulation of ASL pH in CF may negatively impact the innate host defense system."

3.8. Lane Clarke, University of Missouri, Columbia, MO

Lane Clarke started studying cystic fibrosis at the University of North Carolina, Chapel Hill, under the guidance of Richard Boucher and Mike Knowles. Their first paper together [70] showed that cystic fibrosis patients responded to extracellular ATP and UTP, suggesting the presence of functional P2 receptors in the airway. In 1992 Clarke et al [71] showed that in the newly engineered CF mice that there was a lack of chloride transport in the mouse intestine. In 1993 they [72] explained one of many CF mysteries. They found evidence that the channel originally claimed to be the CF channel (the outwardly rectifying anion channel) was regulated by CFTR. This could explain the earlier findings that the rectifying channel was not gated properly by cAMP in CF tissues.

Upon moving to the University of Missouri, Lane Clarke continued his work on epithelia, especially the intestine. With Harline in [73] he published a paper that CFTR was responsible for both chloride and bicarbonate secretion in the mouse duodenum. He also found an chloride/bicarbonate exchanger in the intestine that was regulated by CFTR. He also described an apical H-K ATPase in the mouse colon [74]. It is interesting in two systems, the lungs and the intestine, there exists a mechanism for secreting both base (bicarbonate) and acid (H +). Two years later the Clarke group found yet another mechanism by which CFTR controls the apical pH [75], they found evidence that CFTR regulates a Na+/H+ exchanger.

In 2004 Dr. Clarke published a paper [76] that changed the thinking on how CF disease develops and added a new word, bioavailable, to our vocabulary. They showed that "Paneth cell granules undergo limited dissolution and accumulate within the intestinal crypts of cystic fibrosis (CF) mice." These granules should carry the antimicrobials from the Paneth cells to the intestinal surface. In CF the antimicrobials are secreted into the crypts but are not bioavailable to help kill bacteria. This result influenced people like Jeff Wine where it was hypothesized that the antimicrobials secreted by the airway submucosal glands are not bioavailable on the airway surface where they are needed. In 2009 [77] the Clarke lab identified the anion exchanger that is regulated by CFTR. It was named "Down-regulated in adenoma" (DRA later changed to be SLC26A3) and was responsible for all the basal bicarbonate secretion and ½ of the cAMP stimulated current in the mouse intestine.

Lane Clarke has shown that in the intestine, the CFTR is a member of a large family of proteins that can regulate the pH within the organ. Describing the huge variety of bicarbonate secretors and acid secretors involved in intestinal pH regulation the Clarke's research group unearthed would take a review of its own and will not be attempted here.

3.9. Mike Knowles and Richard Boucher, University of North Carolina, Chapel Hill, NC

Mike Knowles and Ric Boucher first teamed up at the University of North Carolina, Chapel Hill in 1981 [78,79] and adapted technique of measuring the difference in voltage across the nasal epithelium to humans. They quickly applied this new technique to cystic fibrosis where the potential difference in CF was much higher than in normal individuals. Much of the potential difference could be inhibited by amiloride, which blocked the apical sodium channel (ENaC). This led them to conclude, "the greater reduction in potential difference in response to amiloride suggests that absorption of excess salt and perhaps liquid from respiratory epithelial surfaces contributes to the pathogenesis of lung disease in cystic fibrosis." This was the basis for the leading theory of how CF lung disease develops. The airway absorbs too much liquid via increased sodium absorption leading to dehydration of the mucus. The dehydrated mucus becomes plastered to the airway surface and provides a breeding ground for bacteria. This was the theory in the 1980's and is still the theory today, with minor modifications. In another paper [80] they agreed with Paul Quinton that there is loss of chloride permeability in CF, but the cause of CF lungs disease was still the excess fluid absorption. The link between the loss of an anion channel and the activation of a sodium channel was not clear at that point and many researches in the field searched for the link.

In collaboration with Jim Yankaskas [81] they discovered that CF epithelial cells retained the characteristic chloride permeability loss and sodium absorption increase in culture. In 1986 they published a review [82] which is a good summary of the early history of CF. To test the theory that excess sodium absorption was the problem, they did a pilot study [83] of the effect of amiloride on 14 CF patients over 1 year. The loss of forced vital capacity over that year was slowed and the rheology of the sputum improved. Thus it appeared that blocking ENaC might provide a way to help cure or prevent CF lung disease.

In the mid 90's, thanks to a paper published by Smith et al [34], there was a big debate whether the salt concentration in the surface liquid was different between normal and CF cells. Simply put, was the airway like the sweat gland and CF individuals had salty airway fluid? In 1997 Knowles and Boucher [84] published a paper where they measured the ion concentrations. They used filter paper to sample the airway liquid and found no difference in any concentration between normal and CF. Interestingly, they found very little anion gap (supposedly bicarbonate) in CF or normal airways. The only thing odd was the very high concentration of potassium in the fluid (between 15-30 mM).

In 2002 Knowles and Boucher [85] published an excellent review of their view on how CF lung disease develops. The work included many scientists at their institution and other places, too many to cover here. In their model a healthy lung's alveoli secrete large amounts of fluid that the rest of the lung absorbs via sodium absorption. Yet in CF the increased ENaC activity in the airway leads to a dehydration of the airway surface until the fluid level drops below that of the height of the cilia. The mucus becomes dehydrated and stationary, a stable island more easily colonized by bacteria. This does not happen across the entire lung in general as the act of breathing and walking releases ATP onto the surface in many places and opens a second chloride channel, which supports rehydration. However the hydration balance of the CF airway is very precarious. Insults to the airway such as noxious fumes or viruses upset the balance and lead to a patchy distribution of bacterial infection in the lung.

3.10. Jeffrey Wine and Mauri Krouse, Stanford University, Stanford, CA

Dr. Jeffrey Wine switched the whole direction of his research in 1986. Turning from a successful career in crayfish behavior to trying to find the cause and cure for cystic fibrosis. Jeff came to Stanford in the early 1970's as an assistant professor of psychology. In 1981, doctors diagnosed his first daughter Nina with CF, forever changing his personal and professional life. "My daughter could have been born with many diseases and I wouldn't have decided to work on them. But I saw a paper that said CF is an ion channel disease and I knew about ion channels," Wine recalled. Moving from the science of neurons to the function of CFTR in ion channels marked a change in focus that led to 30+ years of contributions to understanding the basic defect in CF. After a sabbatical in Paul Quinton's research lab, just one year, he published his first paper with Behm et al [86] expanding on the previous work of Sato and Quinton. His paper is still important today as it measured the secretion rate in sweat glands and found that CF heterozygotes had ½ the secretion rate of normals whereas CF sweat glands have no secretion to beta-adenergic stimulation.

Some 24 of those years he worked in collaboration with Dr. Mauri Krouse. I joined the Wine lab at the very beginning of its transition to CF work, in 1986, which also was the year when two papers (see section on Mike Welsh) were published claiming to have discovered the chloride channel (an outwardly rectify chloride channel) that was defective in cystic fibrosis. The laboratory of Prof. Wine could not repeat these experiments and found it likely CF was caused by another channel. Jeff Wine led a 5-year campaign to discover the correct anion channel that was the cause of cystic fibrosis. In a meeting of the North American Cystic Fibrosis society in 1990 in Arlington Virginia, Wine and Krouse, with collaborators from Stanford University, submitted an abstract on a small linear chloride channel that was activated by cAMP in canine airway cells. This was followed up with a paper the next year [87] where they showed the small linear anion channel and finding no correlation between the claimed outwardly rectifying chloride channel and levels of CFTR expression. Others at that 1990 meeting had also noted the small linear chloride channel such a M.A. Gray and B. E. Argent from the UK and Dr. Grygorczyk from Canada. In 1991 the CFTR channel was confirmed as a small linear chloride channel by Bear et al when they expressed recombinant CFTR in cells [9]. Once the small CFTR channels identity was confirmed Wine and Krouse teamed with

Christine Haws to be the first to describe a kinetic model for the gating of CFTR [88]. This model has since been modified and expanded, by researchers such as David Sheppard in the UK and TC Hwang in Missouri, but it was the first. This same year a very influential paper from Engelhard et al [30] was published using "in situ hybridization and immunocytochemistry to characterize the cellular distribution of cystic fibrosis (CF) gene expression in human bronchus." They discovered that most of the CFTR in the lung was in the submucosal glands. After reading this paper Jeffrey Wine again changed the course of his lab to almost exclusively study submucosal glands. Within two years he helped discover the now famous submucosal gland cell line (Calu-3) with the labs of Drs. Walt Finkbeiner and Jonathan Widdicombe at UCSF [89]. Again Christine Haws worked to carefully measure the channel properties of CFTR in Calu-3 cells.

Unfortunately the Calu-3 cells represented healthy tissue and there was no CF version of the cell (even though many people have tried the make some), thus Haws, Krouse and Wine [90] used a stably transfected mouse mammary cell line to measure the properties of ΔF508 CFTR. The values they found over 16 years ago are still true today. The channel density of ΔF508 CFTR on the surface is less than 5% of wild type and the open probability is ~ 1/3 of normal CFTR. With the realization that the main form of cystic fibrosis was due to the loss of channels, Prof Wine abandoned patch clamping single cells and concentrated on sheets of cells in the Ussing chamber. Monolayers of Calu-3 cells secreted bicarbonate [31] and most of the unstimulated resting secretion was bicarbonate-dependent [91]. Work with Luckie et al (92) found evidence that in a variety of cells expressing CFTR that bicarbonate may be secreted because mutant non functional CFTR altered the pH surrounding cells.

Using and ingenious method Irokawa [93], and Wine designed a chamber where all the secretion of a sheet of epithelial cells was secreted out a tiny orifice, they called the apparatus the "virtual gland." When Calu-3 cells were tested in the virtual gland the bicarbonate concentration of the fluid secreted to carbachol (a Ca2+ elevating agonist) was the same as the bathing solution (25 mM), but when the cells were stimulated with forskolin (a cAMP elevating agent the opens CFTR) the bicarbonate concentration rose to ~80 mM. Roughly half the secretion was due to bicarbonate secretion in the virtual gland. This was confirmed by Krouse et al [33] in the Ussing chamber with the addition that there existed a H-K ATPase to help neutralize some of the bicarbonate which was secreted. Such a mechanism had been previously reported by Smith and Welsh [27] in airway cells and again by Coakley et al [29] in primary airway cell cultures. In the same year Wu et al [94] published a paper showing an inwardly rectifying potassium channel (Kir4.2) in the apical membrane of Calu-3 cells and also in the apical membrane of freshly dissected airway submucosal glands. This channel may supply the potassium needed by the H-K ATPase.

In recent years the Wine research group has been in the middle of the most exciting topics in the field, new studies on mucus [95], new drugs developed to correct the disease [96] and the hottest topic in the research field today, the CF Pig [97,98].

4. Final context: What's new, what's next?

Everything new these days in the field of cystic fibrosis research seems to have something to do with a pig. The birth announcement for the first CF pig occurred in 2008 [99]. It was a collaboration of over 20 people at the University of Iowa and the University of Missouri. They noted that "these pigs should be of value in producing new models of CF" and they certainly have. While CF mice do not develop lung disease, CF pigs do. The pathology of the newborn pig mirrors that of human infants [100]. They have involvement of the pancreas, intestines (including meconium ileus), liver and gallbladder. In the pig lungs have no initial inflammation or infection. Within months the CF piglets develop infection, inflammation, remodeling and mucus accumulation [101] just like human lungs. The piglets failed to clear/ eradicate bacteria in the lungs suggesting a defective defense system that was apparent within hours after birth. An unexpected finding was reduced levels of insulin-like growth factor were reduced in the CF pig [102]. When human CF infants were tested they found a reduced IGF1 level. This finding might explain why some patients fail to reach their full growth potential even under the best clinical care. It also suggests a new IGF1 supplement therapy for newborns with CF.

A closer look at the lung of CF piglets revealed that there was a loss of both chloride and bicarbonate secretion [103]. They found no increase of sodium or liquid absorption and no change in the depth of the periciliary liquid depth. The defect in sodium transport is the hallmark of the leading hypothesis of how airway lung disease develops. But the authors point out that these neither are not mature pigs nor are they ΔF508 pigs, but rather piglets lacking CFTR. In 2011 a study of ΔF508 pigs was published [104], even though about 6% (compared to normal) CFTR makes it to the cell surface the results are the piglets are almost identical with the earlier knockout experiments. The lungs still display a greatly reduced chloride and bicarbonate secretion. A second unexpected finding was that the teeth of CF piglets are hypomineralized [105]. Both CFTR and an anion exchanger (AE2) expression went up during the enamel maturation stage. They proposed that there is an increased demand for chloride and/or bicarbonate during the development of the teeth.

Just this year the CF pig revealed another important clue to the pathogenesis of CF airway disease. At birth CF lungs are sterile and the infection is due to a defect in a basic defense mechanism so that the bacteria are not eradicated. In a recent Nature paper [36] they found that the pH of the airway surface liquid determines the killing properties of the lungs. Airway surface liquid from normal piglets effectively killed bacteria and if the pH was made more acidic the killing was reduced. The airway surface liquid from CF pigs did not kill bacteria until the pH was made more alkaline. To quote from their abstract "these results directly link the initial host defense defect to the loss of CFTR, an anion channel that facilitates HCO_3^- transport." This paper just might be a new paradigm shift for how a loss of an anion channel leads to CF lung infection.

5. Conclusions

The future is bright for the CF pig. And perhaps the most dramatic finding for those who study pH is the one by Pezzulo et al [36]. They found evidence in CF pig model that reduced airway surface liquid pH impairs bacterial killing in the cystic fibrosis lung. This stands upon an earlier finding by Verkman's group when they found that gland fluid pH is abnormal in early CF, using nasal biopsies from pediatric subjects having minimal CF lung disease before bacteria and immune response could disturb the system [49]. Thus the reduced pH in the thin layer of fluid that lines the lungs may play an important role in the ability of pathogenic bacteria to colonize the airway in cystic fibrosis.

Beyond the alteration of pH, bicarbonate itself may play an important role in the abnormal behavior of mucus in cystic fibrosis. Quinton's new hypothesis [55], that in a healthy person the extracellular bicarbonate functions to chelate calcium from the mucins at the moment of secretion to allow the mucins to fully expand but in CF the mucins don't fully expand and appear as "dehydrated." The possibility that mucus build up in cystic fibrosis patients may largely be caused by bicarbonate disruption, not by salt and fluid imbalance, is intriguing idea from a man who has been correct before.

These results discussed in this review provide evidence for an intrinsic defect in the ability of CF tissues to secrete base [29] or regulate pH, and they come closer to conclusively demonstrating that CF airway surface liquid is abnormally acidic. More data needs to be collected concerning the steady-state pH of the airway surface liquid of humans under physiological conditions. If such a pH difference is eventually established, it will then be necessary to determine if attempts to correct it might improve the health of patients.

Author details

Douglas B. Luckie[1] and Mauri E. Krouse[2]

1 Department of Physiology, Michigan State University, East Lansing, Michigan, USA

2 Flatley Discovery Lab, The Schrafft Center, Charlestown, MA, USA

References

[1] Busch R. On the history of cystic fibrosis. Acta Univ. Carol. 1990;36:13-15.

[2] Di Sant'Agnese, PA, Darling RC, Perrera GA, Shea E. Abnormal electrolyte composition of sweat in cystic fibrosis of the pancreas. Pediatrics 1953;12: 549-563,

[3] Quinton PM. Chloride impermeability in cystic fibrosis. Nature 1983;301:421-422.

[4] Andersen DH. Cystic Fibrosis of the pancreas and its relation to celiac disease. Am J. Dis. Child. 1938;56: 344-399.

[5] Andersen DH, Hodges G. Celiac syndrome V. Genetics of cystic fibrosis of the pancreas with a consideration of the etiology. Am. J. Dis. Child. 1946;72: 62-80.

[6] Kerem B, Rommens JM, Buchanan JA, Markiewicz D, Cox TK, Chakravarti A, Buchwald M, Tsui LC. Identification of the cystic fibrosis gene: genetic analysis. Science 1989;245:1073-80.

[7] Riordan JR, Rommens JM, Kerem B, Alon N, Rozmahel R, Grzelczak, et al. Identification of the cystic fibrosis gene: cloning and characterization of complementary DNA. Science 1989;245:1066-73.

[8] Rommens JM, Iannuzzi MC, Kerem B, Drumm ML, Melmer G, Dean M, et al. Identification of the cystic fibrosis gene: chromosome walking and jumping. Science 1989;245:1059-65.

[9] Bear CE, Li CH, Kartner N, Bridges RJ, Jensen TJ, Ramjeesingh M, Riordan JR. Purification and functional reconstitution of the cystic fibrosis transmembrane conductance regulator (CFTR). Cell. 1992;68(4):809-18.

[10] Linsdell P, Tabcharani JA, Rommens JM, Hou YX, Chang XB, Tsui LC, Riordan JR, Hanrahan JW. Permeability of wild-type and mutant cystic fibrosis transmembrane conductance regulator chloride channels to polyatomic anions. J Gen Physiol. 1997;110: 355–364.

[11] Fuller CM, Benos DJ. Cftr! Am J Physiol 1992;263:C267-86.

[12] Quinton PM. Physiological basis of cystic fibrosis: a historical perspective. Physiol. Rev. 1999;79:S3-S22.

[13] Donaldson SH, Poligone EG, Stutts, MJ. CFTR regulation of ENAC. Methods in Molecular Medicine-Cystic Fibrosis Methods and Protocols II, 2002;70(3)343-364.

[14] Lee MG, Choi JY, Luo X, Strickland E, Thomas PJ, Muallem S. Cystic fibrosis transmembrane conductance regulator regulates luminal Cl-/HCO3- exchange in mouse submandibular and pancreatic ducts. J Biol Chem. 1999;274:14670-7.

[15] Ahmed N, Corey M, Forstner G, Zielenski J, Tsui L-C, Ellis L, Tullis E, Durie P. Molecular consequences of cystic fibrosis transmembrane regulator (CFTR) gene mutations in the exocrine pancreas. Gut 2003;52:1159-1164.

[16] Kopelman H, Corey M, Gaskin K, Durie P, Weizman Z, Forstner G. Impaired chloride secretion, as well as bicarbonate secretion, underlies the fluid secretory defect in the cystic fibrosis pancreas. Gastroenterology 1988;95: 349-355.

[17] Ishiguro H, Steward M, Naruse S. Cystic fibrosis transmembrane conductance regulator and SLC26 transporters in HCO3− secretion by pancreatic duct cells. Acta Physiologica Sinica 2007;59(4): 465-476.

[18] Gray MA, Harris A, Coleman L, Greenwell JR, Argent BE. Two types of chloride channel on duct cells cultured from human fetal pancreas. Am J Physiol. 1989;257(2 Pt 1):C240-51.

[19] Whitcomb DC, Ermentrout GB. A mathematical model of the pancreatic duct cell generating high bicarbonate concentrations in pancreatic juice. Pancreas 2004;29(2):e30-40.

[20] Park M, Ko SB, Choi JY, Muallem G, Thomas PJ, Pushkin A, et al. The cystic fibrosis transmembrane conductance regulator interacts with and regulates the activity of the HCO3- salvage transporter human Na+-HCO3- cotransport isoform 3. J Biol Chem. 2002;Dec 27;277(52):50503-9.

[21] Kaur S, Norkina O, Ziemer D, Samuelson LC, De Lisle RC. Acidic duodenal pH alters gene expression in the cystic fibrosis mouse pancreas. Am J Physiol Gastrointest Liver Physiol. 2004;287(2):G480-90.

[22] Choi JY, Muallem D, Kiselyov K, Lee MG, Thomas PJ, Muallem S. Aberrant CFTR-dependent HCO3- transport in mutations associated with cystic fibrosis Nature. 2001;Mar 1;410(6824):94-7.

[23] Wine JJ. Cystic fibrosis: the 'bicarbonate before chloride' hypothesis. Current Biology 2001;Vol 11 No 12 R463-466.

[24] Knowles M, Gatsy J, Boucher R. Increased bioelectric potential difference across respiratory epithelia in cystic fibrosis. N. Engl J Med. 1981;305(25): 1489-95.

[25] Knowles M, Gatzy J, Boucher R. Relative ion permeability of normal and cystic fibrosis nasal epithelium. J. Clin Invest. 1983;71(5):1410-7.

[26] Smith JJ, Welsh MJ. cAMP stimulates bicarbonate secretion across normal, but not cystic fibrosis airway epithelia. J Clin Invest. 1992;89: 1148-1153.

[27] Smith JJ, Welsh MJ. Fluid and electrolyte transport by cultured human airway epithelia. J Clin Invest. 1993;91(4): 1590–1597.

[28] Poulsen JH, Fischer H, Illek B, Machen TE. Bicarbonate conductance and pH regulatory capability of cystic fibrosis transmembrane conductance regulator. Proc Natl Acad Sci USA. 1994;91:5340-4.

[29] Coakley RD, Grubb BR, Paradiso AM, Gatzy JT, Johnson LG, Kreda SM, O'Neal WK, Boucher RC. Abnormal surface liquid pH regulation by cultured cystic fibrosis bronchial epithelium. Proc Natl Acad Sci USA. 2003;100(26):16083-8.

[30] Engelhardt JF, Yankaskas JR, Ernst SA, Yang Y, Marino CR, Boucher RC, Cohn JA, Wilson JM. Submucosal glands are the predominant site of CFTR expression in human bronchus. Nat. Genet. 1992;2: 240–247.

[31] Lee MC, Penland CM, Widdicombe JH, Wine JJ. Evidence that Calu-3 human airway cells secrete bicarbonate. Am J Physiol. 1998;274(3 Pt 1):L450-3.

[32] Devor DC, Singh AK, Lambert LC, DeLuca A, Frizzell RA, Bridges RJ. Bicarbonate and chloride secretion in Calu-3 human airway epithelial cells. J Gen Physiol. 1999;113(5):743-60.

[33] Krouse ME, Talbott JF, Lee MM, Joo NS, Wine JJ. Acid and base secretion in the Calu-3 model of human serous cells. Am J Physiol Lung Cell Mol Physiol. 2004;287(6):L1274-83.

[34] Smith JJ, Travis SM, Greenberg EP, Welsh MJ. Cystic fibrosis airway epithelia fail to kill bacteria because of abnormal airway surface fluid. Cell. 1996;85(2):229-36.

[35] Welsh MJ, Smith JJ. Stimulation of HCO3- secretion across airway epithelia. JOP. 2001;2(4 Suppl):291-3.

[36] Pezzulo AA, Tang XX, Hoegger MJ, Alaiwa MH, Ramachandran S, Moninger TO, et al. Reduced airway surface pH impairs bacterial killing in the porcine cystic fibrosis lung Nature 2012;487 (7405) 109–113.

[37] Bradbury NA, Jilling T, Berta G, Sorscher EJ, Bridges RJ, Kirk KL. 1992 Regulation of plasma membrane recycling by CFTR. Science. 256(5056): 530-2.

[38] Devor DC, Singh AK, Frizzell RA, Bridges RJ. 1996 Modulation of Cl- secretion by benzimidazolones. I. Direct activation of a Ca(2+)-dependent K+ channel. Am J Physiol. Nov;271(5 Pt 1):L775-84.

[39] Devor DC, Singh AK, Bridges RJ, Frizzell RA. 1996. Modulation of Cl- secretion by benzimidazolones. II. Coordinate regulation of apical GCl and basolateral GK. Am J Physiol. 271(5 Pt 1):L785-95.

[40] Hug MJ, Bridges RJ. pH regulation and bicarbonate transport of isolated porcine submucosal glands. JOP. 2001;2(4 Suppl):274-9.

[41] Kreindler JL, Peters KW, Frizzell RA, Bridges RJ. Identification and membrane localization of electrogenic sodium bicarbonate cotransporters in Calu-3 cells. Biochim Biophys Acta. 2006;1762(7):704-10.

[42] Lee MG, Ahn W, Lee JA, Kim JY, Choi JY, Moe OW, Milgram SL, Muallem S, Kim KH. Coordination of pancreatic HCO3- secretion by protein-protein interaction between membrane transporters. JOP. 2001;2(4 Suppl): 203-6.

[43] Wang Y, Soyombo AA, Shcheynikov N, Zeng W, Dorwart M, Marino CR, Thomas PJ, Muallem S. Slc26a6 regulates CFTR activity in vivo to determine pancreatic duct HCO3- secretion: relevance to cystic fibrosis EMBO J. 2006;25(21):5049-57.

[44] Jayaraman S, Joo NS, Reitz B, Wine JJ, Verkman AS. Submucosal gland secretions in airways from cystic fibrosis patients have normal [Na(+)] and pH but elevated viscosity. Proc Natl Acad Sci USA. 2001;98(14):8119-23.

[45] Jayaraman S, Song Y, Verkman AS. Airway surface liquid pH in well-differentiated airway epithelial cell cultures and mouse trachea. Am J Physiol Cell Physiol. 2001;281(5):C1504-11.

[46] Hara-Chikuma M, Wang Y, Guggino SE, Guggino WB, Verkman AS. Impaired acidification in early endosomes of ClC-5 deficient proximal tubule. Biochem Biophys Res Commun. 2005;329(3):941-6.

[47] Song Y, Thiagarajah J, Verkman AS. Sodium and chloride concentrations, pH, and depth of airway surface liquid in distal airways. J Gen Physiol. 2003;122(5):511-9.

[48] Thiagarajah JR, Song Y, Haggie PM, Verkman AS. A small molecule CFTR inhibitor produces cystic fibrosis-like submucosal gland fluid secretions in normal airways. FASEB J. 2004;18(7): 875-7.

[49] Song Y, Salinas D, Nielson DW, Verkman AS. Hyperacidity of secreted fluid from submucosal glands in early cystic fibrosis. Am J Physiol Cell Physiol. 2006;290(3):C741-9.

[50] Haggie PM, Verkman AS. Defective organellar acidification as a cause of cystic fibrosis lung disease: reexamination of a recurring hypothesis. Am J Physiol Lung Cell Mol Physiol. 2009;296(6):L859-67.

[51] Quinton PM, Reddy MM. CFTR, a Rectifying, Non-Rectifying Anion Channel? J Korean Med Sci. 2000;15(Supp):S17-20.

[52] Reddy MM, Quinton PM. Selective activation of cystic fibrosis transmembrane conductance regulator Cl- and HCO3- conductances. JOP. 2001;2(4 Suppl):212-8.

[53] Muchekehu RW, Quinton PM. A new role for bicarbonate secretion in cervico-uterine mucus release. J. Physiol. 2010;588(Pt 13):2329-42.

[54] Chen EY, Yang N, Quinton PM, Chin WC. A new role for bicarbonate in mucus formation. Am J Physiol Lung Cell Mol Physiol. 2010;299(4):L542-9.

[55] Quinton PM. Role of epithelial HCO3- transport in mucin secretion: lessons from cystic fibrosis. Am Journal of Cell Physiol. 2010;299(6):C1222-33.

[56] Krochmal EM, Ballard ST, Yankaskas JR, Boucher RC, Gatzy JT. Volume and ion transport by fetal rat alveolar and tracheal epithelia in submersion culture. Am J Physiol. 1989;256(3 Pt 2):F397-407.

[57] Ballard ST, Fountain JD, Inglis SK, Corboz MR, Taylor AE. Chloride secretion across distal airway epithelium: relationship to submucosal gland distribution. Am J Physiol. 1995;268(3 Pt 1):L526-31.

[58] Inglis SK, Corboz MR, Taylor AE, Ballard ST. Regulation of ion transport across porcine distal bronchi. Am J Physiol. 1996;270(2 Pt 1):L289-97.

[59] Inglis SK, Corboz MR, Ballard ST. Effect of anion secretion inhibitors on mucin content of airway submucosal gland ducts. Am J Physiol. 1998;274(5 Pt 1):L762-6.

[60] Inglis SK, Corboz MR, Taylor AE, Ballard ST. Effect of anion transport inhibition on mucus secretion by airway submucosal glands. Am J Physiol. 1997;272(2 Pt 1):L372-7.

[61] Trout L, Gatzy JT, Ballard ST. Acetylcholine-induced liquid secretion by bronchial epithelium: role of Cl- and HCO3- transport. Am J Physiol. 1998;275(6 Pt 1):L1095-9.

[62] Trout L, Townsley MI, Bowden AL, Ballard ST. Disruptive effects of anion secretion inhibitors on airway mucus morphology in isolated perfused pig lung. J Physiol. 2003;549(Pt 3):845-53.

[63] Ballard ST, Inglis SK. Liquid secretion properties of airway submucosal glands. J Physiol. 2004;556(Pt 1):1-10.

[64] Poulsen JH, Machen TE. HCO3-dependent pHi regulation in tracheal epithelial cells. Pflugers Arch 1996;432:546-54.

[65] Illek B, Yankaskas JR, Machen TE. cAMP and genistein stimulate HCO3- conductance through CFTR in human airway epithelia. Am J Physiol. 1997;272(4 Pt 1):L752-61.

[66] Illek B, Tam AW, Fischer H, Machen TE. Anion selectivity of apical membrane conductance of Calu 3 human airway epithelium. Pflugers Arch. 1999;437(6):812-22.

[67] Chandy G, Grabe M, Moore HP, Machen TE. Proton leak and CFTR in regulation of Golgi pH in respiratory epithelial cells. Am J Physiol Cell Physiol. 2001;281(3):C908-21.

[68] Fischer H, Widdicombe JH. Mechanisms of acid and base secretion by the airway epithelium. J Membr Biol. 2006;211(3):139-50.

[69] Cho DY, Hwang PH, Illek B, Fischer H. Acid and base secretion in freshly excised nasal tissue from cystic fibrosis patients with ΔF508 mutation. Int Forum Allergy Rhinol. 2011;1(2):123-7.

[70] Knowles MR, Clarke LL, Boucher RC. Activation by extracellular nucleotides of chloride secretion in the airway epithelia of patients with cystic fibrosis. N Engl J Med. 1991;325(8):533-8.

[71] Clarke LL, Grubb BR, Gabriel SE, Smithies O, Koller BH, Boucher RC.Defective epithelial chloride transport in a gene-targeted mouse model of cystic fibrosis. Science. 1992;257(5073):1125-8.

[72] Gabriel SE, Clarke LL, Boucher RC, Stutts MJ. CFTR and outward rectifying chloride channels are distinct proteins with a regulatory relationship. Nature. 1993;363(6426): 263-8.

[73] Clarke LL, Harline MC. Dual role of CFTR in cAMP-stimulated HCO3- secretion across murine duodenum. Am J Physiol. 1998;274(4 Pt 1):G718-26.

[74] Spicer Z, Clarke LL, Gawenis LR, Shull GE. Colonic H(+)-K(+)-ATPase in K(+) conservation and electrogenic Na(+) absorption during Na(+) restriction. Am J Physiol Gastrointest Liver Physiol. 2001;281(6):G1369-77.

[75] Gawenis LR, Franklin CL, Simpson JE, Palmer BA, Walker NM, Wiggins TM, Clarke LL. cAMP inhibition of murine intestinal Na/H exchange requires CFTR-mediated cell shrinkage of villus epithelium. Gastroenterology. 2003;125(4):1148-63.

[76] Clarke LL, Gawenis LR, Bradford EM, Judd LM, Boyle KT, Simpson JE, Shull GE, Tanabe H, Ouellette AJ, Franklin CL, Walker NM. Abnormal Paneth cell granule dissolution and compromised resistance to bacterial colonization in the intestine of CF mice. Am J Physiol Gastrointest Liver Physiol. 2004;286(6):G1050-8.

[77] Walker NM, Simpson JE, Brazill JM, Gill RK, Dudeja PK, Schweinfest CW, Clarke LL. Role of down-regulated in adenoma anion exchanger in HCO3- secretion across murine duodenum. Gastroenterology. 2009;136(3):893-901.

[78] Knowles MR, Carson JL, Collier AM, Gatzy JT, Boucher RC. Measurements of nasal transepithelial electric potential differences in normal human subjects in vivo. Am Rev Respir Dis. 1981;124(4):484-90.

[79] Knowles M, Gatzy J, Boucher R. Increased bioelectric potential difference across respiratory epithelia in cystic fibrosis. N Engl J Med. 1981;305(25):1489-95.

[80] Knowles MR, Stutts MJ, Spock A, Fischer N, Gatzy JT, Boucher RC. Abnormal ion permeation through cystic fibrosis respiratory epithelium. Science. 1983;221(4615): 1067-70.

[81] Yankaskas JR, Knowles MR, Gatzy JT, Boucher RC. Persistence of abnormal chloride ion permeability in cystic fibrosis nasal epithelial cells in heterologous culture. Lancet. 1985;1(8435):954-6.

[82] Knowles MR, Stutts MJ, Yankaskas JR, Gatzy JT, Boucher RC Jr. Abnormal respiratory epithelial ion transport in cystic fibrosis. Clin Chest Med. 1986;7(2):285-97.

[83] Knowles MR, Church NL, Waltner WE, Yankaskas JR, Gilligan P, King M, Edwards LJ, Helms RW, Boucher RC. A pilot study of aerosolized amiloride for the treatment of lung disease in cystic fibrosis. N Engl J Med. 1990;322(17):1189-94.

[84] Knowles MR, Robinson JM, Wood RE, Pue CA, Mentz WM, Wager GC, Gatzy JT, Boucher RC. Ion composition of airway surface liquid of patients with cystic fibrosis as compared with normal and disease-control subjects. J Clin Invest. 1997;100(10): 2588-95.

[85] Knowles MR, Boucher RC. Mucus clearance as a primary innate defense mechanism for mammalian airways. J Clin Invest. 2002;109(5):571-7.

[86] Behm JK, Hagiwara G, Lewiston NJ, Quinton PM, Wine JJ. Hyposecretion of beta-adrenergically induced sweating in cystic fibrosis heterozygotes. Pediatr Res. 1987;22(3):271-6.

[87] Ward CL, Krouse ME, Gruenert DC, Kopito RR, Wine JJ. Cystic fibrosis gene expression is not correlated with rectifying Cl- channels. Proc Natl Acad Sci USA. 1991;88(12):5277-81.

[88] Haws C, Krouse ME, Xia Y, Gruenert DC, Wine JJ. CFTR channels in immortalized human airway cells. Am J Physiol. 1992;263(6 Pt 1):L692-707.

[89] Shen BQ, Finkbeiner WE, Wine JJ, Mrsny RJ, Widdicombe JH. Calu-3: a human airway epithelial cell line that shows cAMP-dependent Cl- secretion. Am J Physiol. 1994;266(5 Pt 1):L493-501.

[90] Haws CM, Nepomuceno IB, Krouse ME, Wakelee H, Law T, Xia Y, Nguyen H, Wine JJ. Delta F508-CFTR channels: kinetics, activation by forskolin, and potentiation by xanthines. Am J Physiol. 1996;270(5 Pt 1):C1544-55.

[91] Singh M, Krouse M, Moon S, Wine JJ. Most basal I(SC) in Calu-3 human airway cells is bicarbonate-dependent Cl- secretion. Am J Physiol. 1997;272(4 Pt 1):L690-8.

[92] Luckie DB, Singh CN, Wine JJ, Wilterding JH. CFTR activation raises extracellular pH of NIH/3T3 mouse fibroblasts and C127 epithelial cells. J Membr Biol. 2001;179(3):275-84.

[93] Irokawa T, Krouse ME, Joo NS, Wu JV, Wine JJ. A "virtual gland" method for quantifying epithelial fluid secretion. Am J Physiol Lung Cell Mol Physiol. 2004;287(4):L784-93.

[94] Wu JV, Krouse ME, Rustagi A, Joo NS, Wine JJ. An inwardly rectifying potassium channel in apical membrane of Calu-3 cells. J Biol Chem. 2004;279(45):46558-65.

[95] Khansaheb M, Choi JY, Joo NS, Yang YM, Krouse M, Wine JJ. Properties of substance P-stimulated mucus secretion from porcine tracheal submucosal glands. Am J Physiol Lung Cell Mol Physiol. 2011;300(3):L370-9.

[96] Van Goor F, Hadida S, Grootenhuis PD, Burton B, Stack JH, Straley KS, Decker CJ, Miller M, McCartney J, Olson ER, Wine JJ, Frizzell RA, Ashlock M, Negulescu PA. Correction of the F508del-CFTR protein processing defect in vitro by the investigational drug VX-809. Proc Natl Acad Sci USA. 2011;108(46):18843-8.

[97] Joo NS, Cho HJ, Khansaheb M, Wine JJ. Hyposecretion of fluid from tracheal submucosal glands of CFTR-deficient pigs. J Clin Invest. 2010;120(9):3161-6.

[98] Cho HJ, Joo NS, Wine JJ. Defective fluid secretion from submucosal glands of nasal turbinates from CFTR-/- and CFTR (ΔF508/ΔF508) pigs.PLoS One. 2011;6(8):e24424.

[99] Rogers C.S., Hao Y., Rokhlina T., Samuel M., Stoltz D.A., Li Y., et al . Production of CFTR-null and CFTR-ΔF508 heterozygous pigs by adeno-associated virus–mediated gene targeting and somatic cell nuclear transfer. J Clin Invest. 2008; 118(4): 1571–1577.

[100] Rogers CS, Stoltz DA, Meyerholz DK, Ostedgaard LS, Rokhlina T, Taft PJ, et al Disruption of the CFTR gene produces a model of cystic fibrosis in newborn pigs. Science 2008;321: 1837–1841.

[101] Stoltz DA, Meyerholz DK, Pezzulo AA, Ramachandran S, Rogan MP, Davis GJ, et al. Sci Transl Med. Cystic fibrosis pigs develop lung disease and exhibit defective bacterial eradication at birth. 2010;2(29):29-31.

[102] Rogan MP, Reznikov LR, Pezzulo AA, Gansemer ND, Samuel M, Prather RS, et al. Pigs and humans with cystic fibrosis have reduced insulin-like growth factor 1 (IGF1) levels at birth. Proc Natl Acad Sci USA. 2010;107(47): 20571-5.

[103] Chen JH, Stoltz DA, Karp PH, Ernst SE, Pezzulo AA, Moninger TO, et al. Loss of anion transport without increased sodium absorption characterizes newborn porcine cystic fibrosis airway epithelia. Cell. 2010 ;143(6):911-23.

[104] Ostedgaard LS, Meyerholz DK, Chen JH, Pezzulo AA, Karp PH, Rokhlina T, et al. The ΔF508 Mutation Causes CFTR Misprocessing and Cystic Fibrosis-Like Disease in Pigs. Sci Transl Med. 2011;3(74): 74ra24.

[105] Chang EH, Lacruz RS, Bromage TG, Bringas P Jr, Welsh MJ, Zabner J, Paine ML. Enamel pathology resulting from loss of function in the cystic fibrosis transmembrane conductance regulator in a porcine animal model. Cells Tissues Organs. 2011;194(2-4):249-54.

Permissions

The contributors of this book come from diverse backgrounds, making this book a truly international effort. This book will bring forth new frontiers with its revolutionizing research information and detailed analysis of the nascent developments around the world.

We would like to thank Prof Maria Puiu, MD, PhD, for lending her expertise to make the book truly unique. She has played a crucial role in the development of this book. Without her invaluable contribution this book wouldn't have been possible. She has made vital efforts to compile up to date information on the varied aspects of this subject to make this book a valuable addition to the collection of many professionals and students.

This book was conceptualized with the vision of imparting up-to-date information and advanced data in this field. To ensure the same, a matchless editorial board was set up. Every individual on the board went through rigorous rounds of assessment to prove their worth. After which they invested a large part of their time researching and compiling the most relevant data for our readers. Conferences and sessions were held from time to time between the editorial board and the contributing authors to present the data in the most comprehensible form. The editorial team has worked tirelessly to provide valuable and valid information to help people across the globe.

Every chapter published in this book has been scrutinized by our experts. Their significance has been extensively debated. The topics covered herein carry significant findings which will fuel the growth of the discipline. They may even be implemented as practical applications or may be referred to as a beginning point for another development. Chapters in this book were first published by InTech; hereby published with permission under the Creative Commons Attribution License or equivalent.

The editorial board has been involved in producing this book since its inception. They have spent rigorous hours researching and exploring the diverse topics which have resulted in the successful publishing of this book. They have passed on their knowledge of decades through this book. To expedite this challenging task, the publisher supported the team at every step. A small team of assistant editors was also appointed to further simplify the editing procedure and attain best results for the readers.

Our editorial team has been hand-picked from every corner of the world. Their multi-ethnicity adds dynamic inputs to the discussions which result in innovative outcomes. These outcomes are then further discussed with the researchers and contributors who give their valuable feedback and opinion regarding the same. The feedback is then collaborated with the researches and they are edited in a comprehensive manner to aid the understanding of the subject.

Apart from the editorial board, the designing team has also invested a significant amount of their time in understanding the subject and creating the most relevant covers. They scrutinized every image to scout for the most suitable representation of the subject and create an appropriate cover for the book.

The publishing team has been involved in this book since its early stages. They were actively engaged in every process, be it collecting the data, connecting with the contributors or procuring relevant information. The team has been an ardent support to the editorial, designing and production team. Their endless efforts to recruit the best for this project, has resulted in the accomplishment of this book. They are a veteran in the field of academics and their pool of knowledge is as vast as their experience in printing. Their expertise and guidance has proved useful at every step. Their uncompromising quality standards have made this book an exceptional effort. Their encouragement from time to time has been an inspiration for everyone.

The publisher and the editorial board hope that this book will prove to be a valuable piece of knowledge for researchers, students, practitioners and scholars across the globe.

List of Contributors

Tomás McKenna, Jean-Ha Baek and Maria Eriksson
Department of Biosciences and Nutrition, Center for Biosciences, Karolinska Institutet, Huddinge, Sweden

Meenal Mehrotra
Department of Pathology and Laboratory Medicine, Medical University of South Carolina, Charleston, SC, USA

Amanda C. LaRue
Research Services, Department of Veterans Affairs Medical Center, Charleston, SC, USA and Department of Pathology and Laboratory Medicine, Medical University of South Carolina, Charleston, SC, USA

Vyacheslav A. Korshunov
Department of Medicine, Aab Cardiovascular Research Institute, University of Rochester School of Medicine and Dentistry, Rochester, NY, USA

Igor A. Dyachenko and Arkady N. Murashev
Pushchino State Natural-Science Institute, Pushchino, Russia
Pushchino Branch, Shemyakin-Ovchinnikov Institute of Bioorganic Chemistry, Pushchino, Russia

Jean-Ha Baek, Tomás McKenna and Maria Eriksson
Department of Biosciences and Nutrition, Center for Biosciences, Karolinska Institutet, Huddinge, Sweden

Zhiguang Yuchi, Lynn Kimlicka and Filip Van Petegem
Department of Biochemistry and Molecular Biology, University of British Columbia, Vancouver, British Columbia, Canada

Maria Puiu, Simona Dumitriu, Adela Chiriţă-Emandi and Smaranda Arghirescu
University of Medicine and Pharmacy "Victor Babes" Timisoara, Romania
Emergency Hospital for Children "Louis Turcanu" Timisoara, Romania

Raluca Grădinaru
University of Medicine and Pharmacy "Victor Babes" Timisoara, Romania

Roya Vakili and Babak Kateby Kashy
Michigan State University, Department of Neurology; Metro Health Neuroscience, Wyoming, MI, USA

Venturina Stagni, Simonetta Santini and Daniela Barilà
Department of Biology, University of Rome "Tor Vergata", Rome, Italy
Laboratory of Cell Signaling, Fondazione Santa Lucia, IRCCS, Rome, Italy

Christopher A. Chapleau and Lucas Pozzo-Miller
Department of Neurobiology, Civitan International Research Center, The University of Alabama at Birmingham, USA

Jane Lane and Alan K. Percy
Department of Pediatrics, Civitan International Research Center, UAB Rett Syndrome Clinic, The University of Alabama at Birmingham, USA

Yoshiaki Nakayama, Naosuke Nakamura and Akira Kurosaka
Laboratory of Neuroglycobiology, Department of Molecular Biosciences, Faculty of Life Sciences, Kyoto Sangyo University, Kyoto, Japan

Daisuke Tsuji and Koji Itoh
Department of Medicinal Biotechnology, Institute for Medicinal Research, Graduate School of Pharmaceutical Sciences, The University of Tokushima, Tokushima, Japan

Maria Puiu
University of Medicine and Pharmacy "Victor Babes" Timisoara - Genetics Department; Emergency Hospital for Children "Louis Turcanu" Timisoara - Genetics Department, Romania

Adela Chirita Emandi and Smaranda Arghirescu
University of Medicine and Pharmacy "Victor Babes" Timisoara - Pediatrics Department; Emergency Hospital for Children "Louis Turcanu" Timisoara - Pediatrics Department, Romania

Wen Xing
State Key Laboratory of Experimental Hematology, Institute of Hematology and Blood Disease Hospital, Chinese Academy of Medical Sciences and Peking Union Medical College, China

Mingjiang Xu and Feng-Chun Yang
Herman B Wells Center for Pediatric Research, Indiana University School of Medicine; Indianapolis, Indiana, USA

Malgorzata Mrugacz
Medical University of Bialystok, Poland

Douglas B. Luckie
Department of Physiology, Michigan State University, East Lansing, Michigan, USA

Mauri E. Krouse
Flatley Discovery Lab, The Schrafft Center, Charlestown, MA, USA